W9-BNZ-572

Teen Health Series

Domestic Violence

SOURCEBOOK

Third Edition

Health Reference Series

Third Edition

Domestic Violence SOURCEBOOK

Basic Consumer Health Information about Warning Signs, Risk Factors, and Health Consequences of Intimate Partner Violence, Sexual Violence and Rape, Stalking, Human Trafficking, Child Maltreatment, Teen Dating Violence, and Elder Abuse

Along with Facts about Victims and Perpetrators, Strategies for Violence Prevention, and Emergency Interventions, Safety Plans, and Financial and Legal Tips for Victims, a Glossary of Related Terms, and Directories of Resources for Additional Information and Support

Edited by
Joyce Brennfleck Shannon

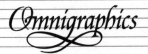

P.O. Box 31-1640, Detroit, MI 48231

Bibliographic Note

Because this page cannot legibly accommodate all the copyright notices, the Bibliographic Note portion of the Preface constitutes an extension of the copyright notice.

Edited by Joyce Brennfleck Shannon

Health Reference Series

Karen Bellenir, *Managing Editor*
David A. Cooke, M.D., *Medical Consultant*
Elizabeth Collins, *Research and Permissions Coordinator*
Cherry Edwards, *Permissions Assistant*
EdIndex, Services for Publishers, *Indexers*

* * *

Omnigraphics, Inc.

Matthew P. Barbour, *Senior Vice President*
Kevin M. Hayes, *Operations Manager*

* * *

Peter E. Ruffner, *Publisher*
Copyright © 2009 Omnigraphics, Inc.
ISBN 978-0-7808-1038-9

Library of Congress Cataloging-in-Publication Data

Domestic violence sourcebook : basic consumer health information about warning signs, risk factors, and health consequences of intimate partner violence, sexual violence and rape, stalking, human trafficking, child maltreatment, teen dating violence, and elder abuse; along with facts about victims and perpetrators, strategies for violence prevention, and emergency interventions, safety plans, and financial and legal tips for victims, a glossary of related terms, and directories of resources for additional information and support / edited by Joyce Brennfleck Shannon. -- 3rd ed.
     p. cm. -- (Health reference series)
  Includes bibliographical references and index.
  Summary: "Provides basic consumer health information about the physical, mental, and social effects of violence against intimate partners, children, teens, parents, and the elderly, along with prevention and intervention strategies. Includes index, glossary of related terms and directory of resources"--Provided by publisher.
  ISBN 978-0-7808-1038-9 (hardcover : alk. paper) 1. Family violence--United States. 2. Victims of family violence--Services for--United States. 3. Sexual abuse victims--Services for--United States. I. Shannon, Joyce Brennfleck.
  HV6626.2.D685 2009
  362.82'92--dc22

2009004386

This book is printed on acid-free paper meeting the ANSI Z39.48 Standard. The infinity symbol that appears above indicates that the paper in this book meets that standard.

Printed in the United States

Table of Contents

Visit www.healthreferenceseries.com to view *A Contents Guide to the Health Reference Series*, a listing of more than 14,000 topics and the volumes in which they are covered

Part VII: Domestic Violence Survivor Assistance

Part VIII: Additional Help and Information

Preface

About This Book

Domestic violence affects people of all ages, and victims include people from every race, ethnicity, religion, and economic situation. Abusers seek to control victims with physical and sexual assault, verbal attacks, threats, isolation, and constant monitoring. To help stop the violence, many communities have instituted a variety of services including education, crisis counseling, safe shelters, legal counsel, financial assistance, and children's aid. While such interventions can help reduce intimate partner violence, elder abuse, and teen dating abuse, many victims may feel powerless and be unaware of how to find the help they need. Furthermore, people who have been abused can experience long-term physical and mental health problems.

Domestic Violence Sourcebook, Third Edition provides updated information about the physical, mental, and social effects of violence experienced by intimate partners, parents, children, teens, and elderly adults. Facts about types of abuse, such as rape and other sexual violence, stalking, and human trafficking, are included, along with information about domestic violence prevention. Guidelines for emergency intervention, safety plans, and identity protection are offered, and facts about financial and legal assistance for victims are provided. The *Sourcebook* concludes with a glossary of related terms and directories of additional resources for families and advocates of people experiencing domestic violence.

How to Use This Book

This book is divided into parts and chapters. Parts focus on broad areas of interest. Chapters are devoted to single topics within a part.

Part I: Domestic Violence Overview explains the warning signs, causes, and statistics of family abuse in the United States. It reviews the negative impact domestic violence has on long-term health and how financial hardship, alcohol abuse, and homelessness can lead to increases in domestic violence prevalence.

Part II: Intimate Partner Violence and Other Forms of Domestic Violence provides information about the risk factors and consequences of violence between intimate partners and related concerns, including sexual assault, rape, stalking, and trafficking in persons. It also discusses how such problems impact the workplace, and it describes special concerns associated with same-sex relationship abuse.

Part III: Victims and Perpetrators describes the diversity of people who may experience domestic violence. It discusses the roles of gender, ethnicity, community structure, and military groupings among people at risk. Perpetrator behavioral tactics and degree of danger and risk indicators are identified, along with common parenting styles among domestic violence perpetrators.

Part IV: Domestic Violence Affects Children and Adolescents gives information about the number of young people affected by family maltreatment and long-term effects they may experience. Dating abuse and date rape among teens are described, and a section about juvenile abusers explains how sibling violence may predict dating violence.

Part V: Elder Abuse describes late-life domestic abuse, including neglect, abandonment, and financial exploitation, as well as physical, sexual, or emotional abuse. The link between caregiver stress and elder abuse is also discussed.

Part VI: Domestic Violence Prevention offers information about respect-based relationships, personal safety, self-defense, and parenting tips. Programs and protocols that have been effective in reducing and preventing domestic violence in homes, classrooms, and the workplace are reviewed. As a further deterrent to domestic abuse, recovery guidelines for adults coping with childhood abuse issues are also included.

Part VII: Domestic Violence Survivor Assistance offers practical advice for victims, families, and advocates about immediate and long-term issues after an incident of abuse. Guidance is provided for immediate actions, calling the police, documenting the abuse, and creating safety plans. Information about longer-term strategies is also provided, including protecting one's identity, internet safety, financial assistance, child custody, and mental health concerns.

Part VIII: Additional Help and Information provides a glossary of terms related to domestic violence and directories for help in finding legal resources, victim assistance hotlines, state address confidentiality programs, and other resources for information about domestic violence.

Bibliographic Note

This volume contains documents and excerpts from publications issued by the following U.S. government agencies: Agency for Healthcare Research and Quality (AHRQ); Centers for Disease Control and Prevention (CDC); National Center on Elder Abuse; National Center for Posttraumatic Stress Disorder; National Institutes of Health (NIH); Substance Abuse and Mental Health Services Administration (SAMHSA); U.S. Department of Health and Human Services (HHS); U.S. Department of Justice (DOJ); U.S. Department of State; and the U.S. Government Accountability Office (GAO).

In addition, this volume contains copyrighted documents from the following individuals, publications, and organizations: AARDVARC.org (Abuse, Rape and Domestic Violence Aid and Resource Collection); Alabama Coalition Against Domestic Violence; Asian and Pacific Islander American Health Forum; *District Chronicles*; Domestic Violence Division of the Nashville Police; Family Violence Prevention Fund; MSU (Michigan State University) Safe Place; National Center for Victims of Crime; National Coalition Against Domestic Violence; National Coalition for the Homeless; National District Attorneys Association; National Domestic Violence Hotline; National Latino Alliance for the Elimination of Domestic Violence; National Network to End Domestic Violence; National Resource Center on Domestic Violence; Nemours Foundation; New Hampshire Department of Justice; North Carolina Coalition Against Domestic Violence; Elizabeth Pantley; RAND Corporation; Rape, Abuse and Incest National Network (RAINN); Regional Research Institute for Human Services–Portland State University; Sage Publications; West Virginia Coalition Against Domestic Violence; and Witness Justice.

Acknowledgements

In addition to the listed organizations, agencies, and individuals who have contributed to this *Sourcebook*, special thanks go to managing editor Karen Bellenir, research and permissions coordinator Liz Collins, and document engineer Bruce Bellenir for their help and support.

About the Health Reference Series

The *Health Reference Series* is designed to provide basic medical information for patients, families, caregivers, and the general public. Each volume takes a particular topic and provides comprehensive coverage. This is especially important for people who may be dealing with a newly diagnosed disease or a chronic disorder in themselves or in a family member. People looking for preventive guidance, information about disease warning signs, medical statistics, and risk factors for health problems will also find answers to their questions in the *Health Reference Series*. The *Series*, however, is not intended to serve as a tool for diagnosing illness, in prescribing treatments, or as a substitute for the physician/patient relationship. All people concerned about medical symptoms or the possibility of disease are encouraged to seek professional care from an appropriate health care provider.

A Note about Spelling and Style

Health Reference Series editors use *Stedman's Medical Dictionary* as an authority for questions related to the spelling of medical terms and the *Chicago Manual of Style* for questions related to grammatical structures, punctuation, and other editorial concerns. Consistent adherence is not always possible, however, because the individual volumes within the *Series* include many documents from a wide variety of different producers and copyright holders, and the editor's primary goal is to present material from each source as accurately as is possible following the terms specified by each document's producer. This sometimes means that information in different chapters or sections may follow other guidelines and alternate spelling authorities. For example, occasionally a copyright holder may require that eponymous terms be shown in possessive forms (Crohn's disease *vs.* Crohn disease) or that British spelling norms be retained (leukaemia *vs.* leukemia).

Locating Information within the Health Reference Series

The *Health Reference Series* contains a wealth of information about a wide variety of medical topics. Ensuring easy access to all the fact sheets, research reports, in-depth discussions, and other material contained within the individual books of the *Series* remains one of our highest priorities. As the *Series* continues to grow in size and scope, however, locating the precise information needed by a reader may become more challenging.

A Contents Guide to the Health Reference Series was developed to direct readers to the specific volumes that address their concerns. It presents an extensive list of diseases, treatments, and other topics of general interest compiled from the Tables of Contents and major index headings. To access *A Contents Guide to the Health Reference Series*, visit www.healthreferenceseries.com.

Medical Consultant

Medical consultation services are provided to the *Health Reference Series* editors by David A. Cooke, M.D. Dr. Cooke is a graduate of Brandeis University, and he received his M.D. degree from the University of Michigan. He completed residency training at the University of Wisconsin Hospital and Clinics. He is board-certified in Internal Medicine. Dr. Cooke currently works as part of the University of Michigan Health System and practices in Ann Arbor, MI. In his free time, he enjoys writing, science fiction, and spending time with his family.

Our Advisory Board

We would like to thank the following board members for providing guidance to the development of this *Series*:

- Dr. Lynda Baker, Associate Professor of Library and Information Science, Wayne State University, Detroit, MI
- Nancy Bulgarelli, William Beaumont Hospital Library, Royal Oak, MI
- Karen Imarisio, Bloomfield Township Public Library, Bloomfield Township, MI
- Karen Morgan, Mardigian Library, University of Michigan-Dearborn, Dearborn, MI

- Rosemary Orlando, St. Clair Shores Public Library, St. Clair Shores, MI

Health Reference Series *Update Policy*

The inaugural book in the *Health Reference Series* was the first edition of *Cancer Sourcebook* published in 1989. Since then, the *Series* has been enthusiastically received by librarians and in the medical community. In order to maintain the standard of providing high-quality health information for the layperson the editorial staff at Omnigraphics felt it was necessary to implement a policy of updating volumes when warranted.

Medical researchers have been making tremendous strides, and it is the purpose of the *Health Reference Series* to stay current with the most recent advances. Each decision to update a volume is made on an individual basis. Some of the considerations include how much new information is available and the feedback we receive from people who use the books. If there is a topic you would like to see added to the update list, or an area of medical concern you feel has not been adequately addressed, please write to:

Editor
Health Reference Series
Omnigraphics, Inc.
P.O. Box 31-1640
Detroit, MI 48231-1640
E-mail: editorial@omnigraphics.com

Part One

Domestic Violence Overview

Chapter 1

Domestic Violence Warning Signs

Warning Signs

There is no way to tell for sure if someone is experiencing domestic violence. Those who are battered, and those who abuse, come in all personality types. Battered women are not always passive with low self-esteem, and batterers are not always violent or hateful to their partner in front of others. Most people experiencing relationship violence do not tell others what goes on at home. So how do you tell? Here are some signs to look for:

Injuries and Excuses

In some cases, bruises and injuries may occur frequently and be in obvious places. When this happens, the intent of the batterer is to keep the victim isolated and trapped at home. When black eyes and other bruising is a result of an assault, the person being battered may be forced to call in sick to work, or face the embarrassment and excuses of how the injuries occurred. In other cases, bruises and other outward injuries never occur. When there are frequent injuries seen by others, the one being battered may talk about being clumsy, or have

This chapter includes text from: "Warning Signs of Domestic Violence," © MSU Safe Place (www.msu.edu/~safe). Reprinted with permission. And, "How can I help a friend or family member who is being abused?" © 2008 National Domestic Violence Hotline (www.ndvh.org). The National Domestic Violence Hotline is available 24 hours per day at 1-800-799-7233.

elaborate stories of how the injuries occurred. The truth about the source of injuries will not usually be told unless the one told could be trusted and/or the one being battered wants help to end the relationship.

Absences from Work or School

When severe beatings or other trauma related to violence occurs, the one being battered may take time off from his/her normal schedule. If you see this happening, or the person is frequently late, this could be a sign of something (such as relationship violence) occurring.

Low Self-Esteem

Some battered women have low self-esteem, while others have a great deal of confidence and esteem in other areas of their life (at work, as a mother, with hobbies, and so forth) but not within their relationship. In terms of dealing with the relationship, a sense of powerlessness and low self-esteem may exist. A battered woman may believe that she could not make it on her own without her partner and that she is lucky to have him in her life.

Accusations of Having Affairs

This is a common tactic used by batterers as an attempt to isolate their partners and as an excuse for a beating. It could include accusations of looking at other men, wanting to be with other men, or having affairs with the man bagging groceries at the local supermarket. Friends of the couple may observe this at times, but what is seen in public is usually only a small fraction of what the battered woman experiences at home.

Personality Changes

People may notice that a very outgoing person, for instance, becomes quiet and shy around his/her partner. This happens because the one being battered "walks on egg shells" when in the presence of the one who is abusive to her. Accusations (of flirting, talking too loudly, or telling the wrong story to someone) have taught the abused person that it is easier to act a certain way around the batterer than to experience additional accusations in the future.

Fear of Conflict

As a result of being battered, some may generalize the experience of powerlessness with other relationships. Conflicts with co-workers, friends, relatives, and neighbors can create a lot of anxiety. For many, it is easier to give in to whatever someone else wants than to challenge it. Asserting one's needs and desires begins to feel like a battle, and not worth the risks of losing.

Not Knowing What One Wants or How One Feels

For adults or children who have experienced violence from a loved one, the ability to identify feelings and wants, and to express them, may not exist. This could result in passive-aggressive behavior. Rather than telling others what you want, you say one thing but then express your anger or frustration in an aggressive manner (such as scratching his favorite car, burning dinner, or not completing a report on time for your boss).

Blaming Others for Everything

The abuse, which usually includes the batterer blaming others for everything that goes wrong, is usually targeted at a partner or ex-partner. For example, a simple drive somewhere could turn into a violent situation if the batterer blames the partner and/or children for getting them lost. Co-workers and relatives may observe this type of behavior, and it may be directed at others as well.

Self-Blame

You may notice someone taking all of the blame for things that go wrong. A co-worker may share a story about something that happened at home and then take all of the blame for whatever occurred. If you notice this happening a lot, it may be a sign that the one who is taking all of the blame is being battered.

Aggressive or Care-Taking Behavior in Children

Children who live in violent homes may take that experience with them to school and to the playground. Often the class bully is a child who sees violence in his home (directed at mom, or at some or all of the children in the home). Children who seem very grown-up and are sensitive and attentive to others' needs may see violence at home as well.

Helping Someone Who Is Being Abused

How can I help a friend or family member who is being abused?

Don't be afraid to let him or her know that you are concerned for their safety. Help your friend or family member recognize the abuse. Tell him or her you see what is going on and that you want to help. Help them recognize that what is happening is not normal and that they deserve a healthy, non-violent relationship.

Acknowledge that he or she is in a very difficult and scary situation. Let your friend or family member know that the abuse is not their fault. Reassure him or her that they are not alone and that there is help and support out there.

Be supportive. Listen to your friend or family member. Remember that it may be difficult for him or her to talk about the abuse. Let him or her know that you are available to help whenever they may need it. What they need most is someone who will believe and listen to them.

Be non-judgmental. Respect your friend or family member's decisions. There are many reasons why victims stay in abusive relationships. He or she may leave and return to the relationship many times. Do not criticize his or her decisions or try to guilt them. He or she will need your support even more during those times.

Encourage him or her to participate in activities outside of the relationship with friends and family.

If he or she ends the relationship, continue to be supportive of them. Even though the relationship was abusive, your friend or family member may still feel sad and lonely once it is over. He or she will need time to mourn the loss of the relationship and will especially need your support at that time.

Help Him or Her to Develop a Safety Plan

Encourage him or her to talk to people who can provide help and guidance. Find a local domestic violence agency that provides counseling or support groups. Offer to go with him or her to talk to family and friends. If he or she has to go to the police, court, or a lawyer, offer to go along for moral support.

Remember that you cannot rescue him or her. Although it is difficult to see someone you care about get hurt, ultimately the person getting hurt has to be the one to decide that they want to do something about it. It's important for you to support him or her and help them find a way to safety and peace.

For More Information

National Domestic Violence Hotline
P.O. Box 161810
Austin, TX 78716
Toll-Free Hotline: 800-799-SAFE (7233)
Toll-Free TTY: 800-787-3224
Website: http://www.ndvh.org

Chapter 2

The Many Faces of Domestic Violence

What is battering?

Battering is a pattern of behavior used to establish power and control over another person with whom an intimate relationship is or has been shared through fear and intimidation, often including the threat or use of violence. Battering happens when one person believes that they are entitled to control another.

Intimate partner violence is intrinsically connected to the societal oppression of women; children; people of color; people with disabilities; people who are lesbian, gay, bisexual and transgender; elders; Jewish people; and other marginalized groups. While oppression functions in similar ways regardless of which group is targeted, different target groups have unique experiences of oppression stemming from their specific historic, cultural, and social experiences and realities. The work to end domestic violence must necessarily include the fight against all oppressions.

Domestic violence may include not only the intimate partner relationships of spousal, live-in partners, and dating relationships, but also familial, elder, and child abuse may be present in a violent home. Abuse generally falls into one or more of the following categories: physical battering, sexual assault, and emotional or psychological abuse, and generally escalates over a period of time.

"The Problem," © 2005 National Coalition Against Domestic Violence (www .ncadv.org). All rights reserved. Reprinted with permission.

9

Victims of abuse may experience punched walls, control of finances, lying, using children to manipulate a parent's emotions, intimidation, isolation from family and friends, fear, shame, criticism, cuts, crying and afraid children, broken bones, confusion, forced sexual contact, manipulation, sexist comments, yelling, rages, craziness, harassment, neglect, shoving, screaming, jealousy and possessiveness, loss of self esteem, coercion, slammed doors, abandonment, silent treatment, rape, destruction of personal property, unwanted touching, name calling, strangling, ripping, slapping, biting, kicking, bruises, punching, stalking, scrapes, depression, sabotaging attendance at job or school, brainwashing, violence to pets, pinching, deprivation of physical and economic resources, public humiliation, broken promises, prevention of seeking medical and dental care, ridicule, restraining, self-medication, forced tickling, threats to harm family and friends, threats to take away the children, threats to harm animals, threats of being kicked out, threats of weapons, or threats of being killed.

Who is battered?

In all cultures, batterers are most commonly male. Rural and urban women of all religious, ethnic, socioeconomic, and educational backgrounds, and of varying ages, physical abilities, and lifestyles can be affected by domestic violence. There is not a typical woman who will be battered—the risk factor is being born female.

Heterosexual males may also be victims of domestic violence as perpetrated by their female partners. They experience the same dynamics of interpersonal violence as female victims including experiences of disbelief, ridicule, and shame that only enhance their silence. However, there are specific cultural groups whose peculiar vulnerabilities may put the members of that population at risk of experiencing violence in their relationships.

Battered immigrant and refugee women in the United States have further complications by issues of gender, race, socioeconomic status, immigration status, and language, in addition to those complications of intimate partner violence. A battered woman who is not a legal resident or whose immigrant status depends on her partner is isolated by cultural dynamics that may prevent her from leaving her husband, seeking support from local agencies that may not understand her culture, or requesting assistance from an unfamiliar American legal system. Some obstacles may include a distrustful attitude toward the legal system, language and cultural barriers (that may at the least be unknown and at the worst hostile), and fear of deportation.

Children witnessing domestic violence and living in an environment where violence occurs may experience some of the same trauma as abused children. Not all children are affected by domestic violence in the same way. Children may become fearful, inhibited, aggressive, antisocial, withdrawn, anxious, depressed, angry, confused; or, suffer from disturbed sleep, problems with eating, difficulties at school, and challenges in making friends. Children often feel caught in the middle between their parents and find it difficult to talk to either of them. Adolescents may act out or exhibit risk-taking behaviors such as drug and alcohol use, running away, sexual promiscuity, and criminal behavior. Young men may try to protect their mothers, or they may become abusive to their mothers themselves. Children may be injured if they try to intervene in the violence in their homes.

Individuals with physical, psychiatric, and cognitive disabilities may not only experience sexual and domestic violence at a higher rate from intimate partners or spouses than the mainstream population, but, unlike the mainstream population, they may also experience mistreatment, abuse, neglect, and exploitation from their caretakers including personal assistants, paid staff, family members, and parents. Examples can be the denial of medications and personal care, the use of psychotropic medication as a restraint, daily and intimate care mistreatment and neglect, inaccessible organizations and facilities, unavailable or disabled assistive technology devices essential for communication and movement, improper use of restraints, and the denial of life-sustaining medical treatment and therapies. Yet, this population gets little attention from the community, the media, or policy makers, allowing the abuse to continue without restraint in isolation and apathy.

Older battered women are a nearly invisible, yet tragically sizable population and uniquely vulnerable to domestic violence. Older women are more likely to be bound by traditional and cultural ideology that prevents them from leaving an abusive spouse or from seeing themselves as a victim. Older women are very often financially dependent on their abusive spouse and do not have access to the financial resources they need to leave an abusive relationship. Many older women find themselves isolated from their family, friends, and community, due to their spouses' neglect and abuse. This is especially true because older women suffer greater rates of chronic illness, which makes them dependent upon their spouses or caregivers and thus reluctant or unable to report abuse.

Rural battered women face lack of resources, isolation, small town politics, few if any support agencies, and poor or little transportation and communication systems, in addition to the other complications of intimate partner violence that are intensified by the rural lifestyle. Sexist, racist, misogynist, anti-Semitic, and homophobic language and actions are often more acceptable in rural communities, and attitudes seem slower to change. The patriarchal "good old boys" network, fundamentalist religious teachings, deep-rooted cultural traditions, and commonly accepted sexual stereotyping can form a chorus of accusations that the battered rural woman is unfaithful in her role as a woman, wife, and mother. The act of leaving the home place, land, and animals that could depend on her may be emotionally wrenching, leaving the battered rural woman surrounded by walls of guilt and self-abasement.

Same-sex battering is one person's use of physical, sexual, or emotional violence, or the threat of violence, or the fear of outing to gain and maintain control over another and sweeps the entire population regardless of culture, race, occupation, income level, and degree of physical or cognitive ability. Although battering is occasionally an isolated act, once it begins, it often continues and escalates in frequency and severity. In addition, the fear of homophobic and hostile law enforcement, judiciary, court personnel, medical and social service providers, and domestic violence programs, may keep lesbian, gay, bisexual, transgender, and intersex victims of same-sex violence from leaving their abusive relationship and seeking help.

Teen dating violence may be one of the major sources of violence in teen life. Even in the best of circumstances, the passage from childhood to adulthood is often one of awkwardness and unease. When that passage is marked with danger and violence that explodes in relationships, then the journey into adulthood becomes even more overwhelming and complex. Given that social, cultural, religious, and family messages about intimacy and relationships between teens can be confusing, misleading, nonexistent, or even unhealthy, many teens find themselves unsure of what to expect and how to behave in dating or intimate relationships. Fear, misconceptions, lack of services, low self-esteem, control by the abuser, peer pressure, and concern about family response all combine to keep battered teens trapped in silence and secrecy.

Chapter 3

Awareness and Attitudes about Domestic Violence

The Office on Violence against Women (OVW), in collaboration with the Polling Company, Inc., conducted two focus groups and a telephone poll of 600 women in June, 2006 to find out how they viewed the crime of domestic violence. This chapter summarizes the results of the survey research.

Understanding Domestic Violence

The majority of survey respondents and focus group participants had a noteworthy command of issues related to domestic violence. When asked directly, most women agreed that domestic violence in the U.S. is a serious problem. Still, the issue did not flow freely when women were asked to cite the most pressing challenges facing women in this country. Further discussion revealed that this is fueled in part by the "out of sight, out of mind" mentality conveniently allowed by domestic violence, whose victims often suffer silently and without conspicuous physical markings. When asked whether domestic violence qualifies more as a criminal issue or a health issue, women were more than four times as likely to say that domestic violence is a criminal issue. The overwhelming consensus among the participants was that any woman could be a victim of abuse regardless of race, age, socioeconomic status, or place of residence.

This chapter includes text from "Awareness and Attitudes about Domestic Violence," U.S. Department of Justice, 2007.

The women studied had more than a general understanding of three different types of abuse:

Verbal Abuse: Nearly three out of four of the women surveyed said that name calling or put-downs on a regular basis constituted domestic violence and 44 percent suggested that even occasional harsh words counted. One in three insisted on something akin to a strict liability standard for the perpetrator, saying that put-downs and criticisms that did not hurt the other person's feelings nonetheless should be considered domestic violence, a sentiment echoed by many women in the focus groups. To these women, verbal battery is a gateway to physical harm and should not be dismissed.

Physical Abuse: The striking and battering of a woman is visible and most commonly associated with violence between intimate partners. That said, nearly all of the women interviewed acknowledged that conduct need not be physical to qualify as domestic violence. Three-fourths of women surveyed agreed that repeated threats to bring harm fit the definition.

Sexual Abuse: Focus group participants did not automatically connect sexual assault and domestic violence. However, nearly nine in ten of the respondents suggested that sexual coercion is included in the term when prompted. Unassisted, only one percent of women surveyed mentioned sexual abuse in their definition of domestic abuse.

More so than a particular word or deed, the women determined that it was pattern and regularity of the behavior that distinguished actual abuse from relational conflict.

In the focus groups, the women implied that the severity of the problem was linked to whether it ultimately should be characterized as domestic violence.

Pointing the Finger of Blame

The majority of survey respondents agreed that the victim was never to blame for staying with an abuser. Instead, they recognized that victims may struggle with an extremely complex emotional, psychological, even monetary calculus before finally deciding to leave their abusers. Shame, low self-esteem, and fear of repercussions from the perpetrator as well as a financial inability to leave can combine to create a figurative prison that grips women. Still, one-third of women reported that some culpability belonged with the victim.

Most thought of the causes of domestic violence as a learned behavior, meaning the perpetrator witnessed this type of conduct in the home while growing up himself, had financial problems, suffered drug and alcohol abuse, or was unable to manage anger. However, these women were also keenly aware that many relationships experience these problems and other stressors, and do not fall into the patterns of domestic violence.

Women Want to Help Others

Of all the solutions and organizations discussed in the focus groups, women responded most positively toward the President's Family Justice Center Initiative and the National Domestic Violence Hotline. Survey respondents felt that shelters, a hotline, and law enforcement were better options than any other. Women wishing to help, but unsure as to the most effective ways to do so, can point a friend or family member in the direction of these resources without endangering themselves or butting in.

Encouraging Women to Get Involved

Nearly all of the focus group participants were personally willing to roll up their sleeves and volunteer to help women caught in the cycle of abuse. However, many of them also confided that when they were faced with an opportunity to assist a victim in the past, it was often after the victim had already hit rock bottom or actively solicited aid on her own.

No Single Solution

Strikingly, no single resource was a runaway favorite amongst women when asked to choose the optimal solution. Types of community assistance (going to a shelter, calling a hotline, or calling the police) were given the distinction of best by more women than any of the other options (staying with a friend or family member, talking to church or religious leaders, talking to a counselor, or talking to a health professional). Nearly one-fourth felt that the solution was a combination of all options.

Chapter 4

Domestic Violence Statistics

Chapter Contents

Section 4.1

Family Violence Statistics

Text in this section is from "Family Violence Statistics,"
Bureau of Justice Statistics, U.S. Department of Justice,
NCJ 207846, June 2005.

Trends in Family Violence

The rate of family violence fell between 1993 and 2002 from an estimated 5.4 victims to 2.1 victims per 1,000 U.S. residents age 12 or older. Throughout the period, family violence accounted for about one in ten violent victimizations.

Reported and Unreported Family Violence

Family violence accounted for 11% of all reported and unreported violence between 1998 and 2002. Of these roughly 3.5 million violent crimes committed against family members, 49% were crimes against spouses, 11% were sons or daughters victimized by a parent, and 41% were crimes against other family members.

The most frequent type of family violence offense was simple assault. Murder was less than half of 1% of all family violence between 1998 and 2002. About three-fourths of all family violence occurred in or near the victim's residence.

Forty percent of family violence victims were injured during the incident. Of the 3.5 million victims of family violence between 1998 and 2002, less than 1% died as a result of the incident.

The majority (73%) of family violence victims were female. Females were 84% of spouse abuse victims and 86% of victims of abuse at the hands of a boyfriend or girlfriend. While about three-fourths of the victims of family violence were female, about three-fourths of the persons who committed family violence were male.

Most family violence victims were white (74%), and the majority were between ages 25 and 54 (65.7%). Most family violence offenders were white (79%), and most were age 30 or older (62%).

18

Fatal Family Violence

About 22% of murders in 2002 were family murders. Nearly 9% were murders of a spouse, 6% were murders of sons or daughters by a parent, and 7% were murders by other family members. Females were 58% of family murder victims. Of all the murders of females in 2002, family members were responsible for 43%.

Children under age 13 were 23% of murder victims killed by a family member, and just over 3% of non-family murder victims. The average age among sons or daughters killed by a parent was seven years, and four out of five victims killed by a parent were under age 13. Among incidents of parents killing their children, 19% involved one parent killing multiple victims.

Eight in ten murderers who killed a family member were male. Males were 83% of spouse murderers and 75% of murderers who killed a boyfriend or girlfriend.

In 2002 family murders were less likely than non-family murders to involve a firearm (50% versus 68%). Parents were the least likely family murderers to use a firearm (28%), compared to spouses (63%) or other family members (51%).

Family Violence Reported to Police

Approximately 60% of family violence victimizations were reported to police between 1998 and 2002. The reporting rate among female victims was not significantly greater than the reporting rate among male victims.

The most common reason victims of family violence cited for not reporting the crime to police was that the incident was a private or personal matter (34%). Another 12% of non-reporting family violence victims did not report the crime in order to protect the offender.

Among the 2.1 million incidents of family violence reported to police between 1998 and 2002, 36% resulted in an arrest.

Family Violence Recorded by Police

Family violence accounted for 33% of all violent crimes recorded by police in 18 states and the District of Columbia in 2000. Of these more than 207,000 family violence crimes, about half (53%, or 110,000) were crimes between spouses.

Among crimes recorded by police, 2% of family violence involved a firearm, compared to 6% of non-family violence. A weapon was used in 16% of family and 21% of non-family violence. About 49% of family violence crimes recorded by police resulted in an arrest. Males comprised 77% of suspected family violence offenders arrested in 2000.

About 6% of all violent crime recorded by police in 2000 involved more than one offender victimizing a lone victim. The exception was stranger crime, in which 14% of incidents involved multiple offenders victimizing a lone victim.

State Prosecution of Family Assault

Of the approximately 1,500 defendants charged with felony assault during May 2000 in the state courts of eleven large counties, about a third were charged with family violence.

Among felony assault defendants charged with family violence in state courts, 84% had at least one prior arrest for either a felony or a misdemeanor (not necessarily for family violence), and 73% had been previously convicted of some type of felony or misdemeanor (not necessarily family violence).

Nearly half of felony assault defendants charged with family violence were released pending case disposition.

Among the 1,500 felony assault cases, the probability of the case leading to conviction (felony or misdemeanor) was greater for family assault defendants (71%) than non-family assault defendants (61%). State courts sentenced 83% of persons convicted of assault (both family and non-family) to either prison or jail.

Among felony assault defendants convicted in state courts:

- 68% of incarceration sentences for family assault were to jail;

- 62% of incarceration sentences for non-family assault were to prison;

- 45% of persons sent to prison for family assault received a sentence of more than two years, compared to 77% of non-family assault offenders sent to prison.

Federal Prosecution of Domestic Violence

Persons suspected of domestic violence made up 4% of the total 18,653 federal suspects referred to U.S. attorneys for alleged violent crimes from 2000 to 2002. Of the 757 suspects referred to U.S. attorneys for domestic violence offenses between 2000 and 2002, most were firearm-related domestic violence offenses rather than interstate domestic violence offenses.

- The Bureau of Alcohol, Tobacco, Firearms and Explosives accounted for 80% of all referrals for firearm-related domestic violence.

- The Federal Bureau of Investigation (FBI) accounted for 72% of all interstate domestic violence referrals.

Federal courts convicted 90% of defendants adjudicated for an interstate domestic violence offense. Among defendants convicted in federal courts:

- 79% of convictions were the product of a guilty plea, and the remaining 21% were the product of conviction following a trial;

- most were male (96%), under age 40 (67%), white (72%), and non-Hispanic (95%);

- four in five defendants had a prior adult conviction.

Of 47 federal defendants sentenced for an interstate domestic violence offense between 2000 and 2002, 91% received a prison term with a median length of 60 months.

Family Violence Offenders in Prison

Of the nearly 500,000 men and women in state prisons for a violent crime in 1997, 15% were there for a violent crime against a family member. Nearly half of all the family violence offenders in state prisons were serving a sentence for a sex offense against a family member. More than three-quarters of parents convicted of a violent crime against their son or daughter were in prison for a sex offense.

Of the crimes for which family violence offenders were in prison:

- most were against a female (78%),

- more than half were against a child under age 18,

- more than a third were against a child under age 13.

About 90% of offenders in state prisons for family violence had injured their victim:

- 50% of family violence victims were raped or sexually assaulted;

- 28% of the victims of family violence were killed;

- 50% of offenders in state prisons for spousal abuse had killed their victims;

21

- Of state prison inmates imprisoned for a crime against their son or daughter, 79% had raped or sexually assaulted the child, and another 10% had killed the child.

Among family violence offenders in state prisons in 1997:

- most were male (93%),
- six out of ten were white, while about a quarter were black,
- about 80% were between ages 25 and 54.

Among offenders whose incarceration in state prisons was for family violence, 23% had used a weapon to commit their crime. The comparable percentage among state prisoners incarcerated for non-family violence was higher with 46% using a weapon to commit their crime.

Family Violence Offenders in Jail

Convicted family violence offenders made up about 22% of the nearly 86,500 convicted violent offenders in local jails in 2002. Most (60%) of these approximately 18,700 jail inmates incarcerated for family violence were in jail for an aggravated assault.

Local jail inmates convicted of family violence reported that:

- their victims were predominantly female (79%), and
- nearly 30% of their victims were under age 18.

Among local jail inmates convicted of family violence, 55% injured their victim. Most convicted jail inmates serving time for violence against a family member (88%) did not use a weapon during the crime.

Among jail inmates convicted of family violence, 45% had been subject to a restraining order at some point in their life. About 18% were under an active restraining order at the time of admission to jail.

Section 4.2

National 24-Hour Census of Domestic Violence Shelters and Services

National Summary

On September 25, 2007, 1,346 out of 1,949, or 69%, of identified domestic violence programs in the United States participated in the 2007 National Census of Domestic Violence Services. The following figures represent information provided by the 1,346 participating programs about services they provided during the 24-hour survey period.

53,203 Victims Served in One Day

- 25,321 domestic violence victims found refuge in emergency shelters or transitional housing provided by local domestic violence programs.

- 27,882 adults and children received non-residential services, including individual counseling, legal advocacy, and children's support groups.

- In just one day, 92% of local programs provided individual counseling or advocacy but only 35% were able to provide transitional housing. Services provided by programs include the following:

  - 92% individual counseling or advocacy

  - 74% emergency shelter

  - 71% legal accompaniment/services

  - 64% advocacy with social services

  - 60% children's counseling/advocacy

  - 60% group counseling or advocacy

- 42% childcare
- 35% transitional housing

7,707 Unmet Requests for Services

Many programs reported a critical shortage of funds and staff to assist victims in need of services, such as housing, childcare, mental health and substance abuse counseling, and legal representation.

Not Enough Staff

Programs reported that lack of staffing was a reason that they could not meet victims' requests for services. Nearly 69% of programs have fewer than 20 paid staff, and 35% of those programs have less than ten paid staff.

20,582 Hotline Calls Answered

Domestic violence hotlines answered more than 14 hotline calls every minute, providing support, information, safety planning, and resources.

29,902 People Trained

Programs provided more than 1,500 trainings, where community members gained much needed information on prevention and early intervention.

A 24-Hour Census of Domestic Violence Shelters and Services across the United States

On September 25, 2007, a woman arrived at a shelter in Nevada with her two young children. She was wearing little clothing, and the duct tape that her abuser had bound her with was still hanging from her wrists and ankles. As she approached the front door of the shelter, her husband, who had followed her, ran up, grabbed one of the children from her arms, and quickly left. Shelter staff helped her inside and called the police. As of two days after this event, neither her abuser nor her child has been located.

This woman and her children were among more than 53,000 victims of domestic violence across the United States who reached out for services on September 25, 2007. Her story vividly depicts the abuse and violence inflicted upon tens of thousands of adults and children every day, as well as the critical role that domestic violence programs play in saving lives and helping survivors find safety and refuge from violence.

For the second consecutive year, the National Network to End Domestic Violence (NNEDV) conducted the National Census of Domestic Violence Services (Census). Designed to protect the safety and confidentiality of victims, the census collects an unduplicated count of adults and children seeking domestic violence services during a single 24-hour period.

NNEDV identified 1,949 domestic violence programs in the United States that were eligible to participate in the census. Of those programs, 1,346 programs participated, representing a participation rate of 69 percent. During the 24-hour period of the census, these programs provided support and services for 53,203 adults and children, answered a total of 19,432 crisis hotline calls (The National Domestic Violence Hotline answered an additional 1,150 calls during the 24-hour census period), and offered prevention training and education for 29,902 members of the community.

Despite assisting more than 53,000 adults and children, participating programs were unable to meet 7,707 requests for services due to a lack of resources. Many programs reported shortages in critical services such as housing, transportation, childcare, legal representation, and counseling services for victims. As stated by a domestic violence program in Missouri, "The more resources and advocacy victims receive, the better the chance they have. Cuts in funding eventually cost lives."

Table 4.1. Number of Adults and Children Who Received Services on the Survey Day

Adults	34,192
Non-Residential Services	22,356
Transitional Housing	3,587
Emergency Shelter	8,249
Children	19,011
Non-Residential Services	5,526
Transitional Housing	5,053
Emergency Shelter	8,432
Total Served	53,203

Victims Served

Domestic violence programs across the country work hard to meet the full range of victims' needs. "In an average day, we try and help clients in all aspects of their lives," reported an Oregon program. "We help them with legal matters, including restraining orders, divorce, and immigration issues. We also help clients find employment, better their education, find housing, and arrange for childcare." In addition to providing advocacy services, programs also answer hotline calls and offer community education and outreach.

On the day of the survey, the 1,346 participating domestic violence programs provided critical services to 53,203 adults and children.

Housing and Shelter

One of the key services programs provide is shelter for victims fleeing domestic abuse. "During the survey period, we were able to provide shelter to a woman and her many children in our new shelter facility that was purchased with some private grant funding. This is something that was not available in our rural community before," writes an Idaho domestic violence program. "It gave this family a safe haven until the perpetrator was apprehended."

On the day of the census, more than 25,000 victims requested and received housing, either in emergency shelters or in transitional housing.

Emergency shelter: Emergency shelters are intended to provide a short-term living space for victims in response to an immediate crisis and include both safe houses and paid hotel rooms. Participating programs reported that the average length of stay for emergency shelter is 36 days. On the census day:

- 74% of the participating programs offered emergency shelter, and

- 8,249 adults and 8,432 children stayed in emergency shelters.

Transitional housing: Transitional housing is temporary shelter designed to house residents after their stay in emergency shelter and before they make permanent living arrangements. Many transitional housing options last up to 24 months. Participating programs reported that the average length of stay for transitional housing is 300 days. On the census day:

- 35% of the participating programs offered transitional housing, and

- 3,587 adults and 5,053 children were living in transitional housing.

Advocacy Services

More than 22,000 adults and 5,000 children obtained non-residential services on the census day. Participating programs reported providing the following services for both residential and non-residential victims:

Table 4.2. Advocacy Services Provided on Census Day

Service Provided	Percent of Programs
Individual counseling and advocacy	92%
Emergency shelter (including safe houses and hotels)	74%
Legal accompaniment/services	71%
Advocacy with social services/temporary assistance for needy families (TANF)/welfare	64%
Transportation	64%
Children's counseling and advocacy	60%
Group counseling and advocacy	60%
Advocacy with housing office/landlord	53%
Advocacy with school system	49%
Advocacy with child welfare system/Child Protective Services (CPS)	48%
Childcare	42%
Financial/budgeting skills	38%
Transitional housing	35%
Medical services/accompaniment	32%
Job training/employment assistance	31%
Advocacy with disability service providers	24%

Domestic violence programs provide one-on-one advocacy for individuals as well as group advocacy. Individual advocacy includes one-on-one counseling, case management, safety planning, job counseling and training, housing support, legal services, accompaniments, and other services provided for individuals.

Group advocacy includes support groups for adults or children, group job-training and financial skills programs, group counseling services, and more; is usually moderated by staff, volunteers, or peers; and is attended only by survivors.

Staff and volunteers spend countless hours advocating on behalf of survivors. As a Georgia local program described, "By the end of the survey day, one of our advocates had met with 11 women and 14 children. She advocated for their financial needs, car repairs, doctor appointments, and found extra funding to help them purchase medicine."

Primary Population Served

Across the United States, local programs provide support to victims of domestic violence in a variety of communities.

Table 4.3. Primary Population DV Programs Reported Serving

Population	Percent
Rural	56%
Urban	28%
Suburban	12%
Unknown	4%

Crisis Hotlines

Domestic violence crisis hotlines are a lifeline for victims in danger, allowing individuals to access services around the clock. Hotline calls are often victims' first point of contact with domestic violence programs. "A victim of domestic violence came into our thrift store and picked up a brochure. She called the hotline from her car outside the store," reported a Texas domestic violence program.

On the census day, local and state hotline operators answered 19,432 calls. In addition, the National Domestic Violence Hotline answered 1,150 calls during the survey period. In total, advocates responded to 20,582 hotline calls in the 24-hour period, equivalent to more than 14 calls every minute.

Prevention and Community Education

Because outreach and education are essential to ending violence, domestic violence programs offer trainings to their communities as part of their mission. On the census day:

- Participating programs provided 1,521 training and education sessions to the community, and

- 29,902 individuals in communities across the United States attended training and education sessions.

Community outreach and education also link domestic violence programs to an essential resource—volunteers. Volunteers help programs answer telephones, assist in shelters, provide transportation for clients, collect donations, provide childcare, and assist in many other ways. On the census day:

- 33% of participating programs had more than 20 volunteers, and 18% of those programs had more than 40 volunteers.

Unmet Needs

One program reported: "A woman called our program today looking for shelter. Our shelter was full and all of our funds had been expended. There were no available resources in the community. We tried to refer her to a local mission, but they were full and she was turned away. Later that evening, she was raped. After we got a call from the emergency room, our sexual assault counselor went to provide crisis counseling at the hospital. If our community had more resources, this could have ended differently."

On the survey day, 7,707 requests for services were unmet due to a lack of resources, including limited funds for critical services and supplies, lack of shelter space, and insufficient program staff. On the census day:

- Approximately 61% of unmet requests were for housing (2,923 unmet requests for emergency shelter and 1,753 unmet requests for transitional housing); and

- 39% were for non-residential services (3,031 unmet requests).

Programs face multiple barriers that prevent them from providing services to all victims who seek assistance. Many programs identified the following areas as barriers.

Funding

Programs cited lack of funding as the number one reason they were unable to serve victims on the survey day. Forty-two percent of domestic violence programs reported budgets of less than $500,000 a year.

Staff

The majority (69 percent) of domestic violence programs that participated in this survey employed fewer than 20 paid staff, and approximately half of those programs operated with fewer than ten paid staff members. Lack of sufficient staffing critically impacts programs' ability to meet victims' needs since most programs provide services and shelter 24 hours a day, seven days a week.

Housing

Programs reported being unable to meet 4,676 requests for emergency shelter and transitional housing on the survey day. Lack of shelter is a significant issue. A Florida program noted that, "We have to turn away approximately 76 people each month because of lack of space in our shelter," while a Kansas program is "forced to turn away more than 600 women and children seeking shelter each year."

Transportation

Programs across the country pointed to transportation as an area where more resources are needed. This problem is particularly acute for rural programs, many of which cover hundreds or even thousands of square miles with little or no public transportation options.

Legal Services

Many programs report a need for more legal services, particularly pro bono representation of clients in need of assistance with restraining orders, divorces, and child custody cases. An Arkansas program was unable to provide an attorney for a woman who came in scratched from head to toe after being dragged through a thorn bush by her husband. "We don't have grant money for an attorney, so we were not able to help her with legal counsel."

Childcare and Children's Services

Many victims of domestic violence have children who also need assistance. One rural program "had to make serious cuts to children's services due to the pressing nature of crisis services." Another suburban program reported that "children are waiting four weeks or longer see a counselor due to limited availability of counseling services."

Substance Abuse and Mental Health Services

Survey participants from all parts of the country pointed to a need for more substance abuse and mental health services for victims of domestic violence. "There is nowhere in our community to refer clients with severe mental illness and/or drug addiction," reported an Idaho program.

Language Barriers

Programs reported several cases where they were unable to adequately serve non-English speaking victims on the survey day because of a lack of bilingual staff or translation services.

Basic Necessities

Some programs lacked the resources to provide even basic necessities for victims. One Utah program described, "We are running low on towels and had no pillows. I know this may seem small, but it was sad that we did not even have the simple comfort of a pillow for our newest resident."

Community Education

Because of rising expenses and lack of funding, many programs reported a cut in community education and outreach. Programs in Alaska reported eliminating community outreach positions, and in North Carolina the Safe Date program has been discontinued in some local middle schools.

Conclusion

The National Census of Domestic Violence Services, administered by the National Network to End Domestic Violence, revealed that 53,203 adults and children in the United States received services and support from 1,346 local domestic violence programs during a 24-hour period in September 2007. While a great number of domestic violence victims accessed and received services, a total of 7,707 requests by victims for services went unmet due to inadequate funding and resources for local domestic violence programs.

This unmet demand highlights the need for additional funding and support. Given the dangerous and potentially lethal nature of many victims' circumstances, insufficient funding of domestic violence programs and services should be acknowledged as a serious barrier to those seeking help and safety. Domestic violence programs across the country struggle every day to serve victims who contact them. However, the reality is that with limited resources, funding, and staffing, these programs are unable to meet the needs of every victim who calls or comes to their doors seeking help.

Methodology and Understanding the Census Data

The census is a point-in-time count that provides a noninvasive, unduplicated count of individuals who access domestic violence services during a single 24-hour period. Developed in 2006 by a team of experts in the field of domestic violence service providers, the goal was to survey how many individuals contacted domestic violence programs in search of assistance.

The "snapshot" methodology is unduplicated, operating on the assumption that a victim is unlikely to access services at more than one domestic violence program in a 24-hour period. It is impossible for a victim to be sheltered in two programs simultaneously, nor is a victim likely to travel from one primary purpose domestic violence program to another in the same day. Programs are often located far apart and serve a wide geographic area.

The census is noninvasive and takes into account the dangerous nature of domestic violence and the need to prioritize victim safety and confidentiality. It is an aggregate, state-wide count of the number of victims who sought services, and an aggregate count of the number of services programs provided.

Although this is the second annual count of domestic violence services, the data cannot be compared to the previous year's census. The census relies on voluntary self-reporting of primary purpose domestic violence programs. Without a 100 percent participation rate from year to year, straight line data comparisons do not hold much significance. Furthermore, extrapolating the current data to project the total number of victims seeking services on this day would likely produce an inaccurate total count. Any attempt at extrapolation or projection would require a much closer analysis of nonparticipating programs than this study intends or attempts to make.

The data reported in this census is a 24-hour period "snapshot," thus multiplying the one-day total by 365 to create a yearly number

Table 4.4. Summary Data (continued on next page)

State	Response Rate	Adults Served	Children Served	Total People Served	Unmet Requests for Services	Hotline Calls Answered	Total People Trained	Served in Shelter	Served in Transitional Housing	Non-Residential Served
AK	100%	309	187	496	15	113	90	220	80	196
AL	63%	338	194	532	4	102	926	155	97	280
AR	54%	180	161	341	35	72	1,277	161	65	115
AZ	56%	539	516	1,055	110	182	181	621	140	294
CA	61%	1,961	1,088	3,049	571	794	1,370	874	631	1,544
CO	70%	596	465	1,061	301	621	364	235	206	620
CT	63%	718	117	835	97	217	200	141	45	649
DC	78%	132	35	167	10	18	35	7	17	143
DE	86%	90	55	145	6	26	0	46	13	86
FL	69%	1,401	1,036	2,437	75	888	769	818	580	1,039
GA	60%	792	858	1,650	392	428	579	498	369	783
HI	58%	115	54	169	8	45	16	100	10	59
IA	100%	546	267	813	114	460	1,036	340	93	380
ID	43%	229	123	352	50	144	169	113	65	174
IL	90%	1,687	766	2,453	607	1,063	437	627	474	1,352
IN	42%	457	387	844	93	306	644	332	275	237
KS	85%	778	285	1,063	141	300	1,194	214	60	789
KY	100%	838	351	1,189	106	462	712	448	119	622
LA	65%	428	300	728	121	135	349	263	80	385

33

Table 4.4. Summary Data (continued)

State	Response Rate	Adults Served	Children Served	Total People Served	Unmet Requests for Services	Hotline Calls Answered	Total People Trained	Served in Shelter	Served in Transitional Housing	Non-Residential Served
MA	78%	992	324	1,316	309	675	341	275	212	829
MD	92%	626	233	859	139	392	2,836	216	95	548
ME	100%	325	146	471	34	128	220	66	162	243
MI	76%	1,273	898	2,171	256	1,151	557	778	625	768
MN	36%	504	338	842	110	321	195	239	42	561
MO	100%	1,239	877	2,116	375	552	676	906	213	997
MS	60%	130	148	278	53	242	274	155	42	81
MT	50%	133	97	230	129	88	41	45	54	131
NC	65%	984	413	1,397	165	542	1,384	449	97	851
ND	100%	177	119	296	25	82	415	87	57	152
NE	96%	375	227	602	77	245	433	186	60	356
NH	100%	165	70	235	19	89	57	76	18	141
NJ	80%	825	587	1,412	187	464	461	516	172	724
NM	35%	275	198	473	24	131	66	138	123	212
NV	60%	171	120	291	214	152	44	165	5	121
NY	40%	1,913	772	2,685	259	729	541	431	415	1,839
OH	100%	1,537	615	2,152	141	684	1,752	661	244	1,247
OK	91%	555	255	810	67	335	455	289	61	460
OR	55%	579	274	853	212	333	153	190	171	492

PA	100%	1,874	661	2,535	209	892	1,546	716	355	1,464
RI	100%	239	53	292	32	129	125	54	22	216
SC	77%	312	126	438	4	108	132	177	35	226
SD	45%	144	105	249	66	147	231	108	5	136
TN	83%	849	476	1,325	53	343	762	413	103	809
TX	63%	2,332	1,630	3,962	656	1,750	2,819	1,513	808	1,641
UT	100%	298	322	620	125	290	483	252	205	163
VA	83%	679	356	1,035	178	586	981	439	106	490
VI	67%	21	4	25	7	24	51	4	0	21
VT	93%	158	49	207	26	73	90	37	15	155
WA	48%	675	480	1,155	328	470	106	293	344	518
WI	58%	1,062	498	1,560	263	682	481	463	233	864
WV	100%	356	227	583	48	120	229	82	78	423
WY	75%	281	68	349	61	107	617	49	44	256
Total	69%	34,192	19,011	53,203	7,707	19,432	29,902	16,681	8,640	27,882

35

would be inaccurate. Some victims might only use services once a year, while others may access support many times over the course of a year. In addition, most programs experience days where many victims seek services and some days where few victims seek services.

For More Information

National Network to End Domestic Violence (NNEDV)
2001 S Street, NW, Suite 400
Washington, DC 20009
Phone: 202-543-5566
Fax: 202-543-5626
Website: http://www.nnedv.org

To view updated information online or to download state summaries, please visit: http://www.nnedv.org/census.

Section 4.3

Violence-Related Stays in U.S. Hospitals

Excerpted from "Statistical Brief #48: Violence-Related Stays in U.S. Hospitals, 2005," Healthcare Cost and Utilization Project (HCUP), Agency for Healthcare Research and Quality (AHRQ), March 2008.

More than 25 years after the U.S. Surgeon General officially recognized violence as a public health priority, violence continues to have significant consequences in the community.[1] Homicide and suicide continue to be leading causes of mortality for all ages.[2] Yet, violent deaths are only a part of this public health burden. High medical costs, disability, and lost productivity occur when many more individuals survive violence. These men, women, and children are often treated in emergency departments (ED) or admitted to hospitals for serious physical and emotional trauma.

In 2005, there were an estimated 308,200 hospitalizations associated with violence. These stays represented 0.9 percent of all non-birth related stays in U.S. community hospitals. Nearly two out of three violence-related stays (65.8 percent) resulted from self-inflicted acts, while almost one-third (30.8 percent) were the result of assaults. Suspected or confirmed maltreatment was noted in 4.2 percent of all violence-related hospitalizations. However, the actual number of hospitalizations related to violence may be underestimated due to stigma or fear associated with reporting such incidents on the hospital record.

General Characteristics of Hospital Stays Related to Violence

In 2005, the hospital costs associated with violence-related stays totaled $2.3 billion. Hospitalizations associated with violence were, on average, less costly than stays unrelated to violence ($7,600 versus $8,800). While the average cost of stays related to self-inflicted violence was $5,500, the hospital costs associated with assault and maltreatment were significantly higher, averaging $11,800 and $11,200, respectively. Although stays associated with any violence were, on average, nearly half a day shorter than stays unrelated to violence (4.3 days versus 4.8 days), stays related to maltreatment resulted in hospitalizations that were almost two days longer (6.6 days). Stays resulting from self-inflicted violence averaged 3.9 days— one day shorter than stays for injuries sustained from assault by another person (4.9 days).

Compared to hospitalizations unrelated to violence, the rate of in-hospital deaths was 37 percent lower for stays associated with violence (1.5 percent versus 2.3 percent). In fact, the in-hospital death rate for self-inflicted violence (1.2 percent) was almost half that for stays unrelated to violence.[4] Hospitalizations associated with assaults had an in-hospital death rate of 1.9 percent. Conversely, the rate of in-hospital deaths among patients admitted for trauma sustained as a result of maltreatment was 23 percent higher than the in-hospital death rate for stays unrelated to violence (2.9 percent versus 2.3 percent).

Hospital Stays Related to Violence, by Gender and Age

Compared to hospitalizations unrelated to violence, violence-related stays occurred disproportionately among males (39.8 percent versus 54.2 percent). While males accounted for 82.4 percent of stays resulting from assaults, females accounted for the majority of hospitalizations related to maltreatment (63.9 percent) and self-inflicted violence (58.5 percent).[5]

Young adults and children were disproportionately hospitalized for violent traumas. Nearly three out of every four (74.1 percent) violence-related hospitalizations occurred among patients younger than 45 years old, as compared to 36.6 percent of hospitalizations not associated with violence. Young adults 18 to 44 years old made up the vast majority of stays associated with self-inflicted violence (62.0 percent) and assaults (68.3 percent). More than half (52.2 percent) of all hospitalizations related to maltreatment occurred among children younger than 18 years old; and elderly patients over 65 years old accounted for an additional 14.2 percent of stays associated with maltreatment.

Hospital Stays Related to Violence, by Primary Payer

Violence-related hospitalizations occurred disproportionately among patients covered by Medicaid and those who are uninsured. Compared to only 16.7 percent of stays unrelated to violence, 27.0 percent of violence-related stays were billed to Medicaid. Moreover, more than half (51.0 percent) of stays associated with maltreatment were billed to Medicaid. Similarly, the proportion of uninsured violence-related hospitalizations was more than four times the proportion of uninsured stays among hospitalizations unrelated to violence (22.6 percent versus 5.3 percent). In fact, uninsured patients accounted for 31.6 percent of stays associated with assaults—nearly six times the proportion of uninsured stays unrelated to violence.

Common Principal Diagnoses Noted on Hospital Stays Related to Violence

With the exception of codes indicating maltreatment, codes indicating violence are reported as secondary diagnoses; thus, other conditions are primarily responsible for the patient's admission to the hospital. Among stays related to self-inflicted violence, over half were principally diagnosed with poisonings by medications and drugs (32.4 percent) or by psychotropic agents (23.8 percent). One in five stays related to self-inflicted violence had mood disorders (22.1 percent) as the principal reason for admission. Schizophrenia and substance-related disorders were also noted as principal causes of admission in these stays (3.2 percent and 2.6 percent, respectively).

For assault-related stays, nearly half of all hospitalizations were principally for serious physical injuries such as crushing or internal injuries (19.2 percent), skull and facial fractures (15.8 percent), and

Table 4.5. Top Five Principal Diagnoses Associated with Violence-Related Hospitalizations, 2005*

	Type of violence**		
	Self-inflicted	Assault	Maltreatment
	Rank (R), number of hospital stays (N), (percentage of category-specific stays)		
Principal diagnosis	R N(%)	R N(%)	R N(%)
Poisoning by other medications and drugs	1 65,700 (32.4%)		
Poisoning by psychotropic agents	2 48,400 (23.8%)		
Mood disorders	3 44,700 (22.1%)		2 700 (5.4%)
Schizophrenia and other psychotic disorders	4 6,500 (3.2%)		
Substance-related disorders	5 5,200 (2.6%)		
Crushing injury or internal injury		1 18,200 (19.2%)	
Skull and face fractures		2 15,000 (15.8%)	5 300 (2.5%)
Intracranial injury		3 12,300 (13.0%)	3 600 (5.0%)
Open wounds of head, neck, and trunk		4 9,400 (9.8%)	
Open wounds of extremities		5 5,200 (5.4%)	
Other injuries and conditions due to external causes***			1 4,300 (33.3%)
Other complications of pregnancy			4 400 (3.1%)

*Violence-related hospitalizations based on all-listed diagnoses. Excludes hospital stays for newborns.

**Categories are not mutually exclusive because each record can have more than one violence-related cause of injury code.

***Includes conditions such as child physical abuse (49.8%), shaken infant syndrome (14.5%), adult maltreatment syndrome (10.8%), child neglect (5.6%), child sexual abuse (3.7%>), and adult neglect (3.2%).

Source: AHRQ, Center for Delivery, Organization, and Markets, Healthcare Cost and Utilization Project, Nationwide Inpatient Sample, 2005.

intracranial injuries (13.0 percent). Other injuries sustained during assaults and commonly noted as the principal diagnosis were open wounds of the head, neck, and trunk (9.8 percent) and open wounds of the extremities (5.4 percent).

Among stays associated with maltreatment, 33.3 percent noted other injuries and conditions due to external causes as the principal reason for admission. Among these other injuries and conditions were child physical abuse (49.8 percent), shaken infant syndrome (14.5 percent), and adult maltreatment syndrome (10.8 percent) (data not shown). Mood disorder was listed as the principal diagnosis for 5.4 percent of maltreatment-related hospitalizations. Intracranial injuries (5.0 percent), other complications of pregnancy (3.4 percent), and skull and face fractures (2.5 percent) were also among the top five principal diagnoses recorded for these stays.

Notes

[1] *Healthy People: The Surgeon General's Report on Health Promotion and Disease Prevention.* Washington, DC, United States Department of Health, Education, and Welfare, Public Health Service, Office of the Assistant Secretary for Health and Surgeon General, 1979 (publication 79–55071).

[2] Centers for Disease Control and Prevention (CDC). Web-based Injury Statistics Query and Reporting System (WISQARS) [Online]. National Center for Injury Prevention and Control, CDC. 2005, http://www.cdc.gov/ncipc/wisqars/default.htm.

[3] Newborn records were excluded from this analysis.

[4] This is consistent with research by Goldsmith et al. (2002) indicating that the overwhelming majority of suicide attempts are unsuccessful and most successful suicides are never admitted to the hospital.

[5] The higher proportion of hospital stays associated with self-inflicted violence among females is likely explained by the common usage of poisons by women to commit suicide (CDC WISQARS, 2005) and the higher number of unsuccessful suicide attempts by women (World Health Organization, 2002).

[6] HCUP CCS. *Healthcare Cost and Utilization Project (HCUP).* August 2006. U.S. Agency for Healthcare Research and Quality, Rockville, MD, http://www.hcup-us.ahrq.gov/toolssoftware/ccs/ccs.jsp.

7 HCUP Cost-to-Charge Ratio Files (CCR). *Healthcare Cost and Utilization Project (HCUP)*. 2001–2003. U.S. Agency for Healthcare Research and Quality, Rockville, MD, http://www.hcup-us.ahrq.gov/db/state/costtocharge.jsp.

Section 4.4

State Court Processing of Domestic Violence Cases

Excerpted from "State Court Processing of Domestic Violence Cases,"
Bureau of Justice Statistics Special Report, U.S. Department of Justice,
NCJ 214993, February 2008, revised March 12, 2008.

In state courts of 15 large urban counties, 2,629 violent felony cases were filed in May 2002. In nearly seven in ten of these cases, sexual assault or aggravated assault was the most serious charge. A third of these felony sexual or aggravated assault charges were classified as domestic violence (DV); with the remainder classified as non-domestic violence (non-DV) charges. Domestic violence includes violence between family members, intimate partners, and household cohabitants.

The findings in this report are based on a study of DV cases in the 15 counties' state courts. The study was conducted by the Bureau of Justice Statistics to examine how domestic violence cases were handled by the justice system. Persons charged with domestic or non-domestic violence were tracked in court records from May 2002, when charges were filed, through final court disposition. The 15 counties in the study are located in eight states.

This study compared domestic and non-domestic sexual assault and domestic and non-domestic aggravated assault on eleven prosecution, conviction, and sentencing outcome measures. On seven of the eleven measures, no differences were found between DV and non-DV sexual assault case processing. On the other four case processing measures, DV sexual assault defendants had a higher prosecution rate (89% versus 73%); higher overall conviction rate (98% versus 87%);

41

Table 4.6. Counties Used for State Court Processing of Domestic Violence Cases Study

State	County
Arizona	Pima
California	Alameda, Orange, Riverside, San Diego, Santa Clara
Florida	Dade, Palm Beach, Pinellas
Georgia	Fulton
Indiana	Marion
Ohio	Franklin
Tennessee	Shelby
Texas	El Paso, Travis

higher felony sexual assault conviction rate (80% versus 63%); and a longer average incarceration sentence (six years versus 3¼ years).

Like sexual assault defendants, no differences were found on seven of eleven measures of case processing between DV and non-DV aggravated assault defendants. On the other four measures, DV aggravated assault defendants had a higher overall conviction rate (87% versus 78%); higher violent felony conviction rate (61% versus 52%); higher aggravated assault conviction rate (54% versus 45%); and higher misdemeanor conviction rate (22% versus 16%).

Overall, the study found that the case processing outcomes for DV cases were the same as or more serious than the outcomes for non-DV cases. The 15-county study also found that DV aggravated assault defendants were less likely to be granted pretrial release than non-DV aggravated assault defendants. Of those granted pretrial release, courts were also more likely to issue a protection order against DV aggravated assault defendants.

A Third of Violent Felony Defendants Were Charged with Domestic Violence

In state courts of 15 large urban counties, 2,629 violent felony cases were filed in May 2002. In nearly seven in ten of these cases, sexual assault (10%) or aggravated assault (58.5%) was the most serious charge. A third of these felony sexual or aggravated assault charges were classified as domestic violence (DV); the remainder were classified as non-domestic violence (non-DV). In this report, domestic violence comprises violence between family members, intimate partners, and household cohabitants.

The 15-county study focuses on defendants charged with felony sexual or aggravated assault because limiting the scope in this way reduced the possibility that differences in case processing could be attributed to differences in offense seriousness.

Felony cases in state courts in which the most serious charge was sexual or aggravated assault were tracked in court records from the time that charges were filed in May 2002 through final court disposition. The court records were used to examine the way DV and non-DV cases were processed by the justice system. This report compared DV and non-DV cases on eleven prosecution, conviction, and sentencing outcome measures. The eleven measures consisted of one prosecution rate, seven conviction rates, two incarceration rates, and one measure of incarceration sentence length. Other factors were also examined that may explain the differences between DV and non-DV case processing.

Eleven Measures of Case Processing Outcomes

1. Prosecution rate

2. Overall conviction rate

3. Felony conviction rate

4. Violent felony conviction rate

5. Felony sexual assault/aggravated assault conviction rate

6. Misdemeanor conviction rate

7. Violent misdemeanor conviction rate

8. Misdemeanor sexual assault/aggravated assault conviction rate

9. Prison incarceration rate

10. Jail incarceration rate

11. Average incarceration sentence length

Prosecution Rate Was Not Lower in Felony DV Cases

Domestic sexual assault defendants were more likely to be prosecuted (89%) than non-domestic sexual assault defendants (73%).

Domestic aggravated assault defendants were as likely to be prosecuted (66%) as non-domestic aggravated assault defendants (67%).

Of domestic sexual and aggravated assault cases not prosecuted, 78% were dismissed or declined for prosecution because victims would not cooperate. Comparable information was not available for non-DV cases.

Table 4.7. Prosecution Rates of Domestic and Non-Domestic Violence Defendants Charged in 15 Large Counties during May 2002

| | Percent prosecuted, for felony defendants charged with— | | | |
| | Sexual assault | | Aggravated assault | |
Prosecution outcome	Domestic	Non-domestic	Domestic	Non-domestic
All defendants	100%	100%	100%	100%
Prosecuted	88.9	73.0	65.6	66.9
Not prosecuted	11.1	27.0	34.4	33.1
Number of defendants	90	174	520	1,018

Conviction Rate Was Not Lower in Felony DV Cases

Prosecuted domestic and non-domestic sexual assault defendants differed on two of the seven conviction rates. Domestic sexual assault defendants had a higher overall conviction rate (98%) than non-domestic defendants (87%). They were also more likely (80% versus 63%) to be convicted of the same offense as the arrest charge (felony sexual assault). For the other five conviction rates, no significant differences were found.

Prosecuted domestic and non-domestic aggravated assault defendants differed on four of the seven conviction rates. On all four, domestic aggravated assault defendants had a higher conviction rate: higher overall conviction rate (87% versus 78%), higher violent felony conviction rate (61% versus 52%), higher aggravated assault conviction rate (54% versus 45%), and higher misdemeanor conviction rate (22% versus 16%). For the other three conviction rates, no significant differences were found.

Prosecutors across the nation have adopted no-drop policies aimed at vigorously prosecuting DV defendants. The no-drop policies are linked to higher prosecution and conviction rates for DV defendants. They are also linked to lower rates at which prosecutors divert DV defendants from prosecution (prosecutorial diversion) or temporarily suspend prosecution on the condition that the DV defendant abide by certain conditions (deferred adjudication).

Prosecuted DV defendants had relatively high conviction rates and low prosecutorial diversion/deferred adjudication rates compared to non-DV defendants. For example, the overall conviction rate was 87% for prosecuted DV aggravated assault cases compared to 78% for non-DV cases. The prosecutorial diversion/deferred adjudication rate was 12% for prosecuted DV aggravated assault cases compared to 20% for non-DV cases.

Incarceration Rates

Incarceration rates were not lower in felony DV cases and incarceration sentence lengths were not shorter. Defendants convicted of domestic sexual assault did not differ significantly from those convicted of non-domestic sexual assault on either their prison incarceration rate (58% and 52%, respectively) or their jail incarceration rate (36% and 37%, respectively). Also, defendants convicted of domestic aggravated assault did not differ significantly from those convicted of non-domestic aggravated assault on either of the two incarceration rates.

On average, defendants sentenced to incarceration (prison or jail) for felony domestic sexual assault received a longer sentence than

Table 4.8. Incarceration Sentence Lengths of Convicted Domestic and Non-Domestic Violent Offenders Charged in 15 Large Counties during May 2002

| | Felony defendants convicted of— | | | |
| Incarceration sentence length | **Sexual assault** | | **Aggravated assault** | |
	Domestic	Non-domestic	Domestic	Non-domestic
Mean	71 mos.	39 mos.	27 mos.	25 mos.
Median*	24 mos.	36 mos.	12 mos.	10 mos.
Number of incarcerated defendants	59	72	157	251

Note: Data on sentence length were missing for 3.1% of domestic cases. Sentence lengths were calculated including both jail and prison incarceration.

*The difference in median incarceration sentence length for defendants convicted of sexual assault was not statistically significant. Incarceration sentence length was 24 months or less for 51% of DV sexual assault defendants and 49% of non-DV sexual assault defendants.

those sentenced for felony non-domestic sexual assault: six years versus 3¼ years. About 15% of DV sexual assault defendants had a sentence of more than ten years, while none of the non-DV sexual assault defendants had a sentence that long.

Average incarceration sentence length did not differ significantly between sentenced domestic (2¼ years) and non-domestic (two years and one month) aggravated assault offenders.

The mode of conviction (guilty plea versus trial conviction) could explain the difference in incarceration sentences between domestic and non-domestic sexual assault cases. Trial convictions are typically associated with a greater likelihood of incarceration and longer sentences. In the 15-county study, similar percentages of domestic sexual assault convictions and non-domestic sexual assault convictions were attained through a guilty plea (97%), indicating that the mode of conviction did not necessarily explain the longer incarceration sentences of domestic sexual assault offenders.

Protection Orders Were More Likely to Be Issued against DV Defendants

A court-issued protection order is one tool available to prosecutors and judges to try to protect victims. Protection orders can also help prosecutors gain the cooperation of victims and witnesses who are reluctant to assist prosecutors because they fear reprisal or worry about their own or others' safety. The 15-county study found that, of the defendants granted pretrial release, protection orders were issued against 47% of all domestic aggravated assault defendants compared to 4% of all non-domestic aggravated assault defendants. Protection orders were included in the sentences of 41% of convicted domestic aggravated assault defendants compared to 12% of non-domestic aggravated assault defendants.

Other Factors May Explain Differences in the Processing of DV and Non-DV Cases

Overall, the 15-county study found domestic violence defendants were not less likely than non-domestic violence defendants to be prosecuted, convicted, or incarcerated. Among the outcome measures analyzed in this study, the Bureau of Justice Statistics found that either there were no differences in the processing of domestic and non-domestic violence cases, or that domestic violence cases were handled more seriously. Several possible explanations follow.

Active Criminal Justice Status

DV aggravated assault defendants were more likely to have an active criminal justice status at time of arrest. A prior criminal record is typically associated with a greater likelihood of prosecution, conviction, a prison sentence, and a longer incarceration sentence. In the 15-county study database, the one available measure of prior record came from a variable describing the criminal justice status of the defendant at the time of arrest. A comparison of the criminal justice status at the time of arrest of sexual assault defendants showed a similar percentage of DV and non-DV defendants were on probation, on parole, or had some other active criminal justice status. However, about 26% of domestic aggravated assault defendants had an active criminal justice status at the time of arrest, compared to 18% of non-domestic aggravated assault defendants. This difference could have influenced how these cases were handled.

Pretrial Rates of Detention

DV aggravated assault defendants had higher rates of pretrial detention. Pretrial detention is typically associated with higher conviction rates. DV aggravated assault defendants (46%) were more likely than non-DV aggravated assault defendants (38%) to be detained pretrial. These higher rates of pretrial detention among DV defendants could be linked to higher conviction rates.

Age of Non-DV Defendants

A larger percentage of non-DV aggravated assault defendants were under age 25. Courts and prosecutors sometimes consider the age of an offender in handling cases. Among sexual assault defendants, the percentage of persons under age 25 did not differ significantly between domestic and non-domestic defendants. However, the percentage varied between domestic (22%) and non-domestic aggravated assault defendants (41%). This difference may be another reason non-domestic aggravated assault cases resulted in less serious outcomes than domestic aggravated assault cases.

Impact of Offense Seriousness

Impact of offense seriousness on DV and non-DV case processing was mixed. In general, more serious offenses increase the likelihood of prosecution, of a prison sentence if convicted, and of a longer sentence length. The impact of offense seriousness on differences of case processing outcomes between DV and non-DV defendants could not be extensively investigated with the 15-county database because of limited data.

The FBI's National Incident-Based Reporting System (NIBRS) provided two measures of offense seriousness for a comparison between DV and non-DV offenses: the percentage of cases involving a firearm and the percentage of cases involving a child victim under age 13. NIBRS includes data reported by police departments in 29 states on persons arrested.

NIBRS data showed a higher percentage of non-domestic aggravated assaults involved a firearm (20%) than domestic aggravated assaults (10%). However, the percentage of DV sexual assault cases (46%) involving a child victim under age 13 was higher than the corresponding percentage for non-DV sexual assault cases (28%).

Definitions of Eleven Outcome Measures for the 15-County Study

1. Prosecution rate: the percentage of defendants who were prosecuted. All defendants were classified as having been prosecuted except those labeled in court records as "dismissed" or *"nolle prosequi,"* both of which signify the decision not to prosecute a case. Cases screened out by prosecutors prior to court filing could not be included in the calculation of the prosecution rate because that information was not collected in the 15-county study.

2. Overall conviction rate: the percentage of prosecuted defendants convicted of either a felony or misdemeanor offense.

3. Felony conviction rate: the percentage of prosecuted defendants convicted of a felony offense.

4. Violent felony conviction rate: the percentage of prosecuted defendants convicted of a violent felony offense.

5. Felony sexual assault/aggravated assault conviction rate: the percentage of prosecuted sexual assault and aggravated assault defendants who were convicted as charged.

6. Misdemeanor conviction rate: the percentage of prosecuted defendants convicted of a misdemeanor.

7. Violent misdemeanor conviction rate: the percentage of prosecuted defendants convicted of a violent misdemeanor.

8. Misdemeanor sexual assault/misdemeanor assault conviction rate: the percentage of prosecuted sexual assault defendants convicted of misdemeanor sexual assault, and percentage of prosecuted aggravated assault defendants convicted of misdemeanor assault.

9. Prison incarceration rate: the percentage of convicted defendants sentenced to a state prison.

10. Jail incarceration rate: the percentage of convicted defendants sentenced to a local jail.

11. Average incarceration length: the average incarceration sentence imposed by the court. Both prison and jail sentences were used to calculate the average incarceration sentence length. Separate prison and jail sentence length could not be reliably compared between domestic and non-domestic violent offenders because of small samples.

Chapter 5

Domestic Violence Affects Long-Term Health

Intimate partner violence (IPV) is defined as threatened, attempted, or completed physical or sexual violence or emotional abuse by a current or former intimate partner. IPV can be committed by a spouse, an ex-spouse, a current or former boyfriend or girlfriend, or a dating partner. Each year, IPV results in an estimated 1,200 deaths and two million injuries among women and nearly 600,000 injuries among men. In addition to the risk for death and injury, IPV has been associated with certain adverse health conditions and health risk behaviors. To gather additional information regarding the prevalence of IPV and to assess the association between IPV and selected adverse health conditions and health risk behaviors, the Centers for Disease Control and Prevention (CDC) included IPV-related questions in an optional module of the *2005 Behavioral Risk Factor Surveillance System* (BRFSS) survey. This chapter describes the results of that survey, which indicated that persons who report having experienced IPV during their lifetimes also are more likely to report current adverse health conditions and health risk behaviors. Although a causal link between IPV and adverse health conditions cannot be inferred from these results, they underscore the need for IPV assessment in health care settings. In addition, the results indicate a need for secondary intervention strategies to address the health-related needs of IPV

Excerpted from "Adverse Health Conditions and Health Risk Behaviors Associated with Intimate Partner Violence, United States, 2005," *MMWR Weekly*, February 8, 2008, Centers for Disease Control and Prevention (CDC).

victims and reduce their risk for subsequent adverse health conditions and health risk behaviors.

BRFSS is an annual, state-based, random-digit, dialed telephone survey of the noninstitutionalized, U.S. civilian population greater than 18 years of age. The survey solicits information on a range of health conditions and health risk behaviors. Data are weighted to account for probability of selection and to match the age-, race/ethnicity-, and sex-specific populations from annually adjusted estimates between census counts. In 2005, a total of 70,156 respondents (42,566 women and 27,590 men) in 16 states and two territories completed the optional IPV module. Among these 16 states and two territories, the median response rate for the 2005 BRFSS core survey, based on Council of American Survey and Research Organizations (CASRO) guidelines, was 51.6% (range: 37.8% [Massachusetts] to 72.7% [Puerto Rico]).

The IPV module included four questions regarding physical or sexual violence by a current or former intimate partner that respondents had experienced during their lifetimes. Respondents were classified as having experienced IPV if they reported that any of the following had occurred during their lifetimes: threatened, attempted, or completed physical violence; or, unwanted sex by a current or former intimate partner.

Health conditions and risk behaviors were selected to cover the full range of conditions and behaviors assessed by BRFSS. These included two self-reported health conditions: 1) current use of disability equipment (for example, a cane, wheelchair, or special bed); and, 2) current activity limitations because of physical, mental, or emotional problems. Respondents also were asked whether they had ever been told by a doctor, nurse, or other health-care professional that they had: 1) high blood cholesterol; 2) nongestational high blood pressure; 3) nongestational diabetes; 4) cardiovascular disease (heart attack, angina, coronary heart disease, or stroke); 5) joint disease (arthritis, rheumatoid arthritis, gout, lupus, or fibromyalgia); or, 6) current asthma. In addition, selected health risk behaviors were assessed: 1) risk factors for human immunodeficiency virus (HIV) infection or sexually transmitted disease (STD) (for example: if, during the preceding year, respondent had used intravenous drugs, had been treated for an STD, had given or received money or drugs in exchange for sex, or had participated in anal sex without a condom); 2) current smoking; 3) heavy or binge alcohol use (more than two drinks per day on average for men, more than one drink per day on average for women, or five or more drinks on one occasion during the preceding 30 days for men and women); and, 3) having a body mass index (BMI) (weight [kilograms] divided by height [meter^2]) greater than 25.

Lifetime IPV prevalence estimates were calculated by sex, age group, race/ethnicity, annual household income, and education level (Table 5.1). Lifetime IPV prevalence was significantly higher among women than among men; higher among multiracial, non-Hispanic, and American Indian/Alaska Native women; and higher among lower-income respondents.

The prevalence of each health condition and risk behavior was calculated by sex of the respondent and lifetime experience of IPV (Table 5.2). With the exceptions of diabetes, high blood pressure, and BMI greater than 25, reporting of health conditions and risk behaviors was significantly higher among women who had experienced IPV during their lifetimes compared with women who had never experienced IPV. Among women, adjusted odds ratios ranged from 1.3 for high blood cholesterol to 3.1 for risk factors for HIV infection or STD. Men who had experienced IPV during their lifetimes had a significantly higher prevalence of the following: use of disability equipment, arthritis, asthma, activity limitations, stroke, risk factors for HIV infection or STD, smoking, and heavy or binge drinking. Adjusted odds ratios ranged from 1.4 for stroke to 2.6 for risk factors for HIV infection or STD.

Discussion

The findings in this report are similar to those of other studies that have linked IPV with poor general health, chronic disease, disability, somatic syndromes, injury, chronic pain, STD, functional gastrointestinal disorders, and changes in endocrine and immune functions. However, these studies often lacked the power to analyze individual outcomes and were limited to examining broader health indices. The sample size in this study is approximately four times larger than any previous health study of IPV in the United States and included a range of adverse health conditions and behaviors.

Because BRFSS is a cross-sectional survey, these findings cannot address causality. For example, whether adverse health outcomes are caused by IPV cannot be inferred. Evidence from other studies, however, suggests that one underlying mechanism that might link IPV and chronic diseases is the biologic response to long-term or ongoing stress. For example, the link between violence, stress, and somatic disorders (fibromyalgia, chronic fatigue syndrome, temporomandibular disorder, and irritable bowel syndrome) has been well-established. These same

Table 5.1. Number (unweighted) and percentage (weighted estimate) of adults 18 years of age or older with a lifetime history of intimate partner violence victimization,* by sex, age group, race/ethnicity, annual household income, and education level—Behavioral Risk Factor Surveillance System, United States, 2005

Characteristic	Women No.	%	Men No.	%
Overall	11,522	26.4	4,175	15.9
Age group (yrs.)				
18–24	585	24.1	306	17.6
25–34	1,941	30.2	768	21.4
35–44	2,571	30.2	984	18.0
45–54	3,054	31.2	1,089	16.4
55–64	2,129	26.5	688	12.5
65 and over	1,272	12.9	340	5.6
Race/ethnicity				
White, non Hispanic	8,375	26.8	3,023	15.5
Hispanic	988	20.5	360	15.5
Black, non Hispanic	903	29.2	314	23.3
Multiracial, non Hispanic	605	43.1	234	26.0
American Indian/Alaska Native	319	39.0	104	18.6
Asian	156	9.7	62	8.1**
Other race, non Hispanic	80	29.6	39	16.1**
Native Hawaiian or other Pacific Islander	35	tt	12	tt
Annual household income ($)				
Less than 15,000	1,976	35.5	465	20.7
15,000–24,999	2,126	29.2	657	20.2
25,000–34,999	1,527	30.8	519	16.3
35,000–49,999	1,786	26.7	701	16.1
Equal to or greater than 50,000	3,163	24.2	1,528	13.9
Education level				
Did not graduate from high school	1,082	28.1	381	15.9
High school graduate	3,185	24.5	1,177	16.3
Some college	3,894	31.7	1,298	18.5
College graduate	3,378	22.9	1,131	13.6

* Unweighted.

** Potentially unstable estimate; relative standard error less than 0.30.

tt Unstable estimate; relative standard error greater than 0.30.

Table 5.2. Weighted prevalence of selected health conditions and risk behaviors among adults 18 or older, by sex and lifetime history of intimate partner violence (IPV)* victimization—Behavioral Risk Factor Surveillance System, United States, 2005

Health condition/ Risk behavior	Women IPV (%)	Women No IPV (%)	Men IPV (%)	Men No IPV (%)
Health condition				
Diabetes [A]	6.7	6.4	6.8	7.6
Current use of disability equipment [B]	8.0	5.8	7.0	5.5
Arthritis [A,C]	36.0	28.6	24.7	23.6
Current asthma [A]	16.0	9.4	8.7	6.1
Current activity limitations [D]	30.7	17.0	24.1	16.7
Stroke [A]	3.2	2.0	2.3	2.4
High blood cholesterol [A]	36.7	34.0	37.3	38.7
High blood pressure [A]	22.6	24.0	24.2	25.8
Heart attack [A]	2.8	2.5	4.2	5.4
Heart disease [A]	4.2	3.0	4.3	5.4
Risk behavior				
Risk factors for human immuno-deficiency virus (HIV) or sexually transmitted diseases (STD) [E]	7.1	2.5	8.2	3.2
Current smoking	33.8	14.9	36.5	19.9
Current heavy or binge drinking [F]	14.5	8.4	36.3	22.8
Current body mass index greater than 25**	55.5	51.5	68.8	68.9

* Includes threatened, attempted, or completed physical violence or unwanted sex by a current or former intimate partner.

[A] Told by a doctor, nurse, or other health care professional that they had the health condition. This refers to lifetime occurrence unless indicated as current.

[B] Use of disability equipment, such as a cane, wheelchair, or special bed.

[C] Includes arthritis, rheumatoid arthritis, gout, lupus, and fibromyalgia.

[D] Activity limitations because of physical, mental, or emotional problems.

[E] Respondents were considered to have risk factors for HIV infection or STD if, during the preceding year, they had used intravenous drugs, had been treated for an STD, had given or received money or drugs in exchange for sex, or had participated in anal sex without a condom.

[F] More than two drinks per day on average for men, more than one drink per day on average for women, or five or more drinks on one occasion during the preceding 30 days for men and women.

** Weight (kilograms) divided by height (meters^2).

stress responses also have been linked to various chronic diseases, including cardiovascular disease, asthma, diabetes, and gastrointestinal disorders. Conversely, adverse health conditions might, in certain cases, lead to increased IPV. Data suggest that women with disabilities experience more IPV than those without disabilities.

The findings in this report are subject to at least three other limitations. First, because BRFSS is a telephone survey of residential households, persons without landline telephones (those with no telephone or with a cellular telephone only) are not represented in the sample. Second, because not all states and territories administered the IPV module, the data might not be representative of the entire U.S. adult population. Finally, although these findings indicated an association between IPV and adverse health conditions and health risk behaviors, not all persons who experience IPV would be expected to experience these conditions and behaviors. The number and range of questions that could be included in the IPV module were limited, and information was not collected on the severity, frequency, and context of IPV experienced by respondents. These important factors likely would influence the observed association between IPV and adverse health conditions and health risk behaviors.

Whether IPV is followed by adverse health conditions or adverse health conditions lead to IPV, both are likely to affect the overall health of affected persons, suggesting that clinicians should consider assessing exposure to IPV when patients have signs or symptoms of stress or other conditions that are consistent with IPV. Such assessment might influence the diagnosis, treatment plan, and ability of the patient to adhere to treatment. Assessing exposure to IPV as part of good clinical practice is included in the recommendations of several medical organizations, including the American Medical Association and the American College of Obstetricians and Gynecologists.

Chapter 6

Impact of Domestic Violence on Reproductive Health and Pregnancy

Reproductive health and pregnancy intersects with domestic violence victims in unique and alarming ways. Intimate partner violence can limit or prevent women from being able to manage their reproductive health and can expose victims to serious sexually transmitted infections and untended pregnancies. Batterers will often control the victim's access to birth control and contraceptive use. When violence is present during a pregnancy, in addition to the immediate trauma to the victim, the abuse can have a negative, long-lasting effect on the mother's health, the developing fetus, and the newborn. Given these facts, it becomes crucial for health care providers to take an active role in screening for abuse.

Did You Know?

- Researchers estimate that 8% of the female population are subjected to physical violence during their pregnancy.[2]

- Up to 70% of women who are abused before pregnancy continue to be abused throughout their pregnancy.[3]

- Physical violence tends to intensify after the abuser learns of the pregnancy.[4]

- Pregnant women who are abused by their partners have a higher risk for alcohol, tobacco, and illicit drug use; depression; and suicide attempts during the pregnancy.[5]

- Although clinical studies have proven the effectiveness of abuse screening by doctors, only 10% of doctors screen for abuse during new-patient visits, and 9% screen for abuse during periodic checkups.[1]

- Up to 50% of adolescent mothers experience intimate partner violence before, during, or just after their pregnancy.[1]

Effects on Reproductive Health

- Studies show that physically and sexually violent experiences increase a woman's risk of human immunodeficiency virus (HIV) and sexually transmitted disease (STD) transmission, the exacerbation of chronic health problems, and negative birth outcomes.[3]

- Abused women are twice as likely to delay prenatal care.[3]

- Several studies have found significant associations between abuse during pregnancy and low birth weights, miscarriages, preterm labor, and cesarean delivery.[3]

- Abused women are more likely than other women to be forced to engage in behaviors that increase their risk of being exposed to STD.[3]

- Women experiencing abuse during or just prior to pregnancy are 60% more likely to have high blood pressure, vaginal bleeding, severe nausea, kidney or urinary tract infections, and hospitalization during pregnancy as compared to non-abused women.[1]

- Children born to abused mothers are 30% more likely than other children to require intensive care upon birth and 17% more likely to be born underweight.[1]

Homicide and Pregnancy

- Homicide is a leading cause of death among pregnant women.[5]

- Pregnant homicide victims are most commonly killed early in their pregnancy; one study estimates that 77% were killed during the first trimester.[6]

- Most homicides of pregnant women were committed with a firearm.[7]

- Pregnant teens between 15 and 19 years of age are more at risk for homicide than any other age group.[7]

Unintended Pregnancies[3]

- Unintended pregnancies may result directly from sexual abuse or from the woman's inability to negotiate contraceptive use with her abuser.

- Women with unintended pregnancies are up to four times more likely to experience physical violence as compared to women with planned pregnancies.

- Two out of three mothers who experience domestic violence at the hands of their partners experienced birth control sabotaged by a partner.

- Among women who are physically abused during their pregnancy, 70% had not intended to become pregnant.

Teen Pregnancies

- One out of four women between the ages of 12 to 18 have been physically or sexually abused, or have been forced to have intercourse with someone they know.[3]

- Studies show that adolescents with a history of abuse are at a greater risk for becoming pregnant as teenagers.[8]

- Female adolescents who are sexually abused are three times more likely to have an unintended pregnancy.[9]

- Teens who are pregnant are at an increased risk of experiencing domestic violence.[1]

- Teens with a history of sexual abuse are most likely to never or rarely use condoms or birth control.[8]

- Studies show a correlation between witnessing intimate partner violence and experiencing other forms of abuse to having sex at a very early age.[8]

- As many as two-thirds of adolescents who become pregnant have been sexually or physically abused at some time in their lives.[1]

Sources

1. Family Violence Prevention Fund. (2007) *The Facts on Reproductive Health and Violence Against Women.*

2. Gazmararian J., et al. (1996) "Prevalence of Violence Against Pregnant Women." *Journal of the American Medical Association.* 275(24).

3. Moore, M. (1999). "Reproductive Health and Intimate Partner Violence." *Family Planning Perspective.* 21(6).

4. Hayes, H.R., and Emshoff, J.G. (1993) "Substance Abuse and Family Violence." *Issues in Children's and Families' Lives.* 7: 281–310.

5. Family Violence Prevention Fund. (2007) *The Facts on Health Care and Domestic Violence.*

6. Krulewitch, C., et al. (2001) "Hidden From View: Violent Deaths Among Pregnant Women in the District of Columbia, 1988–1996." *Journal of Midwifery and Women's Health.* 46:7.

7. Change, J., et al. (2005). "Homicide: A leading cause of injury deaths among pregnant and postpartum women in the United States, 1991–1999." *American Journal of Public Heath.* 95:3.

8. The National Campaign to Prevent Teen Pregnancy (2007). *What It Matters: Teen Pregnancy and Violence.*

9. Center for Impact Research. (2007) *Domestic Violence and Birth Control Sabotage: A Report from the Teen Parent Project.*

For More Information on Reproductive Health and Pregnancy

Family Violence Prevention Fund
383 Rhode Island St., Suite #304
San Francisco, CA 94103-5133
Phone: 415-252-8900
Toll-Free TTY: 800-595-4889
Fax: 415-252-8991
Website: http://www.endabuse.org
E-mail: info@endabuse.org

Guttmacher Institute
125 Maiden Lane, 7th Floor
New York, NY 10038
Toll-Free: 800-355-0244
Phone: 212-248-1111
Fax: 212-248-1951
Website: http://www.guttmacher.org

If You Need Help

National Coalition Against Domestic Violence
P.O. Box 18749
Denver, CO, 80218-0749
Phone: 303-839-1852
Fax: 303-831-9251
TTY: 303-839-1681
Website: http://www.ncadv.org

National Domestic Violence Hotline
P.O. Box 161810
Austin, TX 78716
Toll-Free Hotline: 800-799-SAFE (7233)
Toll-Free TTY: 800-787-3224
Website: http://www.ndvh.org

National Sexual Assault Hotline
Toll-Free: 800-656-HOPE (4673)

Chapter 7

Prevalence of Domestic Violence in the Wake of Disasters

Two questions require attention when considering the implications of domestic violence for postdisaster recovery.

The first question is whether domestic violence increases in prevalence after disasters. There are only minimal data that are relevant to this question. Mechanic et al.[1] undertook the most comprehensive examination of intimate violence in the aftermath of a disaster after the 1993 Mid-western flood. A representative sample of 205 women who were either married or cohabiting with men and who were highly exposed to this disaster acknowledged considerable levels of domestic violence and abuse. Over the nine-month period after flood onset, 14% reported at least one act of physical aggression from their partners, 26% reported emotional abuse, 70% verbal abuse, and 86% partner anger. Whether these rates of physical aggression are greater than normal is not known because studies of domestic violence from previous years and under normal conditions have showed the existence of rates of violence as low as 1% and as high as 12%.

A few studies have produced evidence that supports the assumption of greater domestic violence after disasters. Police reports of domestic violence increased by 46% following the eruption of the Mt. St. Helens volcano.[2] One year after Hurricane Hugo, marital stress was more prevalent among individuals who had been severely exposed to

"Disasters and Domestic Violence," by Fran H. Norris, National Center for Posttraumatic Stress Disorder, May 22, 2007.

the hurricane (for example, life threat, injury) than among individuals who had been less severely exposed, or not exposed at all.[3] Within six months after Hurricane Andrew, 22% of adult residents of the stricken area acknowledged having a new conflict with someone in their household.[4] In a study of people directly exposed to the bombing of the Murrah Federal Building in Oklahoma City, 17% of non-injured persons and 42% of persons whose injuries required hospitalization reported troubled interpersonal relationships.[5]

The second question is whether domestic violence, regardless of the reasons how or why it occurs, influences women's postdisaster recovery. An important finding from the Mechanic et al. (2001) study was that the presence of domestic violence strongly influenced women's postdisaster mental health. Thirty-nine percent of women who experienced post-flood partner abuse developed post-flood posttraumatic stress disorder (PTSD) compared to 17% of women who did not experience post-flood abuse. Fifty-seven percent of women who experienced post-flood partner abuse developed post-flood major depression compared to 28% of non-abused women. Similarly, Norris and Uhl[3] found that as marital stress increased, so too did psychological symptoms such as depression and anxiety. Likewise, Norris et al.[4] found that six and thirty months after Hurricane Andrew, new conflicts and other socially disruptive events were among the strongest predictors of psychological symptoms.

These findings take on additional significance when it is remembered that not only are women generally at greater risk than men for developing postdisaster psychological problems, but women who are married or cohabiting with men may be at even greater risk than single women.[6, 7] In contrast, married status is often a protective factor for men.[8, 9] It also has been found that the severity of married women's symptoms increases with the severity of their husbands' distress, even after similarities in their exposure have been taken into account.[7]

In summary, although the research regarding the interplay of disaster and domestic violence is not extensive, and little of it has been derived from studies of incidents of mass violence, the available evidence does suggest that services related to domestic violence should be integrated into other mental health services for disaster stricken families. Screening for women's safety may be especially important. Helping men find appropriate ways to manage or direct their anger will benefit them and their wives. It will also help their children, as children are highly sensitive to postdisaster conflict and irritability in the family.[7, 10]

Summary of Empirical Findings

- Although there is little conclusive evidence that domestic violence increases after major disasters, research suggests that its postdisaster prevalence may be substantial.

- In the most relevant study, 14% of women experienced at least one act of post-flood physical aggression and 26% reported post-flood emotional abuse over a nine-month period.

- One study reported a 46% increase in police reports of domestic violence after a disaster.

- Other studies show that substantial percentages of disaster victims experience marital stress, new conflicts, and troubled interpersonal relationships.

- There is more conclusive evidence that domestic violence harms women's abilities to recover from disasters.

- In the most relevant study, 39% of abused women developed postdisaster PTSD compared to 17% of other women, and 57% of abused women developed postdisaster depression, compared to 28% of other women.

- Marital stress and conflicts are highly predictive of postdisaster symptoms.

- In light of the fact that, in general, married women are a high-risk group for developing postdisaster psychological problems, it seems advisable to integrate violence-related screenings and services into programs for women, men, and families.

References

1. Mechanic, M., Griffin, M., and Resick, P. (2001). The effects of intimate partner abuse on women's psychological adjustment to a major disaster. Manuscript submitted for publication.

2. Adams, P. R., and Adams, G. R. (1984). Mount Saint Helen's ash fall. *American Psychologist*, 39, 252–260.

3. Norris, F. H., and Uhl, G. A. (1993). Chronic stress as a mediator of acute stress: The case of Hurricane Hugo. *Journal of Applied Social Psychology*, 23, 1263–1284.

4. Norris, F. H., Perilla, J. L., Riad, J. K., Kaniasty, K., and Lavizzo, E. A. (1999). Stability and change in stress, resources,

and psychological distress following natural disaster: Findings from Hurricane Andrew. *Anxiety, Stress, and Coping*, 12, 363–396.

5. Shariat, S., Mallonee, S., Kruger, E., Farmer, K., and North, C. (1999). A prospective study of long-term health outcomes among Oklahoma City bombing survivors. *Journal of the Oklahoma State Medical Association*, 92, 178–186.

6. Brooks, N., and McKinlay, W. (1992). Mental health consequences of the Lockerbie disaster. *Journal of Traumatic Stress*, 5, 527–543.

7. Gleser, G. C., Green, B. L., and Winget, C. N. (1981). *Prolonged psychological effects of disaster: A study of Buffalo Creek*. New York: Academic Press.

8. Fullerton, C.S., Ursano, R.J., Tzu-Cheg, K., and Bharitya, V. R. (1999). Disaster-related bereavement: Acute symptoms and subsequent depression. *Aviation, Space, and Environmental Medicine*, 70, 902–909.

9. Ursano, R. J., Fullerton, C. S., Kao, T. C., and Bhartiya, V. R. (1995). Longitudinal assessment of posttraumatic stress disorder and depression after exposure to traumatic death. *Journal of Nervous and Mental Disease*, 183, 36–42.

10. Wasserstein, S. B., and LaGreca, A. (1998). Hurricane Andrew: Parent conflict as a moderator of children's adjustment. *Hispanic Journal of Behavioral Science*, 20, 212–224.

Chapter 8

Domestic Violence and Financial Hardship

Chapter Contents

Section 8.1

Welfare Recipients Experience Higher Rates of Domestic Violence

Welfare and Domestic Violence: Why It Matters

Individuals receiving welfare experience domestic abuse at higher rates than those with more economic resources, and domestic violence can severely impede a survivors' ability to achieve economic stability.[1, 2] In addition to domestic violence, many welfare recipients face additional barriers to employment, including mental and physical health problems, disabilities, substance abuse, lack of child care, housing instability, and lack of transportation.

Did You Know?

- As many as 30% of women on welfare report domestic violence in a current relationship.[6]

- Many welfare recipients who are current or past survivors of domestic violence were also victims of sexual or physical abuse as children.[9]

- Between 50% and 60% of women receiving welfare have been victims of domestic violence as adults (compared to 22% of women in the general population).[5]

- In a Michigan study, 59% of women on welfare who had experienced severe domestic abuse in the past year had a mental health disorder, compared to 20% of those who reported no severe abuse.[8]

- One study found that abused women on welfare who received job training were about seven times more likely to be working, and those who received job placement services were about four times more likely to be working than women who did not receive job services.[10]

How Abusers Interfere

- Abused women on welfare are ten times more likely to have a current or former partner who would not like them to go to school or work, compared to women on welfare who do not have an abusive partner.[11]

- 44% of women on welfare report that their abusive ex-partners harassed them at work.

- In Pennsylvania, women who sought a protection order because of domestic violence dropped out of the welfare to work program at six times the rate of women who did not.[12]

- In Wisconsin, 63% of women on welfare reported that they had been fired or had to quit a job due to domestic violence.[13]

- Domestic violence is a primary cause of homelessness among women, making it hard for them to retain employment.[14]

Temporary Assistance for Needy Families (TANF) Program

- The Temporary Assistance for Needy Families (TANF) program grants welfare payments to low-income individuals who work and comply with other requirements, but many domestic violence victims are not able to meet requirements because of the abuse they suffer.[3]

- TANF requires victims to interact with their ex-partners to enforce child support agreements and establish paternity, and these requirements can jeopardize the victim's safety.

- Most states have adopted a Family Violence Option (FVO) that exempts domestic violence victims from TANF requirements that may cause abuse to escalate, make it more difficult for the to escape violence, or that result in unfair sanctions against women who fail to meet requirements due to domestic violence.[4]

Welfare Helps Domestic Violence Victims

- Public assistance is often the only way a battered woman can afford to leave an abusive situation and support herself and her children.

- Many women use welfare and work as a way to escape an abusive relationship.[15]

- Shelter programs have reported that a majority of shelter residents use welfare in their efforts to end the violence in their lives.[17]

- Most battered women work or want to work if they can do so safely.[18]

- Job training programs supported by TANF can help women gain the skills necessary to support themselves and their children independently from their abuser.

- In California, 37% of welfare recipients applied for aid entirely because of domestic violence and 18% said that violence contributed to their need for aid.[16]

Federal Exemptions for Victims

The Family Violence Option (FVO) of TANF grants waivers to domestic violence victims that exempt them from having to meet certain eligibility requirements in order to protect confidentiality, support victims' efforts to leave abusive relationships and to protect their safety.[19] Waivers exempt victims from having to meet TANF's five-year time limit to benefits, contact their abuser to enforce child support payments or paternity establishments, and work activity.[20]

- 41 states plus the District of Columbia have adopted the Family Violence Option.[21]

- Six states have equivalent policies that enable victims to get waivers from some or all TANF requirements.[22]

- Three states (Oklahoma, Ohio, and Virginia) have no FVO equivalent policies.[23]

This information was current as of July 2007. For more information about your state laws regarding domestic violence exemptions for welfare recipients, contact your state TANF director. A list of state TANF directors can be found at: http://www.acf.hhs.gov/programs/ofa/tanf-dir.htm.

Many studies have found that the use of FVO waivers by domestic violence victims is far less than the number of victims who report abuse. These studies have concluded that victims do not understand the benefits of the FVO waivers because welfare offices have not properly informed them about the exemptions. For example:

- In California, 25% of women surveyed who identified themselves as victims of violence had received any information from the welfare office about waivers for which they were eligible.

- In Wisconsin, approximately 75% of welfare recipients who identified themselves as victims of violence were not informed about available services, including counseling, housing, or the possibility of using work time to seek help. In addition, while 26.8% reported they were afraid of harassment from their former partner, only 4.9% were told about the good cause exception to the child support cooperation requirement.

- In New York, a study of the New York City welfare agency found it referred less than half of individuals who identified themselves as victims of violence to special domestic violence caseworkers, as required by state law.

These studies have also concluded that women who do not understand FVO waivers fail to use them because:

- they fear that authorities will take away their children if they identify themselves as victims of domestic violence; or,

- they fear retaliation by their partners if they apply for an FVO waiver.

For More Information or If You Need Help

National Domestic Violence Hotline
Toll-Free: 800-799-7233

National Sexual Assault Hotline
Toll-Free: 800-656-4673

Sources

[1, 11–13, 16-17] "Surviving Violence and Poverty: A Focus on the Link between Domestic and Sexual Violence, Women's Poverty and Welfare." 2002. Stand With Sisters.

[2–3, 8, 10] Lyon, Eleanor. 2002. *Welfare and domestic Violence Against Women: Lessons from Research*. National Research Center on Domestic Violence.

[4, 19–20] Cole, Patricia R. 2000. "Welfare and Domestic Violence: Federal and State Laws and Policies," National Center on Domestic and Sexual Violence.

[5, 9, 14, 24] "Violence Against Welfare Recipients: Domestic and Sexual Violence." 2007. Legal Momentum.

[6] Tolman, Richard and Jody Raphael. 2000. "A Review of Research on Welfare and Domestic Violence." *Journal of Social Issues* (Winter).

[7, 15, 18] "The Facts on Welfare and Domestic Violence." 2007. Family Violence Prevention Fund.

[21–23] "Family Violence Option: State by State Summary." 2004. Legal Momentum.

Section 8.2

Economics and Neighborhood Play a Role in Violence

Text in this section is excerpted from "When Violence Hits Home: How Economics and Neighborhood Play a Role," by Michael L. Benson, Ph.D., and Greer Litton Fox, Ph.D. National Institute of Justice, U.S. Department of Justice, September 2004.

How Economics and Neighborhood Play a Role in Domestic Violence

Past research has explored how personality factors and the dynamics of an intimate relationship can lead to violence against women. A National Institute of Justice (NIJ) study takes a broader look at the factors at play in intimate violence. The study reveals that the incidence of violence in the home is exacerbated by economic factors apart from the characteristics of the individuals involved. Researchers found that economic problems or distresses such as losing one's job and specific circumstances such as the length of a relationship interact with the kind of community in which people live to influence the offenders and victims of intimate violence.

The study sheds light on the connections between intimate violence and personal and economic well-being and on how the type of neighborhood in which women live may influence them to stay in or leave abusive relationships. Understanding the links between these factors should help policy makers and practitioners create more targeted prevention and intervention programs and better anticipate when demand for these programs might grow. The findings suggest that service providers who help victims of violence should give priority to women in the most disadvantaged neighborhoods and address their economic circumstances.

The study found:

- Violence against women in intimate relationships occurred more often and was more severe in economically disadvantaged neighborhoods. Women living in disadvantaged neighborhoods were more than twice as likely to be the victims of intimate violence compared with women in more advantaged neighborhoods.

- For the individuals involved, both objective (being unemployed or not making enough money to meet family needs) and subjective (worrying about finances) forms of economic distress increase the risk of intimate violence against women.

- Women who live in economically disadvantaged communities and are struggling with money in their own relationships suffer the greatest risk of intimate violence.

- African-Americans and whites with the same economic characteristics have similar rates of intimate violence, but African-Americans have a higher overall rate of intimate violence due in part to higher levels of economic distress and location in disadvantaged neighborhoods.

The study also showed that even when measures of subjective and objective economic distress were taken into account, women living in disadvantaged neighborhoods still have higher rates of intimate violence. This may be because of the existence of many of the same social problems that increase the risk of street crime in disadvantaged neighborhoods; for example, a lower degree of social capital to respond to criminal behavior that, when longstanding, leads to a greater tolerance for deviant behavior among people living in those neighborhoods.

Effects of Economic Distress

- **Male job instability:** Women whose male partners experienced two or more periods of unemployment over the 5-year study were almost three times as likely to be victims of intimate violence as were women whose partners were in stable jobs.

- **Income levels:** Women living in households with high incomes experienced less violence at the hands of their intimate partners than did women whose households were less financially secure. The results showed a very consistent pattern: As the ratio of household income to needs goes up, the likelihood of violence goes down.

- **Financial strain:** Couples who reported extensive financial strain had a rate of violence more than three times that of couples with low levels of financial strain.

- **Severity of violence:** Women in disadvantaged neighborhoods were more likely to be victimized repeatedly or to be injured by their domestic partners than were women who lived in more advantaged neighborhoods. For instance, about two percent of women in advantaged neighborhoods experienced severe violence, while six percent of women in disadvantaged neighborhoods were the victims of severe violence.

A Volatile Mix

Researchers sought to determine whether the combination of individual economic distress and a community's economic disadvantage increases a woman's risk of intimate violence. Comparing levels of intimate violence among couples experiencing individual economic distress in both advantaged and disadvantaged neighborhoods, researchers found much higher rates of violence among couples in disadvantaged neighborhoods. The rate of intimate violence among financially distressed couples in advantaged neighborhoods is roughly half that of similarly distressed couples in disadvantaged neighborhoods. The highest rates of intimate violence are found among women who live in disadvantaged neighborhoods with men who have had high levels of job instability. In comparison, the rate of intimate violence is lowest among women whose intimate partners have stable employment and live in advantaged neighborhoods. These findings show that individual economic distress and an economically disadvantaged neighborhood work in tandem to increase a woman's risk for violence in an intimate relationship.

Socioeconomics, Race, and Violence

The study found that the rate of intimate violence against women in African-American couples is about twice that for white couples. To find out why, the study looked at the relationship among economic distress, living in a disadvantaged community, and race and ethnicity. The study found that African-Americans are more likely than whites to suffer from economic distress and to live in disadvantaged neighborhoods. The study also found that the individual economic status of African-Americans and Hispanics often does not match the economic status of the neighborhoods in which they live. For instance, 36 percent of African-American couples may be considered economically disadvantaged, but more than twice as many African-Americans (77 percent) live in disadvantaged neighborhoods. Similar patterns are found for Hispanics. By contrast, white couples are much more likely to reside in neighborhoods that mirror their economic status.

To investigate this pattern further, researchers calculated the rates of intimate violence against women among African-Americans and whites while controlling separately for community disadvantage and economic distress. They found that higher rates of intimate violence among African-Americans could be accounted for by their higher levels of economic distress and their greater likelihood of living in disadvantaged neighborhoods. What's more, the rate of violence between intimate partners is virtually identical among African-Americans and whites with high incomes. However, African-Americans with low and moderate incomes do appear to have a significantly higher rate of intimate violence than whites do in those same income categories.

The study also explored the relationship between race and intimate violence by controlling for income and type of community at the same time. Results were mixed, but, in a number of cases, the difference in intimate violence between African-Americans and whites was reduced substantially. The study found that in both advantaged and disadvantaged neighborhoods, African-Americans with high incomes have rates of intimate violence that are close to or less than those for whites. Generally, when African-Americans are compared to whites with similar incomes and neighborhood economic status, the difference in the rate of intimate violence diminishes or is eliminated.

Implications for Practice

For policy makers developing effective prevention and intervention strategies, this study provides important insights into how social changes that cause economic distress influence violence against women in different racial and socioeconomic groups. The stress that accompanies losing a job and seeing personal income shrink can result in severe consequences for individuals, intimate couples, and the communities in which they live.

This study suggests to policy makers and intimate violence service providers that violence against domestic partners does not occur solely because of an offender's psychological makeup or the inability to resolve conflicts constructively in a relationship. Therefore, strategies to address intimate violence should target a broad array of potential areas for intervention and change. At the same time, law enforcement officials could use this information to deal more effectively with intimate violence in the community. Because intimate violence is more likely to occur in disadvantaged neighborhoods, this study suggests that law enforcement officials give increased attention to these neighborhoods and consider employing strategies to prevent and detect intimate partner crimes in vulnerable neighborhoods.

This study found a strong link between intimate violence and the economic well-being of couples and the communities in which they live. This means that economic practices and employment policies may play an important part in women's risk of suffering from intimate violence. It is noteworthy that, in this study, job instability and not employment status itself was a major risk factor for violence against women. The researchers suggest that when policy makers consider the problem of transitory labor demand, they could help address women's risk of intimate partner violence by giving preference to policies and practices that provide job stability rather than those that promote periodic layoffs and rehiring. The researchers also suggest that service providers may want to monitor changes in the local job force because cutbacks could potentially increase the level of intimate violence.

The study also found that the type of community in which women lived played a contributing role in their risk for intimate violence. Women experiencing economic difficulties who live in disadvantaged neighborhoods will continue to experience a greater risk for intimate violence. In light of these findings about how neighborhood types and economic distress increase the risk for intimate violence, service providers may want to consider how they develop interventions. To provide services where women at the greatest risk of intimate violence need them most, service providers could target women who live in the most disadvantaged neighborhoods. Because economic distress has been shown to increase the risk of violence, service providers might choose to address the economic resources of these women and specifically, their need for cash assistance. Based on the findings of this study, financial assistance to women in poverty may lessen their risk of violence.

Section 8.3

Domestic Violence Contributes to Homelessness

When a woman leaves an abusive relationship, she often has nowhere to go. This is particularly true of women with few resources. Lack of affordable housing and long waiting lists for assisted housing mean that many women and their children are forced to choose either abuse at home or life on the streets. Moreover, shelters are frequently filled to capacity and must turn away battered women and their children. An estimated 29% of requests for shelter by homeless families were denied in 2006 due to lack of resources (U.S. Conference of Mayors, 2006).

Domestic Violence as a Contributing Factor to Homelessness

Many studies demonstrate the contribution of domestic violence to homelessness, particularly among families with children. Thirty-nine percent of cities cite domestic violence as the primary cause of family homelessness (U.S. Conference of Mayors, 2007). Two years prior, that figure had been 50% (U.S. Conference of Mayors, 2005). A 2003 survey of 100 homeless mothers in ten locations around the country found that 25% of the women had been physically abused in the last year (American Civil Liberties Union, 2004). State and local studies also demonstrate the impact of domestic violence on homelessness:

- In Minnesota, one in every three homeless women was homeless due to domestic violence in 2003. Forty-six percent of homeless women said that they had previously stayed in abusive relationships because they had nowhere else to go (American Civil Liberties Union, 2004).

- In Missouri, 27% of the sheltered homeless population are victims of domestic violence (American Civil Liberties Union, 2004).

- In San Diego, a survey done by San Diego's Regional Task Force on the Homeless found that 50% of homeless women are domestic violence victims (American Civil Liberties Union, 2004).

- A recent study in Massachusetts reports that 92% of homeless women had experienced severe physical or sexual assault at some point in their life; and 63% were victims of violence by an intimate partner (NAEH Fact Checker, 2007).

Policy Issues

Currently, victims of domestic abuse have unmet needs for both short- and long-term housing. The National Network to End Domestic Violence reports that on a given day, 1,740 people could not be provided emergency shelter and 1,422 could not be provided transitional shelter (National Network to End Domestic Violence, 2007).

Shelters provide immediate safety to battered women and their children and help women gain control over their lives. The provision of safe emergency shelter is a necessary first step in meeting the needs of women fleeing domestic violence.

A sizable portion of the welfare population experiences domestic violence at any given time. Thus, without significant housing support, many welfare recipients are at risk of homelessness or continued violence. In states that have looked at domestic violence and welfare receipt, most report that approximately 50–60% of current recipients say that they have experienced violence from a current or former male partner (Institute for Women's Policy Research, 1997). In the absence of cash assistance, women who experience domestic violence may be at increased risk of homelessness or compelled to live with a former or current abuser in order to prevent homelessness. Welfare programs must make every effort to assist victims of domestic violence and to recognize the tremendous barrier to employment that domestic violence presents.

Long-term efforts to address homelessness must include increasing the supply of affordable housing, ensuring adequate wages and income supports, and providing necessary supportive services.

References

American Civil Liberties Union, Women's Rights Project. "Domestic Violence and Homelessness," 2004. Available at www.aclu.org.

DeSimone, Peter et al. *Homelessness in Missouri: Eye of the Storm?* 1998. Available from the Missouri Association for Social Welfare, 308 E. High St., Jefferson City, MO 65101; 573-634-2901.

Douglass, Richard. *The State of Homelessness in Michigan: A Research Study*, 1995. Available, free, from the Michigan Interagency Committee on Homelessness, c/o Michigan State Housing Development Authority, P.O. Box 30044, Lansing, MI 48909; 517-373-6026.

Homes for the Homeless. *Ten Cities 1997–1998: A Snapshot of Family Homelessness Across America*. Available from Homes for the Homeless and the Institute for Children and Poverty, 36 Cooper Square, 6th Floor, New York, NY 10003; 212-529-5252.

Institute for Women's Policy Research. "Domestic Violence and Welfare Receipt," 1997. *IWPR Welfare Reform Network News, Issue No. 4*. April. Available from Institute for Women's Policy Research, 1400 20th Street, NW, Suite 104, Washington DC 20036; 202-785-5100.

Mullins, Gretchen. "The Battered Woman and Homelessness," in *Journal of Law and Policy, 3* (1994) 1:237–255. Entire issue available from William S. Hein and Co., Inc., 1285 Main St., Buffalo, NY 14209; 800-828-7571.

National Alliance to End Homelessness. 2007. "Fact Checker: Domestic Violence." Washington, DC: National Alliance to End Homelessness. Available at: http://www.naeh.org.

National Network to End Domestic Violence. 2007. "Domestic Violence Counts: A 24-hour census of domestic violence shelters and services across the United States." Washington, DC: National Network to End Domestic Violence.

Owen, Greg et al. *Minnesota Statewide Survey of Persons Without Permanent Shelter; Volume I: Adults and Their Children*, 1998. Available from the Wilder Research Center, 1295 Bandana Blvd., North, Suite 210, St. Paul, MN 55108-5197; 612-647-4600.

U.S. Conference of Mayors. *A Status Report on Hunger and Homelessness in America's Cities: 2005, 2006, 2007*. Available from the U.S. Conference of Mayors, 1620 Eye St., NW, 4th Floor, Washington, DC, 20006-4005; 202-293-7330.

Virginia Coalition for the Homeless. *1995 Shelter Provider Survey*, 1995. Out of Print. Virginia Coalition for the Homeless, P.O. Box 12247, Richmond, VA 23241; 804-644-5527.

Zorza, Joan. "Woman Battering: A Major Cause of Homelessness," in *Clearinghouse Review, vol. 25, no. 4*, 1991. Available from the National

Clearinghouse for Legal Services, 205 W. Monroe St., 2nd Floor, Chicago, IL 60606-5013; 800-621-3256.

Resources

National Clearinghouse for the Defense of Battered Women
125 S. 9th St., Suite 302
Philadelphia, PA 19107
Toll-Free: 800-903-0111 ext. 3
Phone: 215-351-0010
Fax: 215-351-0779
Website: http://www.ncdbw.org

National Coalition Against Domestic Violence
P.O. Box 18749
Denver, CO 80218-0749
Phone: 303-839-1852
Fax: 303-831-9251
TTY: 303-839-1681
Website: http://www.ncadv.org

National Domestic Violence Hotline
P.O. Box 161810
Austin, TX 78716
Toll-Free Hotline: 800-799-SAFE (7233)
Toll-Free TTY: 800-787-3224
Website: http://www.ndvh.org

National Resource Center on Domestic Violence
6400 Flank Dr., Suite 1300
Harrisburg, PA 17112
Toll-Free: 800-537-2238
Toll-Free TTY: 800-553-2508
Fax: 717-545-9456
Website: http://www.nrcdv.org

Section 8.4

Homeless Youth Often Exposed to Abuse

"Homeless Youth," © 2008 National Coalition for the Homeless
(www.nationalhomeless.org). Reprinted with permission.

Definitions and Dimensions

Homeless youth are individuals under the age of eighteen who lack parental, foster, or institutional care. These young people are sometimes referred to as unaccompanied youth.

The number of the homeless youth is estimated by the Office of Juvenile Justice and Delinquency Prevention in the U.S. Department of Justice. Their study, published in 2002, reported there are an estimated 1,682,900 homeless and runaway youth. This number is equally divided among males and females, and the majority of them are between the ages of 15 and 17 (Molino, 2007). According to the U.S. Conference of Mayors, unaccompanied youth account for 1% of the urban homeless population, (U.S. Conference of Mayors, 2007). According to the National Network of Runaway and Youth Services, six percent of homeless youth are gay, lesbian, bisexual, or transgender (GLBT) (Molino, 2007). The number of homeless teenagers who are pregnant is estimated to be somewhere between six and twenty-two percent. (Health Resources and Services Administration [HRSA], 2001) According to the National Alliance to End Homelessness (NAEH), five to seven percent of American youth become homeless in any given year. (NAEH, 2007)

Causes

Causes of homelessness among youth fall into three interrelated categories: family problems, economic problems, and residential instability.

Many homeless youth leave home after years of physical and sexual abuse, strained relationships, addiction of a family member, and parental neglect. Disruptive family conditions are the principal reason that young people leave home: in one study, more than half of the youth interviewed during shelter stays reported that their parents either

81

told them to leave or knew they were leaving and did not care (U.S. Department of Health and Human Services [HHS](a), 1995). In another study, 46% of runaway and homeless youth had been physically abused and 17% were forced into unwanted sexual activity by a family or household member (HHS (c), 1997).

Some youth may become homeless when their families suffer financial crises resulting from lack of affordable housing, limited employment opportunities, insufficient wages, no medical insurance, or inadequate welfare benefits. These youth become homeless with their families, but are later separated from them by shelter, transitional housing, or child welfare policies (Shinn and Weitzman, 1996).

Residential instability also contributes to homelessness among youth. A history of foster care correlates with becoming homeless at an earlier age and remaining homeless for a longer period of time (Roman and Wolfe, 1995). Some youth living in residential or institutional placements become homeless upon discharge—they are too old for foster care but are discharged with no housing or income support (Robertson, 1996). One national study reported that more than one in five youth who arrived at shelters came directly from foster care, and that more than one in four had been in foster care in the previous year (National Association of Social Workers, 1992).

Consequences

Homeless youth face many challenges on the streets. Few homeless youth are housed in emergency shelters as a result of lack of shelter beds for youth, shelter admission policies, and a preference for greater autonomy (Robertson, 1996). Because of their age, homeless youth have few legal means by which they can earn enough money to meet basic needs. Many homeless adolescents find that exchanging sex for food, clothing, and shelter is their only chance of survival on the streets. In turn, homeless youth are at a greater risk of contracting acquired immunodeficiency syndrome (AIDS) or human immunodeficiency virus (HIV)-related illnesses. Estimates for percentages of homeless youth infected with HIV are generally around 5%, but one study in San Francisco found that 17% of homeless youths were infected (HRSA, 2001). It has been suggested that the rate of HIV prevalence for homeless youth may be as much as 2–10 times higher than the rates reported for other samples of adolescents in the United States (National Network for Youth, 1998).

Homeless adolescents often suffer from severe anxiety and depression, poor health and nutrition, and low self-esteem. In one study, the rates of major depression, conduct disorder, and posttraumatic stress syndrome were found to be three times as high among runaway youth as among youth who have not run away (Robertson, 1989).

Furthermore, homeless youth face difficulties attending school because of legal guardianship requirements, residency requirements, improper records, and lack of transportation. As a result, homeless youth face severe challenges in obtaining an education and supporting themselves emotionally and financially.

Program and Policy Issues

Homeless youth benefit from programs that meet immediate needs first and then help them address other aspects of their lives. Programs that minimize institutional demands and offer a range of services have had success in helping homeless youth regain stability (Robertson, 1996). Educational outreach programs, assistance in locating job training and employment, transitional living programs, and health care especially designed for and directed at homeless youth are also needed. In the long term, homeless youth would benefit from many of the same measures that are needed to fight poverty and homelessness in the adult population, including the provision of affordable housing and employment that pays a living wage. In addition to these basic supports, the child welfare system must make every effort to prevent children from ending up on the streets.

Resources

Bass, Deborah. *Helping Vulnerable Youths: Runaway and Homeless Adolescents in the United States*, 1992. Available from the National Association of Social Workers, 750 First Street, NE, Suite 700, Washington DC 20002-4241; 202-408-8600.

Center for Law and Social Policy, *Leave No Youth Behind: Opportunities for Congress to Reach Disconnected Youth*, 2003, pg. 57.

Cwayna, Kevin. *Knowing Where the Fountains Are: Stories and Stark Realities of Homeless Youth*, 1993. Available from Fairview Press, 2450 Riverside Ave., South, Minneapolis, MN 55454; 800-544-8207.

Health Resources and Services Administration, U.S. Department of Health and Human Services. *Program Assistance Letter: Understanding the Health Care Needs of Homeless Youth*, 2001. Available at http:// bphc.hrsa.gov/policy/pal0110.htm.

Institute for Health Policy Studies. *Street Youth at Risk for AIDS*. 1995. University of California, San Francisco.

Jarvis, Sara and Robert Robertson. *Transitional Living Programs for Homeless Adolescents*, 1993. Available from National Technical Assistance Center for Children's Mental Health, Georgetown University Child Development Center, 3307 M St., NW, Suite 401, Washington, DC 20007-8803; 202-687-8635.

Molino, A.C. *Characteristics of Help-Seeking Street Youth and Non-Street Youth*. (2007). National Symposium on Homelessness Research.

National Network for Youth. Toolkit for Youth Workers: Fact Sheet. *Runaway and Homeless Youth*. 1998. Available from the National Network for Youth, 1319 F St., Suite 401, Washington, DC 20004; 202-783-7949.

Pires, Sheila A. and Judith Tolmach Silber. *On Their Own: Runaway and Homeless Youth and the Programs That Serve Them*, 1991. Available from the National Technical Assistance Center for Children's Mental Health, Georgetown University Child Development Center, 3307 M St., NW, Suite 401, Washington, DC 20007-8803; 202-687 8635.

Robertson, Marjorie. *Homeless Youth on Their Own*, 1996. Alcohol Research Group, 2000 Hearst Avenue, Berkeley, CA 94709; 510-642-5208. Available from author.

Robertson, Marjorie. *Homeless Youth in Hollywood: Patterns of Alcohol Use*, 1989. Alcohol Research Group, 2000 Hearst Avenue, Berkeley, CA 94709; 510-642-5208. Available from author.

Roman, Nan P. and Phyllis B. Wolfe. *Web of Failure: The Relationship Between Foster Care and Homelessness*, 1995. Available from the National Alliance to End Homelessness, 1518 K St., NW, Suite 206, Washington, DC 20005-1203; 202-638-1526.

Shinn, Marybeth and Beth Weitzman. "Homeless Families Are Different," in *Homelessness in America*, 1996. Available from the National Coalition for the Homeless, 1012 14th Street, NW, Suite 600, Washington, DC 20005; 202-737-6444, e-mail: info@nationalhomeless.org.

U.S. Conference of Mayors. *A Status Report on Hunger and Homelessness in America's Cities: 2007*. Available from the U.S. Conference of Mayors, 1620 Eye St., NW, 4th Floor, Washington, DC, 20006-4005, 202-293-7330.

U.S. Department of Health and Human Services(a). *Youth with Runaway, Throwaway, and Homeless Experiences... Prevalence Drug Use, and Other At-Risk Behaviors,* 1995. Volume I (the Final Report, including the executive summary) is available; the Executive Summary alone is also available. Order from the National Clearinghouse on Families and Youth, P.O. Box 13505, Silver Spring, MD 20911-3505; 301-608-8098.

U.S. Department of Health and Human Services(b). *Report to the Congress on the Runaway and Homeless Youth Program of the Family and Youth Services Bureau for Fiscal Year 1995,* 1996. Available from the National Clearinghouse on Families and Youth, P.O. Box 13505, Silver Spring, MD 20911-3505; 301-608-8098.

U.S. Department of Health and Human Services (c). *National Evaluation of Runaway and Homeless Youth,* 1997. Available from the National Clearinghouse on Families and Youth, P.O. Box 13505, Silver Spring, MD 20911-3505; 301-608-8098.

Zangrillo, Patricia and Monique Mercer. *Housing and Foster Care: Results of a National Survey,* 1995. Available from the American Public Welfare Association, 810 First St., NE, Suite 500, Washington, DC 20002-4205; 202-682-0100.

Chapter 9

Link between Alcohol Abuse and Domestic Violence

Overview of Alcohol Abuse and Violence against Women

Alcohol is the most widely used and abused substance in the United States. Alcohol abuse and drug abuse create social, health, and other costs of huge proportions. More than 17 million people nationwide have alcohol problems in any given year.

Violence against women is also a major problem. Women of every race, nationality, and income level are the victims of 2.8 million violent crimes each year. By understanding how the two problems are related, society can find ways to treat and prevent both alcohol abuse and domestic violence.

The Link between Alcohol and Violence

Although alcohol abuse and violence often occur together, one does not cause the other. Alcohol or drug use can increase the risk of violence and can affect how often violence occurs and how severe it is. For example, a man with a quick temper or low frustration level may be more likely to act out his anger physically or verbally after he has had alcohol. Alcohol tends to lower a person's inhibitions. In other words, he may act before he thinks. Similarly, after drinking alcohol, a man

---

This chapter includes excerpts from "It Won't Happen to Me: Alcohol Abuse and Violence Against Women," Substance Abuse and Mental Health Services Administration (SAMHSA), November 2003. Updated in November 2008 by Dr. David A. Cooke, M.D., Diplomate, American Board of Internal Medicine.

who tends to express his anger in sexually controlling ways might rape or sexually assault a woman before stopping to think about his behavior. When sober, the same man may be more likely to think first.

Some abusive men use the excuse that substance abuse causes them to be violent. Although many men who abuse alcohol never become violent, nearly half of men who commit acts of violence against their partner also have alcohol abuse problems. They may become violent:

- to release feelings of stress, anger, or frustration;
- to avoid painful issues and shift blame; or
- to feel in control.

Alcohol or drug use is not just a risk factor for potential offenders. For a woman who is drinking, it may also increase her chances of becoming a victim of violence. A woman's judgment may be affected if she is drinking, which could lead her to engage in risky behavior or interfere with her ability to get out of a situation that may be dangerous. So, women that become victims of violence may actually use alcohol before they are ever victimized. They may also begin to use alcohol after the violence as a way of coping with the pain.

The Truth about Alcohol and Violence

Many people do not realize how powerful the effects of alcohol can be on their behaviors, actions, and even brain chemistry. People may drink or use drugs:

- to escape stress, sadness, or depression;
- to appear confident; or
- to numb feelings of guilt, shame, anger, or loneliness.

A number of myths exist about alcohol and its connection to violence. The following list attempts to separate fact from fiction:

Myth: Drinking alcohol gives you more energy.

Fact: Alcohol is actually a depressant. Alcohol slows down the central nervous system. After drinking just a small amount of alcohol, people tend to react more slowly, their judgment can become clouded, and they may be less coordinated.

Myth: Few women in the United States are alcoholics.

Fact: The numbers of men and women affected by alcohol today are roughly equal. However, women tend to abuse prescription drugs much more than men.

Myth: As many men are affected by violence as women.

Fact: More than 85 percent of all victims of intimate partner violence are women.

Myth: Children can't be hurt unless they are victims of violence.

Fact: Children do not have to be physically hurt or even witness violence and substance abuse directly to feel the impact. They see the results. They also may hear parents scream, threaten, break things, or physically abuse. Children exposed to domestic violence may have behavior problems, low self-esteem and depression, as well as poor school performance.

Where to Go for Help

Many who abuse alcohol and are also violent are likely to deny that they have a problem. This denial can make family members feel hopeless. Every community has resources for alcohol prevention and treatment. There is no easy way to get an adult (aged 18 and older) into treatment, but the following are some steps that family and friends can take to help:

- Stop rescuing the person when he or she gets into trouble. The person needs to suffer the consequences of drinking.

- Talk seriously to the person when they are sober, but do so immediately after an incident, so that the event or problem is fresh in their minds. Be specific so there is no confusion.

- Talk to a counselor for information and referrals.

- Be ready to help. Be prepared with information about Alcoholics Anonymous (AA) or community resources. Be willing to accompany the person to an AA meeting or initial meeting with a therapist, if necessary.

The Link between Alcohol and Violence

In the past, society often excused men for committing violent acts against women when they were drunk. Today, however, people no longer accept such behavior as normal. Alcohol and domestic violence have some of the following things in common:

- Both can be passed down from generation to generation.
- Both involve denying and minimizing the problem.
- Both may cause the abuser and the victim to feel isolated.
- Both stem from a need for power and control.

How Violence Begins

Destructive drinking and violence in the home can exist prior to marriage. Bad habits can begin in the teen dating years, sometimes after watching parents exhibit the same behaviors. Whenever destructive drinking and violence occur, one partner will be exerting power and control over the other.

A woman who becomes a victim of abuse is at risk of abusing alcohol and other drugs to escape the pain and shame of abuse. Some abusive partners force the woman to drink or do drugs under the threat of further violence. Most women do not realize that drinking alcohol (in any quantity) puts them at risk for violence.

Alcohol can be connected to domestic violence, although one does not cause the other. Not every man who abuses alcohol becomes violent. Some men are violent whether they drink or not. In cases where alcohol and violence are both present, the family violence may worsen when a man ceases to drink. In response, some women may try to encourage a man to begin drinking again so they can better predict the pattern of abuse.

Cycle of Violence

Domestic violence often runs in cycles. If nothing is done to stop it, violence can repeat itself generation after generation. Violence also occurs cyclically in the stages of a relationship between two people. The stages include the following:

Honeymoon phase: The partners are both on their best behavior; and they share a sense of excitement and newness. Gifts are exchanged. Alcohol may be present only in social or romantic settings. There is no real increase in drinking.

Tension building phase: Over a period of months or a year, a woman feels tension building and notices signs of temper or criticism from her partner. She may try to minimize problems and tends to feel like she is "walking on eggshells." In some, but not all abusive relationships, the man may begin to drink more heavily. As the tension builds, alcohol abuse may become a problem, playing a larger role in verbal attacks and minor violence. Some women may drink to decrease the tension.

Serious battering phase: In this stage, the violence that results may be severe, requiring medical attention for fractures, breaks, and burns. A man who abuses both alcohol and his partner may begin to depend on alcohol to ease his feelings of powerlessness, guilt, and stress. Women also may use alcohol to escape the physical and emotional pain. Following a violent incident, the man's behavior may change dramatically. He becomes charming, which leads to the next phase.

Honeymoon phase: The man feels guilty about the violence and asks for forgiveness. He behaves in ways similar to the early relationship. He tells the woman how much he loves her and how much he needs her. If he has been abusing alcohol, he may stop drinking. Whether or not alcohol is involved, in any abusive relationship, the honeymoon phase eventually leads to the next cycle of violence.

The Importance of Recognizing the Problem

Families experiencing both alcohol and physical abuse have a strong need to deny the problem. People who don't experience the problems directly also need to recognize the problem in their communities. An estimated three million children between the ages of three and seventeen years are at risk of exposure to parental violence each year.

Many people are unaware of the impact that alcohol and domestic abuse have on children. Children may lack hope and feel helpless. They live with fear and shame. Infants can "fail to thrive" or fail to become attached to caregivers. Children may register their trauma in physical ways. They may complain of stomachaches, headaches, and sleep problems. Children may also suffer neglect because their physical and emotional needs are not met. Older children may become aggressive, depressed, or perform poorly in school. In addition, children may become addicted to alcohol or drugs to escape their home life.

Teen Dating Violence

Alcohol plays a large role in abusive relationships among teenagers. More than 60 percent of sexual assaults involve alcohol. In fact, one in four teenagers will experience sexual or nonsexual abuse by the time they finish college or turn 21. Abusive teen relationships follow some of the same patterns as those of older couples. However, the effects of violence on teenage women may include the following:

- Eating disorders

- Use of drugs and alcohol

- Trouble sleeping

- Stress-related physical illnesses

- Depression, suicidal tendencies, increased isolation from friends

- Lack of concentration and lower grades in school

Alcohol, Drugs, and Sexual Assault

Alcohol and Sexual Assault

Sexual assault and rape are sexual acts that are performed against a victim's will. The assault may involve physical force or the threat of physical force, use of guns or other weapons, or pressure. Sexual assault also includes forced touching of the genitals, anus, groin, or breast against a person's will. Rape is forced penetration of the genitals, anus, or oral penetration.

Contrary to popular belief, rapists usually are not strangers to their victims. Friends or acquaintances commit nearly half of all rapes and sexual assaults. In 95 percent of incidents reported on college campuses, the victim knows the person committing the injury.

Those who think sexual assault isn't a problem in the United States don't know the facts. Every two minutes, a woman over the age of 18 is assaulted in the U.S. That amounts to 272,350 sexual assaults per year. And this number represents only the incidents that are reported. More than 80 percent of sexual assault victims do not report to the police.

Drinking has become a popular social activity—even among those who are underage. Alcohol use does not automatically lead to assault. However, alcohol use is the largest risk factor for sexual assault. Women who go to bars or nightclubs alone—especially if they are drinking—increase their risk of assault.

A person's judgment and motor skills decrease when alcohol is consumed. Research has found that when a woman drinks while on a date, she has a greater chance of being sexually assaulted by her date. On school campuses (especially colleges), the larger the quantities of alcohol consumed, the greater the risk is for sexual assault among women on the campus.

Binge drinking has become a problem at many high school and college parties. It is defined, for men, as drinking five or more drinks in a row, and for women, as drinking four or more drinks in a row. Students who binge drink are 21 times more likely than non-binge drinkers to have unplanned and unprotected sex.

Drugs Linked to Date Rape

Other drugs, besides alcohol, have been linked to increased incidences of rape and date rape. Abused mainly by high school and college-age youth, these drugs include the following:

Rohypnol (flunitrazepam): Also known as roofies, rope, roach, and the "Forget-Me Pill." It is not legal in the United States, but it is sold in 50 other countries, including Mexico and Columbia. Two similar drugs have replaced Rohypnol abuse in some parts of the U.S.— Klonopin (clonazepam) and Xanax (alprazolam). The drugs can be easily added to a woman's drink unknowingly because it is colorless, tasteless, and odorless. It causes partial amnesia, so the woman cannot remember anything that occurs for up to eight hours after consuming the drink. Many men add it to a woman's drink with the intention of sexually assaulting her while she is unconscious.

Gamma-hydroxybutyrate acid (GHB): Street names include "Liquid Ecstasy," "Soap," "Easy Lay," and "Georgia Home Boy." Like Rohypnol, GHB makes a victim feel and act drunk and very relaxed. Before 1992, GHB was often sold in health food stores. It became illegal in 2000, but is now legal in the U.S. to treat problems from narcolepsy. It's distribution is tightly restricted. Like Rohypnol, a victim will not taste or see GHB in her drink, nor will she remember any events once she awakens.

Ketamine: A tranquilizer in liquid or powder form used on animals and humans. Street names include "Special K," "Vitamin K," and "Cat Valium." The liquid form can be added to drinks, tobacco, or marijuana. The powder form can also be added to drinks, as well as snorted or smoked. Ketamine causes hallucinations. At high doses, it can cause delirium, loss of memory, and depression.

Myth Versus Reality

There are many myths about sexual assault. People see or hear things on television, in movies, or from family members, and they believe that what they've heard is true. These myths blame the victim and downplay the seriousness of assault. Destroying these myths is the first step toward stopping abuse:

Myth: She got drunk. She deserved it.

Fact: A woman who gets drunk around strangers or friends may show poor judgment, but it does not give a man the right to rape her.

Myth: Rape is about sex.

Fact: Rape is a crime based on the need to control, shame, and harm. Rapists use sexual violence as a weapon.

Myth: She had sex with him before, so it cannot be rape.

Fact: If a woman does not want to have sex with a man—even if she has in the past—and he forces her to, that is rape.

Myth: If a woman drinks, she is more willing to have sex.

Fact: A woman who drinks does not automatically want to have sex. Women drink for many reasons: for the taste, or to relax. Men who believe that alcohol makes a woman more willing to have sex also think a woman who drinks wants to have sex even if she doesn't.

Chapter 10

Religion and Domestic Violence

Issues of religious faith, or the belief in a specific system of principles and practices that give reverence to a higher power, are often central to the experiences of many victims and survivors of domestic violence. Faith communities and secular domestic violence programs are becoming increasingly aware of the need to create an awareness of domestic violence within faith communities, as well as the need for cross-training and education about dynamics of domestic violence and the role that faith plays in individuals' lives. Yet there exist misconceptions between faith communities and secular advocates that have served as barriers to collaboration between these two entities. Faith leaders may fear that secular advocates encourage women to divorce, for example, while secular advocates may fear that faith leaders and community members pressure women to stay in dangerous relationships, using religious beliefs to justify abuse and potentially blaming women for their own victimization (Miles, 2002). Some secular advocates hold the perception that faith leaders, as a part of a larger sociocultural structure, may be reluctant to involve themselves or their communities in responding to domestic violence for various reasons, including denial of the existence or prevalence of domestic violence, a sense of fear and hopelessness, lack of appropriate training, the culture of patriarchy, and the possibility that some of these faith leaders are perpetrators themselves (Miles, 2002).

This material was reprinted/adapted from the publication titled *Religion and Domestic Violence: Information and Resources*, © 2007 National Resource Center on Domestic Violence.

Yet many faith communities are making public statements that denounce domestic violence and the use of religious teachings to justify it. Moving beyond the misconceptions to work together enables secular programs and faith communities to develop supportive networks that provide comprehensive responses to victims and survivors of faith.

Certain interpretations of particular religious tenets are often used by batterers to manipulate and control their partners. The use of these teachings to justify abusive behavior and the imbalance of power within a relationship can further contribute to the feelings of guilt and self-blame many victims experience as a result of the abuse. It is important to note that while women's use of violence toward male partners exists, a close examination of the issue reveals that it is historically, culturally, motivationally, and situationally distinct from male violence toward female partners (Das Dasgupta, 2001). Research shows that the overwhelming majority of domestic violence cases involve male violence against female partners. Although interpretations may be given to religious teachings and traditions that imply the absolute authority of a husband over his wife, many scholars argue that it is inappropriate to use these teachings in their full contexts to support misogynist behavior in marital relationships or sociocultural arenas. The most frequently referenced Judaic, Islamic, and Christian tenets that focus on the nature of heterosexual marriage and the gender roles within that relationship have been included for discussion in this chapter.

Communities of faith play a unique and vital role in the response to and elimination of domestic violence, as they carry the responsibility to protect and nurture the spiritual wellbeing of the community as a whole and its individual members. Victims and survivors of domestic violence may turn to faith leaders for spiritual guidance and support before or in lieu of secular domestic violence services, because of the unique dimension they can add to the sometimes overwhelming experience of seeking help. Similarly, batterers may also turn to faith leaders, perhaps either as a means of legitimizing the abuse or to seek guidance and support in understanding and changing behaviors. Faith leaders may be asked, then, to provide spiritual guidance and counseling to both the victim and the perpetrator. This requires efforts by faith leaders to not only acknowledge domestic violence but also to continually educate themselves and the entire community and to join in creating responses to domestic violence that are safe and supportive for victims and survivors. Yet responses to domestic violence cannot exist without some form of accountability for the batterer. When faith communities make an effort to examine issues of batterer accountability, in addition to those of victim safety and empowerment, they are better able to create a response that meets the needs of individuals and their communities.

Secular programs that are sensitive to the values and beliefs held by victims and survivors of faith can help them identify options and resources that are relevant and specific to their situation. Partnerships and collaborations between secular programs and faith-based groups enable the development of more comprehensive and supportive responses to victims. Through the joint provision of education, resources, and advocacy, communities are bridging the gaps between diverse faith-based and secular responses. This collaborative approach can provide a much more holistic approach to helping victims and survivors of faith that honors individual choice and identity, celebrates survival, and helps victims identify and utilize personal strengths and resources.

Funding, however, is often a barrier to programs and communities seeking to create comprehensive and supportive responses to domestic violence by expanding available resources or developing new programs. With the introduction of the federal faith-based initiatives, efforts have been made to increase faith-based and other community organizations' access to federal funding for the provision of social services.

Interpretations of Religious Doctrine

Throughout history, religious beliefs, traditions, and teachings have been used both to justify and to denounce the use of violence against women. When religious teachings are used to justify domestic violence, they become a tool by which batterers assume and maintain power and control over their partners. The use of these teachings to justify abusive behavior and the imbalance of power within a relationship can also further contribute to the feelings of guilt and self-blame many victims experience as a result of the abuse. Some interpretations of religious texts and teachings imply that husbands have absolute authority over obedient and submissive wives. However, after a careful examination of these teachings in their full context, many religious scholars argue that it is inappropriate to use them to support misogynist behavior within a relationship or to generalize these beliefs to the treatment of women within the larger community.

Judaism

Marriage in the Jewish tradition is viewed as an expression of the holiness of a man and a woman and as necessary for fulfillment, and is based on mutual love and respect (Fortune, 1991). Despite this fact, the core value of *shalom bayis*, or peace in the home (Fortune, 1991), has been interpreted to imply that the sole responsibility of maintaining peace and promoting love, nurturing, and understanding in the family is that of the woman (Jewish Community Help and Abuse Information, n.d.). *Shalom bayis* may be a reason why many Jewish women stay in abusive relationships, in that a victim of domestic violence may be reluctant to seek help because she may feel she failed at her role to maintain the peace in her home; she may be fearful of bringing *shanda*, or shame, on her family and the community (Jewish Women International, 1996). Many people falsely believe that domestic violence does not exist in Jewish homes, and this myth reinforces the silence that allows domestic violence to continue. By bringing attention to the abusive relationship, the victim has not only exposed her imperfect marriage, but she has also exposed the vulnerabilities of her community and may be ostracized or resented for doing so. Many Jewish texts condemn violence against women and can be viewed as resources for Jewish women in abusive relationships. *Judaism and Domestic Violence* outlines several Talmudic and Rabbinic texts that condemn violence against women and set a standard for behavior. Jewish law states that if a man loves his wife as prescribed, his home will be a place of peace (United Synagogue of Conservative Judaism [USCJ], 1995). Rabbi Moshe Isserles commented specifically on what the Jewish attitude is toward a man who strikes his wife: any man who strikes his wife commits a sin and if he does this frequently, it is up to the courts to punish and excommunicate him (USCJ, 1995). Messages such as these not only condemn violence against women, they provide guidelines toward the development of *shalom bayis* in the family.

Islam

For Muslim men and women, the Qur'an is the primary source of their faith and practice. In Islam, the focus of marriage is encapsulated in the following verse of the Qur'an: "...they are a sort of garment for you and you are a sort of garment for them..." (2:188). Qur'anic verse 4:34 is often used to justify physical abuse against a wife if she does not submit to her partner's authority. It states:

> Men shall take full care of women with the bounties Allah has bestowed upon them, and what they may spend out of their possession; as Allah has eschewed each with certain qualities in

relation to the other. And the righteous women are the truly devout ones, who guard the intimacy, which Allah has ordained to be guarded. As for those women whose ill will you have reason to fear, admonish them [first]; then distance yourself in bed, and then tap them; but if they pay you heed, do not seek to harm them. Surely, Allah is indeed the Most High, the Greatest.

This verse may not only be interpreted by batterers to justify physical abuse against their wives, but also to support the belief that the role of men as maintainers and protectors of their wives implies unquestionable obedience to men. Many scholars, however, have interpreted this translation as charging men with the responsibility of financially and physically protecting and caring for their wives and families. Others have noted that the role of protector is synonymous with someone who has the responsibility of safeguarding the interests of another, and not the imposition of authority (Faizi, 2000).

If a wife is deliberately unfaithful (short of adultery) to her husband, instructions are given on how to attempt to resolve this situation. It is the husband's responsibility to first talk to her and then refuse to share her bed. If this fails to resolve the issue, then, only as a last resort before seeking a divorce, a husband may "tap" his wife in a symbolic effort to demonstrate his seriousness in the matter (Alkhateeb, n.d.). Many scholars of the Qur'an have debated over the appropriate translation of the word "tap" as the original Arabic word carries several different meanings (Khan, n.d.). In some texts, it is translated as hit or strike; however, many scholars believe that this is an incorrect translation of the original Arabic word, based on the Prophet's lifelong abhorrence of hitting women (Alkhateeb, n.d.). Additionally, by examining classical commentaries by Muslim jurists, the tap is intended to be a symbolic gesture as with a toothbrush or a folded handkerchief so as not to cause pain (Khan, n.d.). If a woman fears that her husband will be abusive or is unfaithful she has the option of enlisting the support of the community by sitting down with her husband and respected members of the community to draw up a contract with her husband as an ultimatum and an attempt to resolve the issue before she seeks a divorce (Khan, n.d.). In essence, "the Qur'an does not discriminate between the two sexes in any way that undermines their full worth as equal human beings, nor does it give either of them; men or women, priority or superiority over the other in any manner whatsoever, neither does it endorse spouse abuse nor does it encourage spouse battering" (Khan, n.d.).

Christianity

Similar interpretations have been given to Biblical texts that also focus on gender roles within heterosexual marriages. Traditionally, Christian teaching about the roles of husbands and wives within a marriage rely heavily on Ephesians 5:21–33 (Fortune, 1991). Nine of the twelve verses discuss the responsibility of a husband to his wife. The remaining three verses, when taken in isolation, may be interpreted to imply that the husband has absolute authority over the family and this authority cannot be questioned, and that wives, in turn, must demonstrate absolute obedience and summarily submit to abuse from their husbands:

> Wives submit to your husbands as to the Lord. For the husband is the head of the wife, as Christ is the head of the church, his body, of which he is the Savior. Now as the church submits to Christ, so also the wives should submit to their husbands in everything. (Ephesians 5:22–24 in Fortune, 1991)

It is important to note, however, that Ephesians 5:21 begins by saying: "Submit to one another out of reverence for Christ" (Miles, 2002). As was seen in the translation of the Qur'an, certain key words in the Bible also have ambiguous meanings in translation. Several Greek words are commonly understood to be related to the word submission in the Christian scriptures; essentially, however, Ephesians both implicitly and explicitly calls for husbands and wives to "behave responsibly towards one another, align themselves, and to relate to one another in a meaningful and respectful way" (Miles, 2002).

Reverend Marie Fortune (1991) states that the first verse of Ephesians clearly indicates that all Christians are to be mutually subject, or accommodating, to each other, which implies sensitivity, flexibility, and responsiveness of the husband. She goes on to suggest that the husband and wife relationship described in Ephesians 5:23–24 is based on the relationship of Christ to the church. The teaching and ministry of Jesus was one of service to others and to the church, not one of dominance and authority over others. Therefore, a Christian husband who truly believes and understands the teachings of Jesus will not dominate or control his wife, but serve and care for her:

> Husbands, love your wives, just as Christ loved the church and gave himself up for her to make her holy, cleansing her by the washing with water through the word, and to present her to

himself as a radiant church, without stain or blemish or any other wrinkle, but holy and blameless. In this same way, husbands ought to love their wives as their own bodies. He who loves his wife, loves himself. After all, no one ever hated his own body, but feeds and cares for it, just as Christ does the church, for we are members of his body. (Ephesians 5:25–29)

Divorce

Many victims of domestic violence experience serious ethical or religious dilemmas about ending a marriage. Marriage, as discussed earlier, is sanctified in many religious and spiritual traditions throughout the world and is considered by many spiritual traditions to be a cornerstone to social and religious life. Victims of domestic violence may experience many pressures to maintain this kind of relationship, even if it is not based on mutual love and respect. For some women, it is implicit that separating from their partner also means separating from their religious community because of the emphasis placed on maintaining a committed relationship. Many women may also feel that ending the relationship is not an option based on their personal belief that they entered into the relationship as a life-long commitment to themselves and their partner. According to a recent study of Muslim American women's experiences with abuse, for example, study participants lived with abuse for many years and hoped through faith that things would eventually improve, as marriage is an integral part of their religious and social life (Hassouneh-Phillips, 2001).

Many batterers use divorce, or the legal dissolution of a heterosexual marriage, as a powerful tool to manipulate their partners. Muslim batterers, for example, may convince their partners that only the husband may ask for divorce and that a husband may obtain a divorce without any type of legal representation or documentation, contrary to Islamic law, but permitted in some countries.

Divorce in Islam is not as capricious as may be perceived and practiced. Khan (1980) explains, "the process of divorce is spread over a period, during which every effort must be made at smoothing out differences and at reconciliation. If differences become acute, the counsel and help of mediators, one from the wife's people and one from the husband's people, should be sought."

Yet, according to the Qur'an, a Muslim woman has the right to ask for a divorce if she fears cruelty or desertion on the part of her husband (Sultan, 2002). "...But if you fear they cannot observe the limits prescribed by Allah, then it shall be no sin for either of them in what she gives to get her freedom..." (Qur'an 2:230). Some Muslim women, however, may hesitate to divorce due to the heavy emphasis placed on the social importance of marriage in many Muslim communities and the fear that they will displease God or their families, even if the relationship is life threatening (Faizi, 2000). But both the Muslim and the Jewish faiths have always recognized divorce, although it is viewed as a last resort, when all other attempts to restore the relationship have failed and it is determined that the continuation of the relationship is considered to be detrimental to the wellbeing of either party.

Similarly, for Christian women, the promise of 'til death do us part is commonly interpreted to mean that marriage is permanent, even if abuse is present in the relationship (Fortune, 1991). According to Reverend Fortune, mutual respect is a necessary element of a life-long commitment between two people and violence in a life-long relationship transgresses the commitment and fractures the relationship. By seeking safety through a permanent separation from her partner, the victim is acknowledging that the commitment she and her partner made to each other no longer exists, but she is not the one breaking the commitment (Eilts, 1995); rather, it is the abusive behavior that violates the commitment.

Conclusion

A batterer may choose to manipulate his partner's religion and faith as a means to reinforce and maintain power and control over that partner. In fact, many religious communities have made public statements denouncing domestic violence and the use of religious teachings to justify it. The unique role that faith leaders and other community members hold in protecting and nurturing the spiritual wellbeing of their whole community carries the added responsibility to also protect and nurture the safety of individual members. This requires intensive efforts to not only acknowledge domestic violence within their communities but also ongoing education about the issues and the commitment to create appropriate responses that support victims and survivors.

Works Cited

Alkhateeb, S. (n.d.). *Ending Domestic Violence in Muslim Families*. Retrieved May 2003 from: http://themodernreligion.com/index2.html.

Das Dasgupta, S. (2001). *Towards an Understanding of Women's Use of Non-Lethal Violence in Intimate Heterosexual Relationships*. Harrisburg, PA: National Online Resource Center on Violence Against Women (VAWnet), a project of the National Resource Center on Domestic Violence.

Eilts, M. (1995). Saving the family: When is the covenant broken? In *Family Violence and Religion: An Interfaith Resource Guide*. Volcano, CA: Volcano Press.

Faizi, N. (2000). Domestic violence in the Muslim community. *Texas Journal of Women and the Law*, 10, 209–230.

Fortune, M. (1991). A commentary on religious issues. In *Violence in the Family: A Workshop Curriculum for Clergy and Other Helpers*. Cleveland, OH: Pilgrim Press.

Hassouneh-Phillips, D. (2001). Marriage is half faith, the rest is fear Allah: Marriage and spousal abuse among American Muslims. *Violence Against Women, 7*(8), 927–946.

Jewish Community Help and Abuse Information (n.d.). *Jewish Cultural Issues*. Retrieved May 2003 from: http://www.chaicolorado.org/jewish_cultural_issues.htm.

Jewish Women International (1996). *Resource Guide for Rabbis on Domestic Violence*. Washington, DC: Author.

Khan, M.Z. (1980). *Islam: Its Meaning for Modern Man*. London: Routledge and Kegan Paul.

Khan, S. (n.d.). The verse of abuse or the abused verse. In *Dimensions of the Qur'an*. Los Angeles, CA: MVI Publications.

Miles, A. (2002). *Violence in Families: What Every Christian Needs to Know*. Minneapolis, MN: Augsburg Fortress Press.

Sultan, R. (2002). *Divorce in Islam*. Retrieved June 2003 from: http://www.zawaj.com/articles/divorce_reem_sultan.html.

United Synagogue of Conservative Judaism (1995). *Judaism and Domestic Violence* [pamphlet]. New York, NY: Commission on Social Action and Public Policy, United Synagogue of Conservative Judaism.

Chapter 11

Animal Cruelty
and Domestic Violence

Why It Matters

Pets are not immune to domestic violence. Batterers frequently threaten, injure, maim, or kill their partners' or children's pets in conjunction with domestic abuse. Because victims understand the extent of the harm that their abusers will likely inflict upon their pets, many hesitate to leave violent relationships out of concern for the safety of their pets. When batterers abuse victims, victims see the animal cruelty as part of a long history of violence aimed at them and their families.[1] Recognizing this, an increasing number of shelters have added kennels or instituted—"safe haven" animal foster care programs in an effort to protect victims, their children, and their pets.

Did You Know?

- 71% of pet owners entering domestic violence shelters report that their batterer had threatened, injured, or killed family pets.[2]

- One study found that 87% of batterer-perpetrated incidents of pet abuse are committed in the presence of their partners for the purpose of revenge or control.[3]

- Studies show that up to 76% of batterer-perpetrated pet abuse incidents occur in the presence of children.[4]

- 13% of intentional animal abuse cases involve domestic violence.[5]

- Women in domestic violence shelters are 11 times more likely to report animal abuse by their partner than women not experiencing violence.[6]

- 85% of domestic violence shelters report that they commonly encounter women who speak about pet abuse incidents.[6]

- 52% of victims in shelters left their pets with their batterers.[6]

- Criminals and troubled youth have high rates of animal cruelty during their childhood, perpetrators often were victims of child abuse themselves.[7]

- Investigation of animal abuse is often the first point of social services intervention for a family experiencing domestic violence.[8]

The Link between Pet Abuse and Domestic Violence

- Similar to domestic abuse, abusers demonstrate power and control over the family by threatening, harming, or killing animals.[8]

- Domestic violence victims whose batterers abuse their pets report more than twice as many incidents of child abuse as compared to domestic violence victims whose batterers have not abused their pets.[10]

- Batterers threaten, harm, or kill their children's pets in order to coerce them into sexual abuse or to force them to remain silent about abuse.[11]

- Abusers harm pets to punish the victim for leaving, or in attempts to coerce her or him to return.[17]

- Abusers may harm pets to retaliate for acts of self-determination or independence.[9]

- Animal abusers are more likely to be domestic violence abusers, to have been arrested for other violent crimes and drug-related offenses, and engage in other delinquent behavior.[6]

- Many abusers have a history of animal abuse that precedes domestic violence toward their partner.[12]

- Animals may sometimes be used as weapons against domestic violence victims.[6]

The Role of Pets

- Family pets are commonly viewed as family members and companions.

- 55% of domestic violence victims and their children report that their pets are very important sources of emotional support, thus violence toward pets may be especially devastating and viewed as another form of family violence.[13]

- A large majority of women residing in domestic violence shelters report being emotionally close to their pets and experience distress when their animals are abused.[6]

- Studies show that a vast majority of children who witness pet abuse become distressed and emotionally distraught.[6]

- Women without children are more likely to postpone seeking shelter out of concern for their pets' safety as compared to women with children, 33.3% versus 19.5%.[6]

Barriers to Seeking Services

- 65% of women who report prior pet abuse continue to worry about their pets' welfare after entry into a shelter.[6]

- Up to 40% of domestic violence victims are unable to escape their abusers because they are concerned about what will happen to their pets when they leave.[14]

- Only 12% of domestic violence programs can provide shelter for pets and 24% provide referral services to local animal welfare organizations.[15]

- Victims of domestic violence have been known to live in their cars for as long as four months until an opening was available at a pet-friendly safe house or shelter.[16]

Tips for Victims with Pets[9]

- Some shelters allow pets and many others have established— "safe haven" foster care programs for the animal victims of domestic violence.

- If it is not possible to take the animals when the victim leaves the home, try to arrange temporary shelter for the pets with a veterinarian, trusted friend or family member, or local animal shelter.

- When vaccinating pets against rabies and licensing them with the town or county, it is important that registrations are in the victim's name. This will serve as proof that the victim owns the pets.

- Prepare the pets for a quick departure: collect vaccination records, pet license, medical records, and other documents.

- Ask for help from animal care and control officers or law enforcement if pets need to be retrieved from the abuser. Never reclaim animals alone.

Sources

[1] Luke, C., Arluke, A., and Levin, J. (1998). *Cruelty to Animals and Other Crimes: A Study by the MSPCA and Northeastern University.* Boston: MSPCA.

[2] Ascione, F. R., Weber, C. V., and Wood, D. S. (1997). The abuse of animals and domestic violence: A national survey of shelters for women who are battered. *Society and Animals* 5(3), 205–218.

[3] Quinlisk, J. A. (1999). Animal Abuse and Family Violence. In, Ascione, F. R. and Arkow, P., eds.: *Child Abuse, Domestic Violence, and Animal Abuse: Linking the Circles of Compassion for Prevention and Intervention.* West Lafayette, IN: Purdue University Press, pp. 168–175.

[4] Faver and Strand. (2003).

[5] Humane Society of the U.S. (2001). *2000 Report of Animal Cruelty Cases.* Washington, DC.

[6] Ascione, F.R., Weber, C.V., Thompson, T.M., Heath, J., Maruyama, M., and Hayashi, K. (2007). Battered Pets and Domestic Violence: Animal Abuse Reported by Women Experiencing Intimate Violence and by Non-abused Women. *Violence Against Women*, 13(4), 354–373.

[7] Flynn, C.P. (2000). Woman's Best Friend: Pet Abuse and the Role of Companion Animals in the Lives of Battered Women. *Violence Against Women*, 6(2), 162–177.

[8] Arkow, P. (2003). *Breaking the cycles of violence: A guide to multidisciplinary interventions: A handbook for child protection, domestic*

violence, and animal protection agencies. Alameda, CA: Latham Foundation.

[9] *Animal Cruelty/Domestic Violence Fact Sheet* (2007). Humane Society of the United States. http://www.hsus.org/hsus field/.

[10] Ascione, F.R. (2001). Animal Abuse and Youth Violence. *Juvenile Justice Bulletin.* U.S. Department of Justice Office of Juvenile Justice and Delinquency Prevention, Washington, DC.

[11] Loar, L. (1999). "I'll only help you if you have two legs," or, Why human services professionals should pay attention to cases involving cruelty to animals. In Ascione, F.R. and Arkow, P., eds.: *Child Abuse, Domestic Violence, and Animal Abuse: Linking the Circles of Compassion for Prevention and Intervention.* West Lafayette, IN: Purdue University Press, 1999, pp. 120–136.

[12] Weber, C.V. (1999). A Descriptive Study of the Relationship between Domestic Violence and Pet Abuse. ProQuest Information and Learning. *Dissertation Abstracts International: Section B: The Sciences and Engineering, 59(80-B).*

[13] Faver, C.A. and Strand, E.B. (2003). Domestic Violence and Animal Cruelty: Untangling the Web of Abuse. *Journal of Social Work Education.* 39(2), 237–253.

[14] Arkow, P. (1994). Animal abuse and domestic violence: Intake statistics tell a sad story. *Latham Letter 15(2),* 17.

[15] NCADV *National Directory of Domestic Violence Programs*, 2004.

[16] Kogan, L.R., McConnell, S., Schoenfeld-Tacher, R., and Jansen-Lock, P. (2004). Crosstrails: A unique foster program to provide safety for pets of women in safe houses. *Violence Against Women 10,* 418–434.

For More Information or If You Need Help

American Humane Association
63 Inverness Drive East
Englewood, CO 80112
Toll-Free: 800-227-4645
Phone: 303-792-9900
Fax: 303-792-5333
Website: http://www.americanhumane.org
E-mail: info@americanhumane.org

National Child Abuse Hotline
15757 N. 78th St.
Scottsdale, AZ 85260
Toll-Free: 800-4-A-CHILD (22-4453)
Toll-Free TDD: 800-222-4453
Phone: 480-922-8212
Fax: 480-922-7061
Website: http://www.region4wib.org/ChildhelpUSA.htm
E-mail: info@childhelpusa.org

National Domestic Violence Hotline
P.O. Box 161810
Austin, TX 78716
Toll-Free Hotline: 800-799-SAFE (7233)
Toll-Free TTY: 800-787-3224
Website: http://www.ndvh.org

National Sexual Assault Hotline
Rape, Abuse & Incest National Network (RAINN)
2000 L Street, NW, Suite 406
Washington, DC 20036
Toll-Free: 800-656-HOPE (4673)
Phone: 202-544-3064
Fax: 202-544-3556
Website: http://www.rainn.org
E-mail: info@rainn.org

Part Two

Intimate Partner Violence and Other Forms of Domestic Violence

Chapter 12

Understanding Intimate Partner Violence

Intimate partner violence (IPV) is abuse that occurs between two people in a close relationship. The term intimate partner includes current and former spouses and dating partners. IPV exists along a continuum from a single episode of violence to ongoing battering. IPV includes four types of behavior:

- **Physical abuse** is when a person hurts or tries to hurt a partner by hitting, kicking, burning, or other physical force.

- **Sexual abuse** is forcing a partner to take part in a sex act when the partner does not consent.

- **Threats** of physical or sexual abuse include the use of words, gestures, weapons, or other means to communicate the intent to cause harm.

- **Emotional abuse** is threatening a partner or his or her possessions or loved ones, or harming a partner's sense of self-worth. Examples are stalking, name calling, intimidation, or not letting a partner see friends and family.

Often, IPV starts with emotional abuse. This behavior can progress to physical or sexual assault. Several types of IPV may occur together.

"Understanding Intimate Partner Violence Fact Sheet," Centers for Disease Control and Prevention (CDC), 2006.

113

Why is IPV a public health problem?

Many victims do not report IPV to police, friends, or family.[1] Victims think others will not believe them and that the police cannot help.[1]

- Each year, women experience about 4.8 million intimate partner related physical assaults and rapes. Men are the victims of about 2.9 million intimate partner related physical assaults.[1]

- IPV resulted in 1,544 deaths in 2004. Of these deaths, 25% were males and 75% were females.[2]

- The cost of IPV was an estimated $5.8 billion in 1995. Updated to 2003 dollars, that's more than $8.3 billion.[3, 4] This includes medical care, mental health services, and lost productivity (for example, time away from work).

How does IPV affect health?

IPV can affect health in many ways. The longer the abuse goes on, the more serious the effects on the victim.

Many victims suffer physical injuries. Some are minor like cuts, scratches, bruises, and welts. Others are more serious and can cause lasting disabilities. These include broken bones, internal bleeding, and head trauma.

Not all injuries are physical. IPV can also cause emotional harm. Victims often have low self-esteem. They may have a hard time trusting others and being in relationships. The anger and stress that victims feel may lead to eating disorders and depression. Some victims even think about or commit suicide.

IPV is linked to harmful health behaviors as well. Victims are more likely to smoke, abuse alcohol, use drugs, and engage in risky sexual activity.

Who is at risk for IPV?

Several factors can increase the risk that someone will hurt his or her partner. However, having these risk factors does not always mean that IPV will occur.

Some risk factors for perpetration (hurting a partner) include the following:

- Using drugs or alcohol, especially drinking heavily

- Seeing or being a victim of violence as a child
- Not having a job, which can cause feelings of stress

How can we prevent IPV?

The goal is to stop IPV before it begins. Strategies that promote healthy dating relationships are important. These strategies should focus on young people when they are learning skills for dating. This approach can help those at risk from becoming victims or offenders of IPV.

Traditionally, women's groups have addressed IPV by setting up crisis hotlines and shelters for battered women. But, both men and women can work with young people to prevent IPV. Adults can help change social norms, be role models, mentor youth, and work with others to end this violence. For example, by modeling nonviolent relationships, men and women can send the message to young boys and girls that violence is not okay.

How does the Centers for Disease Control and Prevention (CDC) approach IPV prevention?

CDC uses a four-step approach to address public health problems like IPV.

Step 1. Define the problem: Before we can prevent IPV, we need to know how big the problem is, where it is, and whom it affects. CDC learns about a problem by gathering and studying data. These data are critical because they help decision makers use resources where needed most.

Step 2. Identify risk and protective factors: It is not enough to know that IPV affects certain people in a certain area. We also need to know why. CDC conducts and supports research to answer this question. We can then develop programs to reduce or get rid of risk factors.

Step 3. Develop and test prevention strategies: Using information gathered in research, CDC develops and evaluates strategies to prevent IPV.

Step 4. Assure widespread adoption: In this final step, CDC shares the best prevention strategies. CDC may also provide funding or technical help so communities can adopt these strategies.

References

1. Tjaden P, Thoennes N. *Extent, nature, and consequences of intimate partner violence: findings from the National Violence against Women Survey*. Washington (DC): Department of Justice (US); 2000. Publication No. NCJ 181867. Available from: URL: www.ojp.usdoj.gov/nij/pubs-sum/181867.htm.

2. Department of Justice, Bureau of Justice Statistics. *Homicide trends in the United States* [online]. [cited 2006 Aug 28]. Available from URL: www.ojp.usdoj.gov/bjs/homicide/intimates.htm.

3. Centers for Disease Control and Prevention (CDC). *Costs of intimate partner violence against women in the United States*. Atlanta (GA): CDC, National Center for Injury Prevention and Control; 2003. [cited 2006 May 22]. Available from: URL: www .cdc.gov/ncipc/pub-res/ipv_cost/ipv.htm.

4. Max W, Rice DP, Finkelstein E, Bardwell RA, Leadbetter S. The economic toll of intimate partner violence against women in the United States. *Violence and Victims* 2004; 19(3): 259–72.

Chapter 13

Intimate Partner Violence Statistics

Intimate partner violence has been declining. Nonfatal violence has declined since 1993 from six victims per 1,000 persons age 12 or older in 1993 to just over two victims per 1,000 persons age 12 or older in 2005. Homicides of intimates declined: male victims declined from 1,300 in 1976 to under 400 in 2005; and, female victims declined from 1,600 victims in 1976 to 1,100 victims in 2005. Nonfatal violence has declined since 1993, regardless of the relationship between the victim and the offender.

Victim Characteristics

Gender

Females are more likely than males to experience nonfatal intimate partner violence. On average between 2001 and 2005, nonfatal intimate partner victimizations represented:

- 22% of nonfatal violent victimizations against females age 12 or older; and,

- 4% of nonfatal violent victimizations against males age 12 or older.

Excerpted from "Intimate Partner Violence in the United States," by Shannan Catalano, Ph.D., Bureau of Justice Statistics (BJS) Statistician, U.S. Department of Justice, 2007.

Table 13.1. Victim/offender relationship in nonfatal violent victimizations, by victim and gender, 2001–2005 (average annual rate per 1,000 persons age 12 or older)

Victim/offender relationship	Female Rate	Percent	Male Rate	Percent
		100%		100%
Intimate	4.2	21.5	0.9	3.6
Other relative	1.7	8.9	1.2	4.6
Friend/acquaintance	7.0	36.2	8.6	34.3
Stranger	6.5	33.4	14.4	57.4

For homicides, intimate partners committed 30% of homicides of females, and 5% of homicides of males.

Table 13.2. Homicide victim/offender relationship by victim gender, 1976–2005 (percent of homicide victims by gender)

Victim/offender relationship	Female	Male
Total	100%	100%
Intimate	30.1	5.3
Other family	11.7	6.7
Acquaintance/known	21.8	35.5
Stranger	8.8	15.5
Undetermined	27.7	37.1

Trends for nonfatal intimate partner victimization differ by gender. The rate of nonfatal intimate partner victimization for females was about four victimizations per 1,000 persons age 12 or older in 2005, down from about ten in 1993; males remained stable between 2004 and 2005.

Age

For females of most age categories, nonfatal intimate partner victimization declined over time.

- In general, females ages 12 to 15 and age 50 or older were at the lowest risk of nonfatal intimate partner violence.
- During 2005, females ages 35 to 49 were at a greater risk of nonfatal intimate partner violence than older females.

With the exception of males and females age 65 or older, average annual rates from 2001 through 2005 for nonfatal intimate partner victimization were higher for females than males within each age category.

- Females ages 20 to 24 were at the greatest risk of nonfatal intimate partner violence.

- In general, males ages 12 to 15 and age 65 or older experienced the lowest rates of nonfatal intimate partner violence.

Marital Status

Rates of nonfatal intimate partner violence for females who were married, divorced, separated, or never married were lower in 2005 than in 1993. Females who were separated reported higher rates than females of other marital status; married females reported the lowest rates of nonfatal intimate partner violence.

On average from 2001 to 2005, both females and males who were separated or divorced had the greatest risk of nonfatal intimate partner violence while persons who were married or widowed reported the lowest risk of violence.

Most intimate homicides involved spouses, although in recent years the number of deaths by boyfriends and girlfriends was about the same.

Race

Between 1993 and 2005, rates of nonfatal intimate partner violence decreased for white females, white males, and black females.

Between 2004 and 2005, rates of intimate partner violence remained stable for:

- white females at 3.1 per 1,000 persons age 12 or older;

- black females at 4.6 per 1,000 persons age 12 or older; and,

- white males at 0.7 per 1,000 persons age 12 or older.

The average annual rate of nonfatal intimate partner violence from 2001 to 2005 was:

- generally higher for American Indian and Alaskan Native females, and

- similar for black females and white females.

Between 1993 and 2005, the rate of nonfatal intimate partner victimizations declined for:

- Hispanic females by two-thirds, and
- by over half for non-Hispanic females.

On average from 2001 to 2005, rates of intimate partner violence were similar for both Hispanic and non-Hispanic females and males.

Intimate homicide rate has fallen for blacks in every relationship category, while the rate for whites has not changed for all categories.

Income

From 2001 to 2005, for nonfatal intimate partner victimization:

- females living in households with lower annual incomes experienced the highest average annual rates of intimate partner violence; and,
- females remained at greater risk than males within each income level.

Home Ownership

From 2001 to 2005, for nonfatal intimate partner violence:

- average annual rates were higher for persons living in rental housing than other types of housing regardless of the victim's gender;
- females residing in rental housing were victimized at an average annual rate more than three times the rate of females living in owned housing; and,
- males residing in rental housing were victimized by an intimate partner about three times the rate of males living in owned housing.

Children Exposed to Intimate Partner Violence

On average between 2001 and 2005, children were residents of the households experiencing intimate partner violence in 38% of the incidents involving female victims, and 21% of the incidents involving male victims.

Table 13.3. Average annual number and percentage of households experiencing nonfatal intimate partner violence where children under age 12 resided, by gender of victims, 2001–2005

Households with intimate partner violence victims	Annual average Number	Percent
All households with	615,795	100%
Children	216,490	35.2
No children	303,615	49.3
Unknown	95,685	15.5
Female victim households with	510,970	100%
Children	194,455	38.1
No children	235,940	46.2
Unknown	80,580	15.8
Male victim households with	104,820	100%
Children	22,040	21.0
No children	67,680	64.6
Unknown	15,105	14.4

Note: The National Crime Victimization Survey (NCVS) does not ask about the extent to which young children may have witnessed the violence.

Offender Characteristics

Gender

Nonfatal intimate partner violence is most frequently committed by individuals of opposite genders. On average from 2001 to 2005:

- about 96% of females experiencing nonfatal intimate partner violence were victimized by a male and about 3% reported that the offender was another female; and,

- about 82% of males experiencing nonfatal intimate partner violence were victimized by a female and about 16% of males reported that the offender was another male.

Age

On average, from 2001 to 2005, most victims of nonfatal intimate partner violence report that the age of the offender was similar to their own age.

Table 13.4. Average annual percent of nonfatal intimate partner victimizations by age of victim and offender, 2001–2005

Age of victim	Age of offender						
	12–14	15–17	18–20	21–29	30 or older	Mixed ages	Don't know
12–14	16.7%	75.5%			7.8%		
15–17		58.9	23.4%	10.8%		3.4%	3.5%
18–20		3.9	37.5	46.3	6.1	3.0	3.3
21–29			4.5	65.7	26.0	1.6	2.2
30 and older	0.2		0.1	8.7	88.7	0.3	2.0

In blank spaces, the information is not provided because the small number of cases is insufficient for reliable estimates.

Note: Detail may not add to 100% due to rounding.

Race

Similar to other types of nonfatal violent victimization, nonfatal intimate partner violence is primarily with the victim and offender being of the same race.

- About 84% of white victims were victimized by white offenders.
- About 93% of black victims were victimized by black offenders.

Circumstances

Type of Crime

For nonfatal intimate partner violence, as for violent crime in general, simple assault (as opposed to rape/sexual assault, aggravated assault, or robbery) is the most common type of violent crime. The long-term trend for female victims of nonfatal intimate partner violence shows that between 1993 and 2005 the rate of simple assault declined by about two-thirds and the rate of aggravated assault declined by two-thirds. On average between 2001 and 2005, females experienced higher rates of nonfatal intimate partner violence than males in each type of crime.

Time

Nonfatal intimate partner violence is more likely to occur between the hours of 6 p.m. and 6 a.m. Females and males experienced nonfatal intimate partner victimization at similar times during the day and night.

Place

Between 2001 and 2005, the majority of nonfatal intimate partner victimizations occurred at home with approximately two-thirds of females and males were victimized at home; and about 11% of female and 10% of male victims of nonfatal intimate partner violence were victimized at a friend's or neighbor's home.

Table 13.5. Average annual number and percent distribution of location of incident for nonfatal intimate partner violence, by gender of victim, 2001–2005

	Average annual	
	Number	**Percent**
Female victims	510,970	100%
Victim's home	319,945	62.6
Near victim's home	48,075	9.4
Friend/neighbor's home	56,920	11.1
Commercial place	17,305	3.4
Parking lot or garage	21,535	4.2
School	9,750	1.9
Open area/street/public place	23,575	4.6
Other	13,870	2.7
Male victims	104,820	100%
Victim's home	63,075	60.2
Near victim's home	9,915	9.5
Friend/neighbor's home	10,660	10.2
Commercial place	6,245	6
Parking lot or garage	4,295	4.1
School	570	0.5*
Open area/street/public place	4,730	4.5
Other	5,330	5.1

*Based on 10 or fewer sample cases.

Note: Detail may not add to totals due to rounding.

Alcohol and Drugs

On average between 2001 and 2005:

• the presence of any alcohol or drugs was reported by victims in about 42% of all nonfatal intimate partner violence;

• victims reported that approximately 8% of all nonfatal intimate partner victimizations occurred when a perpetrator was under the influence of both alcohol and drugs;

• female and male victims of nonfatal intimate partner violence were equally likely to report the presence of alcohol during their victimization; and,

• female and male victims of nonfatal intimate partner violence both reported their attacker was under the influence of drugs in about 6% of all victimizations.

Note: Responses are based on perception of victim as to whether offender used alcohol or drugs.

Presence of Weapons

On average between 2001 and 2005, for nonfatal intimate partner violence:

• male victims were more likely than female victims to face an offender armed with a weapon;

• female victims were more likely than male victims to face an offender armed with a firearm; and,

• about 6% of female and 10% of male victims faced an offender armed with a sharp weapon, such as a knife.

The number of female and male nonfatal intimate partner victims killed with guns has fallen. For female victims, the number of intimate partner victims killed by other weapons has remained stable.

Location of Residence (Urban, Suburban, Rural)

On average between 2001 and 2005:

• males and females living in urban areas reported the highest levels of nonfatal intimate partner violence;

Table 13.6. Average annual number and percent distribution of type of weapon used in incidents where victim faced an armed offender, by gender, 2001–2005

	Average annual number and percent of weapons used in nonfatal intimate partner violence			
	Female		Male	
	Number	Percent	Number	Percent
Total intimate partner victims	510,970	100%	104,820	100%
No weapon present	411,140	80.5	71,825	68.5
Weapon present	79,715	15.6	29,430	28.1
Firearm	18,485	3.6	515	0.5
Sharp weapon	28,625	5.6	10,350	9.9
Blunt objects	32,605	6.4	18,560	17.7
Do not know if offender had weapon	20,120	3.9	3,565	3.4

Note: The firearms category includes handguns, other guns, and incidents where the gun type was unknown. Sharp objects include knives and any other sharp objects. Blunt objects include other weapon types and those classified as a blunt object. The "other" weapon category refers to items not generally considered weapons but that were used as a weapon such bottles, rocks, and sticks.

- males and females residing in rural and suburban areas were equally likely to experience nonfatal intimate partner violence; and,

- intimate homicides made up a larger percentage of murders in rural areas than in suburban or urban areas.

Injury and Treatment

On average since 2001, for nonfatal intimate partner violence, about one-third of female and male victims reported that they were physically attacked; and, approximately two-thirds of female and male victims stated that they were threatened with attack.

Type of Attack

On average between 2001 and 2005, for nonfatal intimate partner violence about two-thirds of female and male victims reported they were hit, slapped, or knocked down; and male victims were more likely than female victims to be grabbed, held, or tripped.

Table 13.7. Average annual percent of threats, by type, in nonfatal intimate partner violence crime, by gender, 2001–2005

Type of threat	Percent of victims of nonfatal intimate partner violence, 2001–2005	
	Female	Male
Threatened to kill	26.9%	15.1%*
Threatened to rape	0.5*	—
Threatened with harm	59.3	55.3
Threatened with a weapon	17.6	22.9
Threw object at victim	7.5	7.4*
Followed/surrounded victim	5.9	1.8*
Tried to hit, slap, or knock down victim	14.1	12.6*

*Based on 10 or fewer sample cases.

Note: Detail may not add to total because victims may have reported more than one type of threat.

—Information is not provided because the small number of cases is insufficient for reliable estimates.

Table 13.8. Average annual percent of attacks, by type, in nonfatal intimate partner violent crime, 2001–2005

Type of attack	Percent of victims of nonfatal intimate partner violence who were attacked	
	Female	Male
Raped	7.2%	0.8%*
Sexual assault	1.9	0.9
Attacked with firearm	0.5*	—
Attacked with knife	2.5	8*
Hit by thrown object	2.1	4.5*
Attacked with other weapon	0.8*	1.8*
Hit, slapped, knocked down	62.7	62.2
Grabbed, held, tripped	54.9	26

*Based on 10 or fewer sample cases.

—Information is not provided because the small number of cases is insufficient for reliable estimates.

Note: Detail may not add to total because victims may have reported more than one type of attack.

Injury

On average between 2001 and 2005, half of all females experiencing nonfatal intimate partner violence suffered an injury from their victimization. Of female victims about 5% were seriously injured and about 44% suffered minor injuries; and about 3% were raped or sexually assaulted.

Table 13.9. Average annual number and percent of injuries sustained by female victims as a result of nonfatal intimate partner violence, 2001–2005

Intimate partner victim	Average annual	
	Number	Percent
Total	510,970	100%
Not injured	248,805	48.7%
Injured	262,170	51.3%
Serious injury	25,710	5%
Gunshot wound	595	0.1*
Knife wounds	4,940	1*
Internal injuries	3,440	0.7*
Broken bones	12,155	2.4
Knocked unconscious	3,730	0.7*
Other serious injuries	855	0.2*
Rape/sexual assault without additional injuries	13,350	2.6
Minor injuries only	222,670	43.6
Injuries unknown	435	0.1*

*Based on 10 or fewer sample cases.

Note: Total may not add to 100% due to rounding.

On average between 2001 and 2005, more than one-third of male victims of nonfatal intimate partner violence were injured; 4% were seriously injured and 36% suffered minor injuries.

Table 13.10. Average annual number and percent of injuries sustained by male victims as a result of nonfatal intimate partner violence, 2001–2005

	Average annual	
	Number	**Percent**
Total intimate partner victims	104,820	100%
Not injured	61,285	58.5%
Injured	43,540	41.5%
Serious injury	4,335	4.1*
Minor injuries only	38,050	36.3
Rape/sexual assault without other injuries	580	0.6*
Injuries unknown	570	0.5%*

*Based on 10 or fewer sample cases.

Note: Detail may not add to totals due to rounding.

Table 13.11. Average annual percent of medical treatment sought as a result of nonfatal intimate partner violence, by gender, 2001–2005

	Average annual	
	Female	**Male**
Not injured	48.7%	58.5%
Injured	51.3%	41.5%
Injured, not treated	32.8	27.9
Treated for injury	18.5	13.1
At scene or home	8.3	9.8
Doctor's office or clinic	1.3	0.6*
Hospital	8.7	2.8*
Not admitted	8.4	2.8*
Admitted	0.3	—
Other locale	0.2	—
Don't know	—	0.5%*

*Based on 10 or fewer sample cases.

— Information is not provided because the small number of cases was insufficient for reliable estimates.

Note: Detail may not add to totals due to rounding.

Medical Care

On average between 2001 and 2005 for nonfatal intimate partner violence:

- less than one-fifth of victims reporting an injury sought treatment following the injury;

- about 8% of female and 10% of male victims were treated at the scene of the injury or in their home; and,

- females experiencing an injury were more likely than their male counterparts to seek treatment at a hospital.

Chapter 14

Intimate Partner Violence Risk Factors and Consequences

Chapter Contents

Section 14.1

Risk Factors for Intimate Partner Violence

"IPV Prevention Scientific Information: Risk and Protective Factors," Centers for Disease Control and Prevention (CDC), September 2007.

Risk factors are associated with a greater likelihood of intimate partner violence (IPV) victimization or perpetration. They are contributing factors and may or may not be direct causes. Not everyone who is identified as at risk becomes involved in violence.

Some risk factors for IPV victimization and perpetration are the same. In addition, some risk factors for victimization and perpetration are associated with one another; for example, childhood physical or sexual victimization is a risk factor for future IPV perpetration and victimization.

A combination of individual, relational, community, and societal factors contribute to the risk of becoming a victim or perpetrator of IPV. Understanding these multilevel factors can help identify various opportunities for prevention.

Individual Factors

- Low self-esteem
- Low income
- Low academic achievement
- Young age
- Aggressive or delinquent behavior as a youth
- Heavy alcohol and drug use
- Depression
- Anger and hostility
- Antisocial personality traits
- Borderline personality traits

- Prior history of being physically abusive
- Having few friends and being isolated from other people
- Unemployment
- Emotional dependence and insecurity
- Belief in strict gender roles (for example, male dominance and aggression in relationships)
- Desire for power and control in relationships
- Perpetrating psychological aggression
- Being a victim of physical or psychological abuse (consistently one of the strongest predictors of perpetration)
- History of experiencing poor parenting as a child
- History of experiencing physical discipline as a child

Relationship Factors

- Marital conflict–fights, tension, and other struggles
- Marital instability—divorces or separations
- Dominance and control of the relationship by one partner over the other
- Economic stress
- Unhealthy family relationships and interactions

Community Factors

- Poverty and associated factors (for example, overcrowding)
- Low social capital—lack of institutions, relationships, and norms that shape a community's social interactions
- Weak community sanctions against IPV (such as, unwillingness of neighbors to intervene in situations where they witness violence)

Societal Factors

- Traditional gender norms (for example, women should stay at home, not enter workforce, and be submissive; men support the family and make the decisions)

Section 14.2

Consequences of Intimate Partner Violence

Excerpted from "IPV Prevention Scientific Information: Consequences,"
Centers for Disease Control and Prevention (CDC), September 2007.

In general, victims of repeated violence over time experience more serious consequences than victims of one-time incidents. The following list describes some, but not all, of the consequences of IPV.

Physical

In 2005, 329 males and 1,181 females were murdered by an intimate partner (Bureau of Justice Statistics 2007).

As many as 42% of women and 20% of men who were physically assaulted since age 18 sustained injuries during their most recent victimization. Most injuries, such as scratches, bruises, and welts, were minor.

More severe physical consequences of IPV may occur depending on severity and frequency of abuse. These include the following:

- Bruises
- Knife wounds
- Pelvic pain
- Headaches
- Back pain
- Broken bones
- Gynecological disorders
- Pregnancy difficulties like low birthweight babies and perinatal deaths
- Sexually transmitted diseases including human immunodeficiency virus (HIV) and acquired immunodeficiency syndrome (AIDS)

- Central nervous system disorders
- Gastrointestinal disorders
- Heart or circulatory conditions

Children may become injured during IPV incidents between their parents. A large overlap exists between IPV and child maltreatment. One study found that children of abused mothers were 57 times more likely to have been harmed because of IPV between their parents, compared with children of non-abused mothers.

Psychological

Physical violence is typically accompanied by emotional or psychological abuse. IPV—whether sexual, physical, or psychological—can lead to various psychological consequences for victims:

- Depression
- Antisocial behavior
- Suicidal behavior in females
- Anxiety
- Low self-esteem
- Inability to trust men
- Fear of intimacy
- Symptoms of posttraumatic stress disorder
  - Emotional detachment
  - Sleep disturbances
  - Flashbacks
  - Replaying assault in mind

Social

Victims of IPV sometimes face the following social consequences:

- Restricted access to services
- Strained relationships with health providers and employers
- Isolation from social networks

Health Behaviors

Women with a history of IPV are more likely to display behaviors that present further health risks (for example, substance abuse, alcoholism, suicide attempts) than women without a history of IPV.

IPV is associated with a variety of negative health behaviors. Studies show that the more severe the violence, the stronger its relationship to negative health behaviors by victims.

- Engaging in high-risk sexual behavior
- Unprotected sex
- Decreased condom use
- Early sexual initiation
- Choosing unhealthy sexual partners
- Multiple sex partners
- Trading sex for food, money, or other items
- Using harmful substances
- Smoking cigarettes
- Drinking alcohol
- Drinking alcohol and driving
- Illicit drug use
- Unhealthy diet-related behaviors
- Fasting
- Vomiting
- Abusing diet pills
- Overeating
- Overuse of health services

Cost to Society

- Costs of intimate partner violence (IPV) against women in 1995 exceeded an estimated $5.8 billion. These costs included nearly $4.1 billion in the direct costs of medical and mental health care and nearly $1.8 billion in the indirect costs of lost productivity (CDC 2003). This is generally considered an underestimate because the costs associated with the criminal justice system were not included.

- When updated to 2003 dollars, IPV costs exceeded $8.3 billion, which included $460 million for rape, $6.2 billion for physical assault, $461 million for stalking, and $1.2 billion in the value of lost lives.

- Victims of severe IPV lose nearly 8 million days of paid work—the equivalent of more than 32,000 full-time jobs—and almost 5.6 million days of household productivity each year (CDC 2003).

- Women who experience severe aggression by men (for example: not being allowed to go to work or school, or having their lives or their children's lives threatened) are more likely to have been unemployed in the past, have health problems, and be receiving public assistance.

Chapter 15

Intimate Partner
Violence Impacts Family
and the Workplace

Chapter Contents

Section 15.1

Intimate Partner Violence in the Workplace

Why It Matters

With more than one million people reporting a violent assault by an intimate partner every year in the United States, domestic violence should be a concern for every employer.[1] Domestic violence endangers companies' most important asset: their employees. Intimate partner violence affects employee health and safety, decreases productivity, and increases employer health care costs. Employers may be hesitant to address domestic violence in the workplace because of uncertainty about preventive roles, a desire to respect employee privacy and the need for guidance.[2] However, employers who do address this issue can provide real help to victims and prevent associated risks.[3]

Did You Know?

- A 2005 national survey found that 21% of full-time employed adults were victims of domestic violence.[4]

- 44% of respondents to a recent survey have personally experienced domestic violence's impact on the workplace, most frequently because a co-worker was a victim.[5]

- One study found that over 75% of domestic violence perpetrators used workplace resources to express remorse or anger towards, check-up on, pressure, or threaten their victim.[6]

- One study of female domestic violence victims found that 44% were left without transportation when the abuser disabled their car or hid their car keys, inhibiting their ability to attend work.[7]

Costs

- The Centers for Disease Control and Prevention estimate that the annual cost of lost productivity due to domestic violence equals $727.8 million.[8]

- The national health care costs of domestic violence (often absorbed by employers) are high, with direct medical and mental health care services for victims amounting to $4.1 billion.[9]

- Employers who fail to protect their employees may be liable. Jury awards for inadequate security suits average $1.2 million nationwide and settlements average $600,000.[10]

State Laws

- Twenty-one states have enacted mandatory or suggested workplace policies that require employers to assist victims of domestic violence by granting leave to victims who need to address their situation, the use of prevention programs, and the prohibition of discrimination against an employee for being a victim of domestic violence.

- Similar laws are pending in several other states.

- For more information on laws regarding domestic violence in the workplace in your state, visit http://www.legalmomentum.org, or contact your state legislator.

Job Performance and Productivity

- In a survey of 7,000 women, 37% said domestic violence had a negative impact on their job performance.[11]

- Domestic violence victims lose nearly 8 million days of paid work— the equivalent of more than 32,000 full-time jobs—and nearly 5.6 million days of household productivity as a result of violence.[12]

- Women who have been raped or sexually assaulted report diminished work functioning.[13]

- Researchers from the University of Arkansas found that women who were victims of recent domestic violence had 26% more time lost to absenteeism and tardiness than non-victims.[14]

- Approximately one-quarter of the one million women stalked each year report missing work as a result of the stalking, missing an average of 11 days.[15]

How Employers Respond

- In one study, 66% of corporate leaders identified domestic violence as a major social issue.[16]

- Over 70% of workplaces in the U.S. have no formal program or policy that addresses workplace violence.[17]

- Only 4% of all workplaces train employees on domestic violence and its impact on the workplace.[18]

- A 2007 national study found that 61% of American men think employers should be doing more to address domestic violence.[19]

- In one survey of senior corporate executives, 91% said that domestic violence affects both the private and working lives of their employees.[20]

- 50% of all employers with 1,000 or more employees had an incident of workplace violence within the 12 months prior to completing a 2006 survey on workplace violence prevention.[21]

- Only 12% of corporate leaders surveyed in 2002 think that corporations should play a major role in addressing domestic violence. Most believe domestic violence prevention is the responsibility of the family, social service organizations, and the police.[22]

What You Can Do to Help

- Urge your employer and companies in your community to establish employee assistance programs for victims of domestic violence, dating violence, sexual assault, and stalking.

- Companies can seek assistance from national groups, such as Corporate Alliance to End Partner Violence (CAEPV) to receive assistance on how to address intimate partner violence in the workplace.

- Urge your state legislators and member of Congress to pass laws that protect domestic violence and sexual assault victims from discrimination in the workplace.

Domestic Violence and the Workplace Resources

Coalition of Labor Union Women
815 16th St. NW, 2nd Floor S.
Washington, DC 20006

Phone: 202-508-6969
Fax: 202-508-6968
Website: http://www.cluw.org
E-mail: getinfo@cluw.org

Corporate Alliance to End Partner Violence
2416 E. Washington St., Suite E
Bloomington, IL 61704
Phone: 309-664-0667
Fax: 309-664-0747
Website: http://www.caepv.org
E-mail: caepv@caepv.org

Family Violence Prevention Fund
383 Rhode Island St., Suite #304
San Francisco, CA 94103-5133
Phone: 415-252-8900
Toll-Free TTY: 800-595-4889
Fax: 415-252-8991
Website: http://www.endabuse.org/workplace
E-mail: info@endabuse.org

National Coalition Against Domestic Violence
P.O. Box 18749
Denver, CO, 80218-0749
Phone: 303-839-1852
Fax: 303-831-9251
TTY: 303-839-1681
Website: http://www.ncadv.org

Safe@Work Coalition
Website: http://www.safeatworkcoalition.org

Sources

[1, 14] _Costs of Intimate Partner Violence Against Women in the United States._ 2003. Centers for Disease Control and Prevention, National Centers for Injury Prevention and Control. Atlanta, GA.

[2] _Domestic Violence and the Workplace._ 2002. Partnership for Prevention.

[3] _Strategic Employer Responses to Domestic Violence._ 2007. Family Violence Prevention Fund. Available at http://www.endabuse.org/workplace.

[4, 12, 18, 19] *The Survey of Workplace Violence Prevention.* October, 2006. Bureau of Labor Statistics.

[5, 6, 21, 22] Corporate Alliance to End Partner Violence. 2007. "Workplace Statistics." Available at http://www.caepv.org/getinfo/facts_stats .php? factsec=3.

[7, 13, 17] *The Facts on the Workplace and Domestic Violence Against Women.* 2007. Family Violence Prevention Fund.

[8, 9, 10, 15] Family Violence Prevention Fund. *Seven Reasons Employers Should Address Domestic Violence.*

[11] *Employment Discrimination Against Victims of Domestic and Sexual Violence.* 2007. Legal Momentum.

[16] Anne O'Leary Kelly and Carol Reeves. 2007. "The Effects and Costs of Intimate Partner Violence for Work Organizations." *Journal of Interpersonal Violence,* Vol. 22, No. 3, 327–344.

[20] *Father's Day Survey.* 2007. Family Violence Prevention Fund.

Section 15.2

Family and Employment Consequences of Intimate Partner Violence

Excerpted from "Family and Employment Consequences of Intimate Partner Violence: A Longitudinal Analysis," U.S. Department of Justice, March 2005.

Violence against women by their male intimate partners has gone from acceptable practice to a hidden taboo, to a topic on which there is much public discourse, policy, and concern. Yet, little is known about its affect upon women's work and family lives. Many have attempted to document the prevalence of intimate partner violence, and some have examined the short-term consequences. However, with the exception of homicide studies (the most extreme consequence), little research addresses the months and years following assault. We know very little about the role played by intervening authorities or how a woman's own actions at the time of assault influence her likelihood of divorce or residential mobility, labor force trajectory, and the risk of subsequent assault.

This section addresses the three primary research questions (and two secondary questions) from the *Family and Employment Consequences of Intimate Partner Violence: A Longitudinal Analysis* study:

1. Are intimate partner violence victims more likely than other women (including victims and non-victims) to divorce or move out of their home within six months of a reported assault?

    *   Do injury, self-defense, and help seeking influence the chances that a victim divorces or separates, moves alone, or that her household moves?

2. Are intimate partner violence victims more or less likely than other women to leave or enter the labor force within six months of a reported assault?

    *   Do injury, self-defense, and help seeking affect the likelihood of changes in victims' labor force status?

3. What factors are associated with reports of repeat assault?

Results

The answer to the first research question is a resounding "yes." Married victims of intimate partner violence appear to be more likely than other married women to divorce or experience household moves. Unmarried partner violence victims are more likely than other women to move. Additionally, they are more likely to move than are other violent crime victims. However, the only evidence that a violent crime victim's actions during an assault influence domestic outcomes is with unmarried victims. Unmarried victim's self-defensive actions are slightly related to a higher likelihood that they move. Additionally, their calls to the police following an intimate assault are associated with marginally lower odds of moving.

The findings addressing the second research question suggest that crime victimization is indeed associated with a woman's entry into the labor force. However, investigating all women, it was found that victims of intimate partner violence have patterns that look more like those of non-victims than those of other victims. Yet, when analyses are restricted to victims of violent crime, recent intimate partner victimization does, indeed, show up as a risk factor for entering the labor force. Thus, it appears when compared to all who were violently victimized, those whose assaults were perpetrated by a partner are the most likely victims to seek employment after an assault. This is not surprising, given that they may need to find work as part of a strategy for becoming more independent of a violent partner. Few incident characteristics are associated with entering the labor force. The important exception is having been injured to the extent that medical care was sought. Both seeking medical help and entering the labor force may represent a victim's urgency toward ending the violence. These models also revealed that demographic characteristics are less important in predicting victim's labor force entries than they are for the total sample of all women.

The findings for labor force exits reveal that victimization history has little influence on an employed woman's odds of leaving work. Additionally, it was found that a violent crime victim's experiences and actions at the time of assault do not matter.

Finally, in response to the third research question, important associations were found between an intimate partner violence victim's responses to assault and her likelihood of being re-victimized by an intimate. Actions taken in self-defense appear to increase the risk of sustaining a later assault, while exiting the labor force decreases those odds. Also, we find that a victim's own help-seeking behavior seems to have no affect on her chances of re-victimization, yet when others call the police, or when arrests are made future, violence appears to be deterred.

The analyses offer more straightforward support for the hypothesis of "retaliation" than for "exposure reduction," since self-defense seems to lead to more, not less, violence. However, when someone other than the victim initiates the reduction in exposure, such as when another calls the police or when the police make an arrest, the "exposure reduction" hypothesis is supported.

In sum, the findings do suggest that violent crime victimization and intimate partner violence, specifically, are important predictors of changes in household composition and employment status.

Chapter 16

Intimate Partner Violence and Lesbian, Gay, Bisexual, and Transgender Relationships

Dynamics of Domestic Violence

Same-gender and gender-variant relationships often exist in an atmosphere of secrecy, isolation, or conversely, invasive scrutiny. In their everyday lives, lesbian, gay, bisexual, and transgender (LGBT) persons constantly assess if it is safe, worth the time and aggravation, or indeed, anyone else's business before correcting others' assumptions, outing themselves, and explaining their relationship.

The failure of communities to acknowledge domestic and sexual violence in same gender or gender variant relationships provides the LGBT batterer with multiple means with which to abuse his or her victim. Abusers can take advantage of the beliefs that women do not perpetrate violence and that men engage only in mutual combat. Both myths place victim/survivors at increased risk. And police often arrest both parties, effectively reinforcing the abuser's blame of the victim. At another level, information about LGBT violence is used to reinforce the concept that lesbians, gay men, bisexual, and transgender people are immoral, unstable, and therefore undeserving of ordinary human rights. An abuser can use these attitudes to shame a victim into silence.

Isolation, another common tactic, is possibly even more potent in LGBT relationships because it is not just about being kept from the

This material was reprinted from the publication titled *Lesbian, Gay, Bisexual and Trans (LGBT) Communities and Domestic Violence: Information and Resources* © 2007 National Resource Center on Domestic Violence. Reprinted with permission.

sociability and support of significant people in the community by the abuser. It can include being outed and then rejected by some of those same people. Isolation also increases the interdependence of partners and heightens a victim's fears about losing the relationship. Cut off from family and friends, a victim/survivor suffers not only from loss of identity and support, but also from an invisibility imposed by a culture that has difficulty acknowledging domestic violence, LGBT people, and same-gender or gender-variant relationships.

Among LGBT elders and youth, especially transgender people who may be particularly vulnerable, ageism also exacerbates the effects of isolation and becomes a factor for an abuser to exploit. LGBT people over the age of 60 are almost twice as likely to live alone as elders in the general population (Swan, 2005). Their experience and living circumstances often leaves them particularly vulnerable to the physical domination and/ or financial exploitation of a younger partner, family member, or trusted loved one. Conversely, youth abused and forced to leave home by family intolerance may be reluctant to leave an abusive relationship fearing that with nowhere to go, they may end up on the streets.

A LGBT person grows up knowing that society thinks their love is disgusting, that they are perverted, or at the very least not valued and are, therefore, an acceptable target of discrimination and violence. Much of this is internalized, but even if not internalized, others in the community believe it. This fosters an environment that provides an abuser with unique and potent opportunities for manipulating, threatening, intimidating, and terrorizing an intimate partner. LGBT victim/survivors must overcome obstacles including concerns about community and systems response; lack of culturally sensitive support and services; and fear of seeking support because of the disbelief or disapproval of friends, family, colleagues, children, employers, and others in their community and society at large (Boulder County Safehouse, 2002).

Intervention and Prevention Services

Historically, domestic violence discussions focus on the rights and protections of adults and adult relationships, assumed to be heterosexual. Although teen dating violence is currently a focus of many intervention and prevention programs and services, little of this attention is directed towards the needs of LGBT teens. In addition, it may be that homelessness and violent physical assault when coming out is even more of a pressing issue for LGBT youth than dating violence. According to a report from the National Gay and Lesbian Task Force and the National Coalition for the Homeless (2007), "available research suggests

148

that between 20 percent and 40 percent of all homeless youth identify as lesbian, gay, bisexual, or transgender (LGBT)" and one study found that "more than one-third of youth who are homeless or in the care of social services experienced a violent physical assault when they came out, which can lead to youth leaving a shelter or foster home because they actually feel safer on the streets."

Access to Services

Many parallels can be drawn between intimate partner violence in same-gender or gender-variant relationships and violence in heterosexual relationships. Lesbians working in mainstream programs, however, recognized violence in their own relationships and those of other LGBT friends and realized early on that the causes of domestic violence were more complex with the LGBT community. This work was problematic for some programs because it called to question women's use of violence, and seemed to refute the early analysis of the cause of domestic violence. Most mainstream domestic violence programs began with a focus on serving young, middle-class white women with children. Programs that began by serving mainstream communities often try to reach out to members of LGBT communities, but struggle with understanding the particular needs of most marginalized groups. Mainstream programs often attempt to do outreach in LGBT communities by placing ads in community publications, distributing brochures, or hanging posters depicting couples who appear to be same-sex or gender variant in shelters and public spaces. These are important things to do, but if the mainstream program does not actively engage with the LGBT communities they wish to serve about the nature of their needs, the efforts of the program often prove ineffective.

In an effort to avoid inappropriate approaches, programs sometimes rely on staff or volunteers who identify as LGBT to be the resident experts on the experiences of all LGBT people. The assumption that an individual can represent and speak for all people from a diverse set of communities is often a set-up for failure for the identified staff person or volunteer and for the program attempting outreach. In the process, the people seeking services are often not served well.

Advocates within LGBT communities are working to promote more community-centered approaches. Conversations between program advocates and people seeking services integrate a more complete analysis of the violence into the intake process to determine what services are appropriate for each partner.

Providing shelter to same-gender or gender-variant survivors has been another problematic area for mainstream programs. Shelters have long been the domains of heterosexual female victim/survivors. However, due to a broader understanding of the interconnection of oppressions and an increased awareness of the need for safe space for LGBT victim/survivors, an increasing number of mainstream programs are offering space in safe homes, rooms in existing shelters, or accommodations at hotels or motels for male and bisexual victims.

Safety for members of the trans community is also beginning to be addressed. Yet in many regions of the United States, safe shelter options are severely limited or nonexistent for gender-variant victim/survivors. While it has been somewhat easier for lesbian and bisexual women to seek and receive shelter or other supports, they often feel the need to conceal their own sexual orientation or gender identity or that of their abuser in order to assure admittance.

In response to the needs of victim/survivors and the people who abuse them, members of many LGBT communities have begun to raise awareness of these needs, both within their own communities and in mainstream society. LGBT advocates have begun to create and implement services that move away from traditional models relying on criminal justice and shelter services that are separate from the community in which the victim/survivor lives.

Within some LGBT communities, attention is turning to harm-reduction models and finding safer spaces within the community. Survivors are encouraged to act as their own agents by identifying ways to be safe, for example, changing locks to the home, getting rid of weapons and ammunition, or fitting a room with a secure lock and a working phone to serve as a more secure temporary refuge. Realizing that no place is guaranteed safe, however, survivors often go to friends for help.

Advocates working within LGBT communities are using social gatherings to educate people on the dynamics of domestic violence and how to provide refuge for a friend. The core belief for many doing intervention and prevention work within LGBT communities today is that safety comes with self-determination for victim/survivors, community accountability for those who batter, and consciousness raising for all community members. When victim/survivors have community support and resources, they are more able to make choices about ways to be safe without relying upon unfriendly institutions. Advocates working within LGBT communities emphasize developing and maintaining supportive, loving, and equitable relationships. The goal is to help couples create strategies for building positive relationships. Advocates are also working to assure that there is an expectation and responsibility within each community for the community to respond to intimate partner violence among its members and to honor its obligation to stop it.

Chapter 17

Partner Violence Precedes Many Homicides and Child Maltreatment

Two studies released by the Centers for Disease Control and Prevention (CDC) in April 2008 found that many people who die violently experience intimate partner violence and/or relationship problems beforehand, and tens of thousand of newborns and infants experience abuse or neglect.

Partner Violence Precedes Many Homicides

Nearly one in five homicides (19 percent) is precipitated by intimate partner violence, according to a report from the CDC's National Violent Death Reporting System (NVDRS). Fifty-two percent of female homicides, and nine percent of male homicides, are precipitated by intimate partner violence. In addition, 32 percent of suicides are precipitated by a problem with an intimate partner.

The new study provides a detailed analysis of 2005 data from 16 states on all types of violent death, as well as information about the circumstances surrounding these deaths. It finds that there are some 50,000 violent deaths in the United States each year. Most of those deaths are suicides (more than 56 percent), while nearly 30 percent are homicides and deaths involving legal interventions, and another 13 percent are of undetermined intent.

Overall, men are more likely than women to die violently, and American Indians/Alaska Natives and African Americans have higher rates of violent death than whites and Hispanics. The rate of violent death is highest for people age 20 to 24, and the home is the most common location for all types of violent death.

There were about 200 violent incidents in which a homicide was followed by the suicide of the suspect in the 16 states in 2005. In those cases, 168 of the 225 murder victims were female, and 180 of the suspects who committed homicide and then suicide were male. The highest percentage of both homicide and suicide victims in these cases were age 35 to 44.

The report says that programs designed to enhance social problem-solving and coping skills, and skills dealing with stressful life events, have potential to reduce violence since relationship problems and intimate partner violence are precipitating factors in many types of violent death. It also recommends prevention programs aimed at addressing mental health problems and increasing education about the warning signs for violence.

The CDC's NVDRS is a comprehensive reporting system that collects and centralizes data on violent deaths from death certificates, coroner or medical examiner reports, and law enforcement reports. The states participating in the study are Alaska, Colorado, Georgia, Kentucky, Maryland, Massachusetts, New Jersey, New Mexico, North Carolina, Oklahoma, Oregon, Rhode Island, South Carolina, Utah, Wisconsin, and Virginia. The National Violence Prevention Network is working to expand the study to every state.

Child Abuse and Neglect

In 2006, 91,278 infants under a year old experienced nonfatal abuse or neglect, including nearly 30,000 who experienced maltreatment in their first week of life. According to "Nonfatal Maltreatment of Infants," 86 percent of the abuse and neglect cases involving the 29,881 newborns were reported to child protective services by professionals, most often medical staff or social service workers.

That same year, state and local child protective service workers substantiated that 905,000 children (under age 18) were victims of abuse or neglect.

"The concentration of reports of neglect in the first few days of life, and the preponderance of reports from medical professionals during the same period, suggest that neglect was often identified at birth," it notes. "One hypothesis for the concentration of maltreatment and neglect reports in the first few days of life is that the majority of reports resulted from maternal or newborn drug tests." Prenatal substance abuse test results are routinely reported to child protective service agencies as neglect. Many women, and pregnant women in particular, struggle to find drug treatment programs that will serve them.

"Establishing safe, stable, and nurturing relationships between children and adults is the vaccine against child abuse and neglect," National Center for Injury Prevention and Control Director Ileana Arias, Ph.D. said during an audio news conference. "We must support programs that inform and provide support for parents, families, and health professionals on how to ensure protected and nurturing environments for children." She said maltreatment is the third leading cause of death for children under age one in this country.

Growing up in a violent home may be a terrifying and traumatic experience that can affect every aspect of a child's life, growth, and development. Children who suffer from abuse and neglect are often at risk for poor health outcomes and may be more likely than other children to engage in risky behaviors during adolescence and adulthood.

"Nonfatal Maltreatment of Infants" defines physical abuse to include beating, kicking, biting, burning, and shaking, and neglect to include abandonment, maternal drug use or failing to meet basic needs like housing, food, clothing, and access to medical care.

The CDC and the Administration for Children and Families analyzed data from the National Child Abuse and Neglect Data System (NCANDS), which has been collecting annual data since 1993. The report is the first published national analysis of substantiated nonfatal maltreatment of infants using NCANDS data. Researchers were able to examine data from 45 states.

Chapter 18

Sexual Assault in Abusive Intimate Partner Relationships

A recent study funded by the National Institute of Justice (NIJ) on women who had been physically assaulted by an intimate partner found that two-thirds of the women had also been sexually assaulted by that partner.[1] In addition to a victim's physical and psychological injuries, her older children were found to be at increased risk for depression.

Researchers Judith McFarlane and Anne Malecha from Texas Woman's University collected data from 148 women who sought assistance from the judicial system after being physically assaulted by an intimate partner.[2] The women, who were interviewed first in 2001, were contacted again in 2003 with questions about forced sex.[3] Researchers looked at the incidence and consequences of sexual assault in intimate relationships and compared the findings with data collected from women who were physically but not sexually assaulted by their partners. The researchers identified risk factors for women in abusive relationships that could be used to develop referral and safety programs for victims and their children.

Impact of Reporting on Revictimization

Most research supports the claim that sexual assault is common in physically abusive relationships. McFarlane and Malecha found

"Sexual Assault in Abusive Relationships," by Lauren R. Taylor and Nicole Gaskin-Laniyan, Ph.D., National Institute of Justice, U.S. Department of Justice, NCJ 216525, January 2007.

that 68 percent of the abused women reported having been sexually assaulted by their intimate partners. Sexual assault occurred repeatedly within these intimate relationships—almost 80 percent of sexually assaulted women reported more than one incident of forced sex.

Most of the women in the study did not report the assault or seek assistance after the first rape—just six percent contacted the police after the first rape, and eight percent applied for a protective order. But women seeking assistance from the courts were less likely to be revictimized. Specifically, women who contacted the police following the first rape were 59 percent less likely to be raped by an intimate partner again, whether or not the abuser was arrested. Women who applied for a protective order after the first rape were 70 percent less likely to be raped again, whether or not the order was obtained. Most women waited several years after the first sexual assault before applying for a protective order, with Caucasians waiting the longest (on average eight years), followed by Latina women (five years), and African American women (three years).

Physical and Emotional Tolls of Intimate Partner Sexual Abuse

Sexual assault by intimate partners has a profound effect on victims and their children. Researchers McFarlane and Malecha also found that the sexually assaulted women in the study had worse mental and physical health than women who had been physically but not sexually abused. The women had more posttraumatic stress disorder (PTSD) symptoms, more pregnancies resulting from rape, and more sexually transmitted diseases.[4] Foreign-born women in the study were found to have a high risk of developing PTSD and also to have fewer social supports. In addition, 27 percent of the women surveyed began or increased their use of alcohol, illicit drugs (usually cocaine), or nicotine after they were sexually assaulted by an intimate partner.

Women who had been sexually assaulted by an intimate partner were also more likely to threaten or attempt suicide than women who were physically but not sexually abused. Twenty-two percent of sexually assaulted women said they had threatened or attempted suicide within 90 days of applying for a protection order, compared with four percent of women who were physically abused.

Sexually abused women in the study were also more likely to have had their abusers harass them at work and threaten them with murder. Researchers did not find significant differences in these risk factors across ethnicity or race of the women.

What Children Witness

The effect of sexual assault in an abusive relationship permeates a household. Almost 90 percent of children of women in the study who were physically assaulted or both physically and sexually assaulted were exposed to these incidents against their mothers. By the age of three years, 64 percent of the children had witnessed the abuse; 30 percent of them received counseling. Older children (aged 12 to 18 years) of sexually abused mothers showed more depression and had appreciably more behavioral problems than children of mothers who had not been sexually assaulted.

Steps for Change

When a woman is sexually assaulted by an intimate partner, her health—mental and physical—is compromised. Her children's risk for depression is also heightened.

Workers in the justice, health, and social service fields can take steps to help victims of intimate partner sexual assault. The researchers recommend that these professionals do the following:

- Receive training on the frequency and health and safety consequences of intimate partner sexual assault.

- Assess clients for type and frequency of sexual assault.

- Assess victims to determine if they are at risk for PTSD, substance use, and suicide.

- Inform women who have been sexually assaulted by their partner about their higher risk of being murdered by that partner.

- Inform sexually abused immigrant women about their potential increased risk for PTSD.

- Instruct mothers about the potential effects of partner abuse on their children.

This information, delivered with the appropriate referrals and safety planning information, could lead to greater protection for abused women and their children.

Notes

1. Sexual assault is defined as forced vaginal, oral, or anal sex.

2. All sought protective orders from the courts. Thirty-three percent were African American, 26 percent were Caucasian, and 41 percent were Latina. Twenty-eight percent were also immigrants. There were no significant demographic differences between the women who had been raped and those who had been physically abused but not raped.

3. Researchers initially interviewed 150 women in 2001. Because two of the women died in the interim, only 148 were interviewed in 2003.

4. Twenty percent of the women in the sample had rape-related pregnancies, and 15 percent contracted sexually transmitted diseases.

Chapter 19

Sexual Violence

Chapter Contents

Section 19.1

Facts about Sexual Violence

This section includes text from the following Centers for Disease Control and Prevention (CDC) documents: "Sexual Violence Prevention Scientific Information: Definitions," December 2008; "Facts at a Glance: Sexual Violence," Spring 2008; "Understanding Sexual Violence," 2007; and, "Sexual Violence Prevention Scientific Information: Risk and Protective Factors," December 2008.

Sexual Violence Prevention Definitions

Sexual violence (SV) is any sexual act that is forced against someone's will. These acts can be physical, verbal, or psychological. There are four types of sexual violence; all types involve victims who do not consent, or who are unable to consent or refuse to allow the act.

- **A completed sex act** is defined as contact between the penis and the vulva or the penis and the anus involving penetration, however slight; contact between the mouth and penis, vulva, or anus; or penetration of the anal or genital opening of another person by a hand, finger, or other object.

- **An attempted (but not completed) sex act.**

- **Abusive sexual contact** is defined as intentional touching, either directly or through the clothing, of the genitalia, anus, groin, breast, inner thigh, or buttocks of any person.

- **Non-contact sexual abuse** is defined as abuse that does not involve physical contact. Examples of non-contact sexual abuse include voyeurism; intentional exposure of an individual to exhibitionism; pornography; verbal or behavioral sexual harassment; threats of sexual violence; and taking nude photographs of a sexual nature of another person.

Why is a consistent definition important?

A consistent definition is needed to monitor the incidence of SV and examine trends over time. In addition, it helps determine the magnitude of SV and compare the problem across jurisdictions. A consistent definition also helps researchers measure risk and protective factors for victimization or perpetration in a uniform manner. This information ultimately assists prevention and intervention efforts.

Facts about Sexual Violence

Adults

In a nationally representative survey of 9,684 adults:

- 10.6% of women reported experiencing forced sex at some time in their lives,

- 2.1% of men reported experiencing forced sex at some time in their lives, and

- 2.5% of women surveyed and 0.9% of men surveyed said they experienced unwanted sexual activity in the previous 12 months.

College Age

- 20% to 25% of women in college reported experiencing an attempted or a completed rape in college.

Children and Youth (17 years or younger)

In a nationally representative survey:

- 60.4% of female and 69.2% of male victims were first raped before age 18;

- 25.5% of females were first raped before age 12, and 34.9% were first raped between the ages of 12–17;

- 41.0% of males were first raped before age 12, and 27.9% were first raped between the ages of 12–17.

A 2005 survey of high school students found that 10.8% of girls and 4.2% of boys from grades 9–12 were forced to have sexual intercourse at some time in their lives.

Perpetrators

In a nationally representative survey, in the first rape experience:

- female victims reported perpetrators were intimate partners (30.4%), family members (23.7%), and acquaintances (20%); and

- male victims reported perpetrators were acquaintances (32.3%), family members (17.7%), friends (17.6%), and intimate partners (15.9%).

Health Disparities

- Among high school students, 9.3% of black students, 7.8% of Hispanic students, and 6.9% of white students reported that they were forced to have sexual intercourse at some time in their lives.

- Among 8,000 women surveyed in 1995–1996, 17.9% of non-Hispanic whites, 11.9% of Hispanic whites, 18.8% of African Americans, 34.1% of American Indian/Alaska Natives, 6.8% of Asian/Pacific Islanders, and 24.4% of women of mixed race experienced an attempted or a completed rape at some time in their lives.

Non-Fatal Injuries and Medical Treatment

- Among sexual violence victims raped since their 18th birthday, 31.5% of women and 16.1% of men reported a physical injury as a result of a rape, and 36.2% of the injured female victims received medical treatment.

- Based on national emergency department data, sexual assaults represented 10% of all assault-related injury visits to the emergency department by females in 2006.

Understanding Sexual Violence

Sexual violence (SV) refers to sexual activity where consent is not obtained or freely given. Anyone can experience SV, but most victims are female. The person responsible for the violence is typically male and is usually someone known to the victim. The person can be, but is not limited to, a friend, coworker, neighbor, or family member.

Why is sexual violence a public health problem?

SV is a significant problem in the United States.

- Among high school students surveyed nationwide, about 8% reported having been forced to have sex. Females (11%) were more likely to report having been forced to have sex than males (4%).

- An estimated 20% to 25% of college women in the United States experience attempted or complete rape during their college career.

- In the United States, one in six women and one in 33 men reported experiencing an attempted or completed rape at some time in their lives.

These numbers underestimate the problem. Many cases are not reported because victims are afraid to tell the police, friends, or family about the abuse. Victims also think that their stories of abuse will not be believed and that police cannot help them. Victims may be ashamed or embarrassed. Victims may also keep quiet because they have been threatened with further harm if they tell anyone.

How does sexual violence affect health?

SV impacts health in many ways. Some ways are serious and can lead to long-term health problems. These include chronic pain, headaches, stomach problems, and sexually transmitted diseases. In addition, rape results in about 32,000 pregnancies each year.

SV can have an emotional impact as well. Victims often are fearful and anxious. They may replay the attack over and over in their minds. They may have problems with trust and be wary of becoming involved with others. The anger and stress that victims feel may lead to eating disorders and depression. Some even think about or attempt suicide.

SV is also linked to negative health behaviors. For example, victims are more likely to smoke, abuse alcohol, use drugs, and engage in risky sexual activity.

How can we prevent sexual violence?

The ultimate goal is to stop SV before it begins. Efforts at many levels are needed to accomplish this. Some examples include the following:

- Engaging high school students in mentoring programs or other skill-based activities that address healthy sexuality and dating relationships

- Helping parents identify and address social and cultural influences that may promote attitudes and violent behaviors in their kids

- Creating policies at work, at school, and in other places that address sexual harassment

- Developing mass media (for example, radio, television, magazines, newspapers) messages that promote norms, or shared beliefs, about healthy sexual relationships

Risk Factors for Sexual Violence Perpetration

Risk factors are associated with a greater likelihood of sexual violence (SV) perpetration. They are contributing factors and may or may not be direct causes. Not everyone who is identified as "at risk" becomes a perpetrator of violence. A combination of individual, relational, community, and societal factors contribute to the risk of becoming a perpetrator of SV. Understanding these multilevel factors can help identify various opportunities for prevention.

Individual Factors

- Alcohol and drug use
- Coercive sexual fantasies
- Impulsive and antisocial tendencies
- Preference for impersonal sex
- Hostility towards women
- Hyper-masculinity
- Childhood history of sexual and physical abuse
- Witnessed family violence as a child

Relationship Factors

- Association with sexually aggressive and delinquent peers
- Family environment characterized by physical violence and few resources
- Strong patriarchal relationship or familial environment
- Lack of emotional support in the family environment

Community Factors

- Lack of employment opportunities
- Lack of institutional support from police and judicial system
- General tolerance of sexual violence within the community
- Weak community sanctions against sexual violence perpetrators

Societal Factors

- Poverty
- Societal norms that support sexual violence
- Societal norms that support male superiority and sexual entitlement
- Societal norms that maintain women's inferiority and sexual submissiveness
- Weak laws and policies related to gender equity
- High tolerance levels of crime and other forms of violence

Protective Factors

Protective factors may lessen the likelihood of sexual violence victimization or perpetration by buffering against risk. These factors can exist at individual, relational, community, and societal levels.

Section 19.2

Men and Sexual Trauma

Excerpted from "Men and Sexual Trauma," by Julia M. Whealin, Ph.D.,
National Center for Posttraumatic Stress Disorder, May 22, 2007.

At least 10% of men in our country have suffered from trauma as a result of sexual assault. Like women, men who experience sexual assault may suffer from depression, posttraumatic stress disorder (PTSD), and other emotional problems as a result. However, because men and women have different life experiences due to their different gender roles, emotional symptoms following trauma can look different in men than they do in women.

Who are the perpetrators of male sexual assault?

Those who sexually assault men or boys differ in a number of ways from those who assault only females. Boys are more likely than girls to be sexually abused by strangers or by authority figures in organizations such as schools, churches, or athletics programs. Those who sexually assault males usually choose young men and male adolescents (the average age is 17 years old) as their victims and are more likely to assault many victims, compared to those who sexually assault females. Perpetrators often assault young males in isolated areas where help is not readily available. For instance, a perpetrator who assaults males may pickup a teenage hitchhiker on a remote road or seek some other way to isolate his intended victim. As is true about those who assault and sexually abuse women and girls, most perpetrators of males are men. Specifically, men are perpetrators in about 86% of male victimization cases. Despite popular belief that only gay men would sexually assault men or boys, most male perpetrators identify themselves as heterosexuals and often have consensual sexual relationships with women.

What are some symptoms related to sexual trauma in boys and men?

Particularly when the assailant is a woman, the impact of sexual assault upon men may be downplayed by professionals and the public.

However, men who have early sexual experiences with adults report problems in various areas at a much higher rate than those who do not.

Emotional disorders: Men and boys who have been sexually assaulted are more likely to suffer from PTSD, other anxiety disorders, and depression than those who have never been abused sexually.

Substance abuse: Men who have been sexually assaulted have a high incidence of alcohol and drug use. For example, the probability for alcohol problems in adulthood is about 80% for men who have experienced sexual abuse, as compared to 11% for men who have never been sexually abused.

Encopresis: One study revealed that a percentage of boys who suffer from encopresis (bowel incontinence) had been sexually abused.

Risk-taking behavior: Exposure to sexual trauma can lead to risk-taking behavior during adolescence, such as running away and other delinquent behaviors. Having been sexually assaulted also makes boys more likely to engage in behaviors that put them at risk for contracting human immunodeficiency virus (HIV) (such as having sex without using condoms).

How does male gender socialization affect the recognition of male sexual assault?

- Men who have not dealt with the symptoms of their sexual assault may experience confusion about their sexuality and role as men (their gender role). This confusion occurs for many reasons. The traditional gender role for men in our society dictates that males be strong, self-reliant, and in control. Our society often does not recognize that men and boys can also be victims. Boys and men may be taught that being victimized implies that they are weak and, thus, not a man.

- Furthermore, when the perpetrator of a sexual assault is a man, feelings of shame, stigmatization, and negative reactions from others may also result from the social taboos.

- When the perpetrator of a sexual assault is a woman, some people do not take the assault seriously, and men may feel as though they are unheard and unrecognized as victims.

- Parents often know very little about male sexual assault and may harm their male children who are sexually abused by downplaying or denying the experience.

What impact does gender socialization have upon men who have been sexually assaulted?

Because of their experience of sexual assault, some men attempt to prove their masculinity by becoming hyper-masculine. For example, some men deal with their experience of sexual assault by having multiple female sexual partners or engaging in dangerous "macho" behaviors to prove their masculinity. Parents of boys who have been sexually abused may inadvertently encourage this process.

Men who acknowledge their assault may have to struggle with feeling ignored and invalidated by others who do not recognize that men can also be victimized. Because of ignorance and myths about sexual abuse, men sometimes fear that the sexual assault by another man will cause them to become gay. This belief is false. Sexual assault does not cause someone to have a particular sexual orientation. Because of these various gender-related issues, men are more likely than women to feel ashamed of the assault, to not talk about it, and to not seek help from professionals.

Are men who were sexually assaulted as children more likely to become child molesters?

Another myth that male victims of sexual assault face is the assumption that they will become abusers themselves. For instance, they may have heard that survivors of sexual abuse tend to repeat the cycle of abuse by abusing children themselves. Some research has shown that men who were sexually abused by men during their childhood have a greater number of sexual thoughts and fantasies about sexual contact with male children and adolescents. However, it is important to know that most male victims of child sexual abuse do not become sex offenders.

Furthermore, many male perpetrators do not have a history of child sexual abuse. Rather, sexual offenders more often grew up in families where they suffered from several other forms of abuse, such as physical and emotional. Men who assault others also have difficulty with empathy, and thus put their own needs above the needs of their victims.

Is there help for men who have been sexually assaulted?

It is important for men who have been sexually assaulted to understand the connection between sexual assault and hyper-masculine, aggressive, and self-destructive behavior. Through therapy, men often learn to resist myths about what a "real man" is and adopt a more re-alistic model for safe and rewarding living.

It is important for men who have been sexually assaulted and who are confused about their sexual orientation to confront misleading societal ideas about sexual assault and homosexuality.

Men who have been assaulted often feel stigmatized, which can be the most damaging aspect of the assault. It is important for men to discuss the assault with a caring and unbiased support person, wheth-er that person is a friend, clergyman, or clinician. However, it is vital that this person be knowledgeable about sexual assault and men.

A local rape crisis center may be able to refer men to mental-health practitioners who are well-informed about the needs of male sexual assault victims.

Summary

There is a bias in our culture against viewing the sexual assault of boys and men as prevalent and abusive. Because of this bias, there is a belief that boys and men do not experience abuse and do not suf-fer from the same negative impact that girls and women do. However, research shows that at least 10% of boys and men are sexually as-saulted and that boys and men can suffer profoundly from the expe-rience. Because so few people have information about male sexual assault, men often suffer from a sense of being different, which can make it more difficult for men to seek help. If you are a man who has been assaulted and you suffer from any of these difficulties, please seek help from a mental-health professional who has expertise work-ing with men who have been sexually assaulted.

Section 19.3

Sexual Exploitation
by Helping Professionals

Sexual exploitation by a helping professional: Sexual contact of any kind between a helping professional (doctor, therapist, teacher, priest, professor, police officer, lawyer, and so forth) and a client/patient.

- It is difficult for a client/patient to give informed consent to sexual contact or boundary violations because the helping professional holds a great deal of power over that client/patient.

- 90% of sexual boundary violations occur between a male provider and a female client/patient (Plaut, S.M., 1997, p. 79).

- Such behavior is regarded as unethical and, in every licensed profession, can be grounds for malpractice and possible loss of license.

There are three major types of sexual involvement between a client/patient and a professional:

1. Sexual activity in the context of a professional treatment, evaluation, or service.

2. Sexual activity with the implication that it has therapeutic benefit.

3. A sexually exploitative relationship.

Why it is not acceptable behavior:

- The helping professional starts from a position of great power over the client/patient and is expected to respect and maintain professional boundaries.

- The professional has a responsibility to protect the interests of the client/patient and not to serve his/her own needs.

- The client/patient has put his/her trust in that professional and the betrayal of that trust can have devastating consequences.

Within the Therapeutic Relationship

- Clients in therapy are the most susceptible because the client is already vulnerable and trusts the therapist to help her/him feel better.

- Therapy relationships are particularly intimate, with clients sharing their innermost thoughts, feelings, and experiences.

Issue of Transference

- **Transference:** The way in which a client transfers negative/positive feelings about others to the therapist. Transference in and of itself is not a bad thing. In fact, it is necessary in all therapeutic relationships.

- **Countertransference:** When the therapist projects his or her own feelings back onto the client.

- **Problem:** When the therapist is unable to recognize transference and countertransference reactions and, instead, responds in a sexual manner.

Common Reactions

- Sexual dysfunction
- Anxiety disorders
- Depression
- Increased risk of suicide
- Feelings of guilt, shame, anger, confusion, worthlessness
- Loss of trust

Very Low Report Rate

- It is estimated that only 4–8% of survivors of sexual exploitation by helping professionals report the exploitation (Gartrell, N., et al., 1987 per TAASA, p. 168, 2004).

- Often there is reluctance to report because of anticipated or real pain associated with pursuing the case, or fear that she or he won't be believed.

- It often takes several years for the client to recognize that she or he has been harmed.

Three Ways to Take Action

1. **Licensing board complaints:** Standards vary by state and profession. Possible punishments include suspension or revocation of a license or rehabilitation programs. In these cases the client's confidentiality is protected in any public reports of the proceedings.

2. **Civil lawsuits:** Client hires his or her own attorney and sues the therapist directly. Usually this is the only way to receive payment for damages. Procedures are public, and the burden of proof is on the client.

3. **Criminal proceedings:** An option in some states. In these cases, the state prosecutes (state versus therapist). The best possible outcome is a criminal sanction (probation, incarceration).

References

Plaut, S. Michael. "Boundary violations in professional-client relationships: overview and guidance for prevention." *Sexual and Marital Therapy*, 12, 1, 1997.

Plaut, S. Michael. "Understanding and Managing Professional-Client Boundaries." *Handbook of Clinical Sexuality for Mental Health*. Stephen B. Levine (ed). New York: Brunner-Routledge, 2003.

Texas Association Against Sexual Assault. *Sexual Assault Advocate Training Manual*, 2004.

Chapter 20

Stalking

Chapter Contents

Section 20.1

Are You Being Stalked?

Facts about Stalking

What Is Stalking?

While legal definitions of stalking vary from one jurisdiction to another, a good working definition of stalking is a course of conduct directed at a specific person that would cause a reasonable person to feel fear.

Stalking in America

- 1,006,970 women and 370,990 men are stalked annually in the U.S.

- One in 12 women and one in 45 men will be stalked in their lifetime.

- 77% of female victims and 64% of male victims know their stalker.

- 87% of stalkers are men.

- 59% of female victims and 30% of male victims are stalked by an intimate partner.

- 81% of women stalked by a current or former intimate partner are also physically assaulted by that partner.

- 31% of women stalked by a current or former intimate partner are also sexually assaulted by that partner.

- 73% of intimate partner stalkers verbally threatened victims with physical violence, and almost 46% of victims experienced one or more violent incidents by the stalker.

- The average duration of stalking is 1.8 years.

- If stalking involves intimate partners, the average duration of stalking increases to 2.2 years.

- 28% of female victims and 10% of male victims obtained a protective order. 69% of female victims and 81% of male victims had the protection order violated.

Source: Tjaden and Thoennes, (1998). "Stalking in America," National Institute of Justice (NIJ).

Impact of Stalking on Victims

- 56% of women stalked took some type of self-protective measure, often as drastic as relocating (11%). [Tjaden and Thoennes, (1998). "Stalking in America," NIJ.]

- 26% of stalking victims lost time from work as a result of their victimization, and 7% never returned to work. [Tjaden and Thoennes.]

- 30% of female victims and 20% of male victims sought psychological counseling. [Tjaden and Thoennes.]

- The prevalence of anxiety, insomnia, social dysfunction, and severe depression is much higher among stalking victims than the general population, especially if the stalking involves being followed or having one's property destroyed. [Blaauw et. al., (2002). "The Toll of Stalking," *Journal of Interpersonal Violence.*]

RECON *Study of Stalkers*

- Two-thirds of stalkers pursue their victims at least once per week, many daily, using more than one method.

- 78% of stalkers use more than one means of approach.

- Weapons are used to harm or threaten victims in one out of five cases.

- Almost one-third of stalkers have stalked before.

- Intimate partner stalkers frequently approach their targets, and their behaviors escalate quickly.

Source: Mohandie et al., "The RECON Typology of Stalking: Reliability and Validity Based upon a Large Sample of North American Stalkers." *Journal of Forensic Sciences* 2006.

Stalking and Intimate Partner Femicide (Murder of a Woman)

- 76% of intimate partner femicide (murder) victims had been stalked by their intimate partner.

- 67% had been physically abused by their intimate partner.

- 89% of femicide victims who had been physically abused had also been stalked in the 12 months before the murder.

- 79% of abused femicide victims reported stalking during the same period that they reported abuse.

- 54% of femicide victims reported stalking to police before they were killed by their stalkers.

Source: McFarlane et al., (1999). "Stalking and Intimate Partner Femicide," *Homicide Studies*.

Stalking on Campus

- 13% of college women were stalked during one six to nine month period.

- 80% of campus stalking victims knew their stalkers.

- Three in ten college women reported being injured emotionally or psychologically from being stalked.

Source: Fisher, Cullen, and Turner, (2000). "The Sexual Victimization of College Women," NIJ and Bureau of Justice Statistics (BJS).

State Laws[1]

- Stalking is a crime under the laws of all 50 states, the District of Columbia, and the federal government.

- 15 states classify stalking as a felony upon the first offense.

- 34 states classify stalking as a felony upon the second offense and/or when the crime involves aggravating factors.[2]

- Aggravating factors may include: possession of a deadly weapon; violation of a court order or condition of probation/parole; victim under 16; same victim as prior occasions.

[1] Last updated October 2005.

[2] In Maryland, stalking is always a misdemeanor.

For a compilation of state, tribal, and federal laws visit http://www.ncvc.org/src.

The Stalking Resource Center

The Stalking Resource Center is a program of the National Center for Victims of Crime. Their dual mission is to raise national awareness of stalking and to encourage the development and implementation of multidisciplinary responses to stalking in local communities across the country.

They can provide you with:

- Training and Technical Assistance

- Protocol Development

- Resources

- Help in collaborating with other agencies and systems in your community

Are You Being Stalked?

Stalking is a series of actions that make you feel afraid or in danger. Stalking is serious, often violent, and can escalate over time. Stalking is a crime.

A stalker can be someone you know well or not at all. Most have dated or been involved with the people they stalk. About 75 percent of stalking cases are men stalking women, but men do stalk men, women do stalk women, and women do stalk men.

Some things stalkers do:

- Follow you and show up wherever you are

- Repeatedly call you, including hang-ups

- Damage your home, car, or other property

- Send unwanted gifts, letters, cards, or e-mails

- Monitor your phone calls or computer use

- Use technology, like hidden cameras or global positioning systems, to track where you go

- Drive by or hang out at your home, school, or work

- Threaten to hurt you, your family, friends, or pets

- Find out about you by using public records or online search services, hiring investigators, going through your garbage, or contacting friends, family, neighbors, or co-workers

- Other actions that control, track, or frighten you

You are not to blame for a stalker's behavior.

Things You Can Do

Stalking is unpredictable and dangerous. No two stalking situations are alike. There are no guarantees that what works for one person will work for another, yet you can take steps to increase your safety.

- If you are in immediate danger, call 911.

- Trust your instincts. Don't downplay the danger. If you feel you are unsafe, you probably are unsafe.

- Take threats seriously. Danger generally is higher when the stalker talks about suicide or murder, or when a victim tries to leave or end the relationship.

- Contact a crisis hotline, victim services agency, or a domestic violence or rape crisis program. They can help you devise a safety plan, give you information about local laws, refer you to other services, and weigh options such as seeking a protection order.

- Develop a safety plan, including things like changing your routine, arranging a place to stay, and having a friend or relative go places with you. Also, decide in advance what to do if the stalker shows up at your home, work, school, or somewhere else. Tell people how they can help you.

- Don't communicate with the stalker or respond to attempts to contact you.

- Keep evidence of the stalking. When the stalker follows you or contacts you, write down the time, date, and place. Keep e-mails, phone messages, letters, or notes. Photograph anything of yours the stalker damages and any injuries the stalker causes. Ask witnesses to write down what they saw.

- Contact the police. Every state has stalking laws. The stalker may also have broken other laws by doing things like assaulting you or stealing or destroying your property.

- Consider getting a court order that tells the stalker to stay away from you.

- Tell family, friends, roommates, and co-workers about the stalking and seek their support. Tell security staff at your job or school. Ask them to help watch out for your safety.

If You're Stalked

You might have the following reactions:

- Feel fear of what the stalker will do
- Feel vulnerable, unsafe, and not know who to trust
- Feel nervous, irritable, impatient, or on edge
- Feel depressed, hopeless, overwhelmed, tearful, or angry
- Feel stressed, including having trouble concentrating, sleeping, or remembering things
- Have eating problems, such as appetite loss, forgetting to eat, or overeating
- Have flashbacks, disturbing thoughts, feelings, or memories
- Feel confused, frustrated, or isolated because other people don't understand why you are afraid

These are common reactions to being stalked.

If Someone You Know Is Being Stalked, You Can Help

Listen. Show support. Don't blame the victim for the crime. Remember that every situation is different and allow the person being stalked to make choices about how to handle it. Find someone you can talk to about the situation. Take steps to ensure your own safety. For more ideas on how you can help, contact:

Stalking Resource Center
Toll-Free: 800-FYI-CALL (394-2255)
Toll-Free TTY: 800-211-7996
Phone: 202-467-8700
Website: http://www.ncvc.org
E-mail: src@ncvc.org

Important: If you are in immediate danger, call 911.

Section 20.2

Technology and Stalking

Cynthia Southworth, Jerry Finn, Shawndell Dawson, Cynthia Fraser, and Sarah Tucker. Intimate Partner Violence, Technology, and Stalking. VIOLENCE AGAINST WOMEN 13: 842–856, © 2007. Reprinted by Permission of SAGE Publication.

Intimate Partner Violence, Technology, and Stalking

During the past decade, domestic violence advocacy organizations have heard stories from increasing numbers of survivors whose abusers are using technology to stalk them. These stories, and others that resulted in news coverage or court cases, illustrate the various ways that stalkers and abusers use technology to control and harm their victims. As a result, several national survivor advocacy projects, including Safety Net: The National Safe and Strategic Technology Project and the Stalking Resource Center, were created to respond to the use of technology in intimate partner stalking. This chapter examines the use of technology in intimate partner stalking and describes experiences of survivors and the need for advocacy-centered responses, including training, legal remedies, and changes in public policy and technology industry practices. Because people surviving abuse differently identify themselves, the terms victim and survivor are interchangeably used. Stalker, abuser, and offender are also interchangeably used to refer to perpetrators of intimate partner violence—a category encompassing domestic violence, sexual violence, and stalking that targets a current or former spouse, boyfriend, girlfriend, or significant other (Greenfeld and Rand, 1998).

Intimate partner violence often includes a range of behaviors that utilize psychological threat and intimidation and physical victimization. Domestic violence has been conceptualized as creating a pattern in which the central issue is control to create dependence, promote social isolation, and inhibit a victim's reality testing (Rogers, Castleton, and Lloyd, 1996; Walker, 1984). This pattern of control includes limiting the use of technologies intended to promote better communication. Thus, abusers often limit victims' access to transportation, monitor telephone calls and letters, and engage in stalking to track the victim's whereabouts (Brewster, 2003). As technology has expanded to include cellular telephones, internet communications, global positioning system (GPS) devices, wireless video cameras, and other digitally based devices, abusers have used these tools to frighten, stalk, monitor, and control their victims. The technology is new to many advocates and victims, necessitating that advocates learn about and address these high-tech tactics, but always in the larger context of a victim's stalking experience. The rapid expansion and availability of new information technologies poses new threats to both victims and domestic violence service providers. Increasing advocates' understanding of stalking with technology will assist them in assessment and safety planning with survivors.

Stalking with Technology

The term cyberstalking has been used to describe a variety of behaviors that involve (a) repeated threats and/or harassment, (b) by the use of electronic mail or other computer-based communication, (c) that would make a reasonable person afraid or concerned for his or her safety (D'Ovidio and Doyle, 2003; Fisher, Cullen, and Turner, 2000). Westrup (1998) suggests the definition should also include behaviors that are perceived as unwelcome and intrusive. Research on cyberstalking has identified many forms of computer and telecommunication-based harassment, including the following:

- Monitoring e-mail communication either directly on the victim's computer or through "sniffer" programs

- Sending e-mail that threatens, insults, or harasses

- Disrupting e-mail communications by flooding a victim's e-mail box with unwanted mail or by sending a virus program

- Using the victim's e-mail identity to send false messages to others or to purchase goods and services

- Using the internet to seek and compile a victim's personal information for use in harassment (Finn and Banach, 2000; Kranz, 2001; Ogilvie, 2000; Spitzberg and Hoobler, 2002)

According to the National Institute of Justice, more than one million women are stalked annually (Tjaden and Thoennes, 1998). Because so many cases are unreported, the actual number of women stalked is likely much higher. Recognition of intimate partner relationships is important to the discussion of stalking and cyberstalking because 59% of female stalking victims were stalked by an intimate partner and 81% of women who were stalked by a current or former intimate partner were also physically assaulted by that partner (Tjaden and Thoennes, 1998). There are no studies that accurately document the extent of cyberstalking; however, the number of reports related to online harassment is increasing (Fremouw, Westrup, and Pennypacker, 1997; Lee, 1998). A nonprofit organization, Working to Halt Online Abuse (WHOA, 2004), reports that it receives approximately 50 to 100 requests a week for guidance and support to stop cyberstalking. A study of college students revealed that 9.6% reported that they had received repeated e-mails from a significant other (spouse, boyfriend or girlfriend, partner) that "threatened, insulted or harassed" (Finn, 2004).

Thus far, research on the use of technology in stalking has focused on cyberstalking. The term is, however, too limited because a number of other information technologies are also being used to intimidate and control victims. Consequently, there is a need for a broad-based definition of cyberstalking in legal and research undertakings (Bahm, 2003). The term stalking with technology will be used in this research to indicate stalking with any of a wide variety of information-based technologies.

The Use of Technology to Stalk: Stories from Survivors

No study has specifically addressed the use of technology in intimate partner stalking. The Stalking Resource Center (2003) and the Safety Net Project (Safety Net, 2004), however, have reported news stories and anecdotal experiences related to victims. These self-reported experiences and news stories indicate that technology is regularly and pervasively used in stalking and underscore the need for more resources and research (Southworth, 2002). Based on these stories, the following are technologies that should be taken into account by domestic violence advocates and researchers when considering education, safety planning, prevention, and research activities.

Telephone Technologies and Global Positioning Systems (GPS)

Most stalking victims regularly use telephones, and some stalkers are adept at tapping telephone lines, reviewing telecommunication devices for the deaf (TTY or TDD) histories, intercepting calls made on cordless telephones, or using cellular telephone features to obtain sensitive information about their victims.

Caller Identification (Caller ID)

San Antonio—A 23-year-old man has been charged with murdering a former girlfriend after using a Caller ID service to track her down. ("Man Charged," 1995, p. A33)

Abusers have used caller ID, a telephone service that reveals the telephone number, name, and location of callers, to locate victims in hiding. Caller ID is supported by a telephone line linked to an electronic device that captures information about incoming calls and stores it in the display unit for future use. New caller ID devices offer not only the name and number of the caller but also the exact address of the telephone. Older caller ID devices only provided the telephone number, though internet telephone directories make it possible to track the exact location of a victim. Moreover, many survivors have unlisted and unpublished phone numbers but still find their personal information published in online directories. Web Wise Women (Safety Net, 2004) explains that many businesses sell customer information to these online services and suggests several strategies to prevent victim information from being posted on the internet. These include educating women about per-call (*67) or permanent call ID blocking, checking with organizations and businesses to be sure that personal information is not published or sold, and requesting that their names be removed when they are found on a database.

Fax Machines

While hiding from an abusive partner, a woman needed to get papers to her abuser. She sent them to him via her attorney from the shelter's fax machine. Her attorney faxed the papers to the abuser's attorney, who gave the papers to the abuser— and no one ever cut off the fax header. The abuser got the phone number and location of the victim and she had to move again. (Safety Net, 2004, p. 15)

Fax machines print information, such as the sender's name and fax number, on the top of every page and thus provide location information to a stalker. New fax machines also contain caller ID, creating additional safety challenges for survivors. Women should be educated to use a fax machine that only prints the date and/or page number or to use a public fax machine such as one from a Kinko's or UPS Store.

TTY and TTD

A prosecutor was working with a victim who was deaf. The prosecutor got a call on his TTY phone and it was supposedly from the victim who said, "If you don't drop the charges against my boyfriend I'm going to kill myself." Help was sent immediately to the victim's home, but to their surprise, she was sleeping the entire time. The abuser impersonated the victim in an attempt to persuade the prosecutor to withdraw charges. (Safety Net, 2004, p. 21)

TTY telephones are text telephones used by the hearing impaired. Deaf and hearing impaired victims have benefited from these devices and the greater accessibility of other electronic communication. However, abusers are also using these devices to impersonate and monitor victims. For example, TTY devices record an exact history of every conversation, which can facilitate the abuser's ability to monitor conversations.

Calling Cards

An advocate was being stalked by an abuser who threatened her life because she helped his wife obtain a protection order. He obtained her information from the Department of Motor Vehicles for one dollar, and continues to harass her with phone calls and messages. Thus far, law enforcement has been unable to confirm the caller and his location because the abuser is using a prepaid phone card. (Safety Net, 2004, p. 28)

Increasingly, stalkers are using the anonymity of prepaid calling cards to harass their victims. If the calling card is not activated with a credit card, linked to a discount card, or billed to a person's long-distance carrier, it is difficult to trace someone making calls with a prepaid card.

Cordless Telephones

A victim advocate in a rural state picked up her cordless phone and heard the conversation of her nearest neighbor who lived over a mile away. She realized how easy it would be for abusers to eavesdrop on their victims' most private conversations. (Safety Net, 2004, p. 23)

Cordless telephones can be used as listening devices, and conversations can be intercepted by baby monitors, some walkie-talkies, and other cordless telephones. In addition, a strategically placed radio scanner in a parked car can pick up a cordless telephone call from a nearby home (Privacy Rights Clearinghouse, 2002).

Cellular and Wireless Telephones

Although many survivors benefit from telephone donation programs, cellular and wireless telephones pose some challenges as well. Similar to cordless telephones, conversations on older, less sophisticated, analog cellular telephones may be intercepted by radio scanners. Although more recent digital wireless telephones are more private, digital cellular telephones may switch to analog mode when used in remote areas without digital coverage. According to the Privacy Rights Clearinghouse, analog cellular services have been available for 25 years, transmit through the air using radio waves, and are accessible across 95% of the country. Digital services, available since 1995, convert the signal into the ones and zeros of computer code and are harder to intercept.

Though considered a lifeline to many victims, a cellular telephone can (inadvertently or intentionally) become a listening device. Many users have bumped their cellular telephone, had it call the last person dialed, and unknowingly broadcast their interactions. Cellular telephones can be converted into a listening device using a basic setting available on most telephones. In addition, a family's cellular telephone billing records can provide a survivor's entire calling history to an abusive partner.

The wireless industry is currently developing a directory of all cellular telephone customers, but customers will only be added if they choose to "opt-in" for this service. An opt-in practice is more responsive to the safety needs of intimate partner and other stalking survivors than an opt-out approach and reflects the increasing interest of the Cellular Telecommunications and Internet Association and others in the industry to create policies that proactively respond to the needs of survivors.

GPS and Location Services

A Wisconsin article reported that a woman found it impossible to escape her ex-boyfriend. He would follow her as she drove to work or ran errands. He would inexplicably pull up next to her at stoplights and once tried to run her off the highway. When he showed up at a bar she was visiting for the first time, on a date, [she] began to suspect [her ex-boyfriend] wasn't operating on instinct alone. The article reported that the stalker put a global positioning tracking device between the radiator and grill of the survivor's car. (Orland, 2003)

GPS devices are small devices that use satellite navigational technology to give precise worldwide positioning and pinpoint locations. Originally designed for the U.S. Department of Defense, this technology has been adapted and is now affordable and available for consumer use. These devices vary as much by price as they do by size and appearance, including appearing as a small black box, a portable unit, or even a small chip in a wristband. Stalkers have used these devices to track their victim's location via real-time web site updates or fee-based online monitoring services.

Stalkers can also manipulate telephone-based instant messenger services and location services associated with wireless telephone service plans to track their intimate partners. In 2001, the Federal Communications Commission mandated that by 2005 all wireless carriers must install GPS into cellular telephones to facilitate 911 emergency responses. Enhanced 911 is designed to provide the telephone number and exact location of a wireless telephone 911 caller. Although carriers are still rolling out this new feature and it is not yet available in most communities, some wireless providers are offering optional location services that allow subscribers to see the location of family members through a "buddy list." This technology can be useful to victims of stalking because law enforcement and emergency personnel services can more easily locate them. On the other hand, it also inadvertently increases surveillance options for abusers and stalkers ("Cell Phone Tech," 2004).

Computer and Internet Technology

A New England woman planned to escape her violent husband. She secretly found a new home for herself and her two daughters and sent an e-mail to a friend asking for help moving. She thought she had deleted the e-mail, though it sat in her e-mail program's "deleted mail folder." Her husband found the e-mail, learned that she was planning to flee for safety, and killed her. (Safety Net, 2004, p. 69)

Stalkers have adapted new computer and internet tools to monitor and control their victims. Initially, abusers used low-tech monitoring options such as looking at web site browser history and reading deleted e-mail, but now stalkers are increasingly using more sophisticated but broadly available spy ware software and hardware.

Spy Ware Software and Keystroke Logging Hardware

In September 2001, a Michigan man was charged with installing spy software on the computer of his estranged wife. He installed a commercially available software program on her computer at her separate residence. Without her knowledge, the program sent him regular e-mails reporting all computer activity, including all e-mails sent and received and all web sites visited. He was charged with using a computer to commit a crime, eavesdropping, installing an eavesdropping device, and unauthorized access. He pled guilty to eavesdropping and using a computer to commit a crime and received two years probation. (Wendland, 2001)

Computer monitoring software—spy ware—was originally developed to monitor children's internet use. Spy ware has multiple definitions. One refers to the "ad ware" that marketing companies use to learn internet searching habits of users. Another definition refers to personal surveillance of computer and internet activities, such as the monitoring that occurred in the 2001 Michigan case. Stalkers and abusers can use these programs to monitor the activities of their victims. Spy ware can be installed by having physical access to the computer or through remote installation by hiding the program as an e-mail attachment. There are hundreds of different software programs available for purchase and freely accessible on the internet. These programs vary, but most record all computer activities. Many programs take pictures of the computer screen every few seconds, thus recording attempts to hide computer histories and e-mail from an abuser.

In addition to software programs, hardware devices called "keystroke loggers" that plug into the keyboard and back of the computer are readily available. These tiny devices contain small hard drives that record every key typed, including all passwords, PIN numbers, web sites, and e-mail. Software programs intended to identify spy ware are not able to identify many software monitoring programs or any hardware loggers. The best prevention is for victims to use a safer computer at such places as a public library.

Hidden Cameras

The Supreme Court of New Jersey found that the defendant's video surveillance of the victim (his estranged wife) in her bedroom presented a prima facie case of stalking and harassment under the New Jersey Domestic Violence Act. The defendant acted "purposefully or knowingly" against a "specific person." He "repeatedly maintained a visual proximity" to the victim. Based on the prior history of violence and threats, a reasonable person in the victim's situation, knowing what the victim knew about her estranged husband, would have feared bodily injury as a result of the defendant's conduct. This case was remanded on due process grounds, but the finding of stalking was affirmed. (H.E.S. v. J.C.S., 2003)

Cameras have become more powerful, affordable, smaller, and easier to disguise. Tiny wireless high-resolution cameras can be hidden in smoke detectors, children's lamps, or behind a pin-sized hole in a wall. These minicameras can be wired or wireless and can be installed anywhere and activated remotely. Web cameras provide continuous viewing or can record to a computer hard drive for later viewing. According to the Privacy Rights Clearinghouse (2002), inexpensive wireless cameras are relatively easy to install and monitor by voyeurs nearby who intercept the wireless signal. Images can be picked up as far as 300 yards from the source, depending on the strength of the signal and the sensitivity of the receiver.

Online Databases and Information Brokers

In Texas, a domestic violence survivor whose ex-husband was soon to be released from jail discovered that information about her house, including a photo and map, had been posted online in county property tax assessments. When the victim approached the tax assessment office to have her information removed, she was told that only law enforcement and court officers had the privilege to opt-out of this sort of public online publication of personal information. (Safety Net, 2004, p. 92)

Corporations, courts, and government agencies are selling, sharing, and publishing sensitive information about citizens worldwide. Stalkers are using these publicly available free web sites and paid information brokers to obtain personal information. In addition to the technology concerns survivors have about the activities of stalkers, survivors are also encountering technology policy barriers that compromise their safety and privacy. Givens (2002) has outlined privacy and safety concerns about open records on the internet. Survivors have found that within their own communities, critical conversations about privacy and victim safety are being left out of community decisions to publish information that is considered to be part of a public record. A person's consent is not sought when others seek to post sensitive or personal information and oftentimes they are not notified when the information is posted to the web. Many courts are beginning to publish both indexes of court records and the full documents and case files on the web, often without providing any notice to citizens or options to restrict web access for victims. For example, as of April 2004, in Montgomery County, Pennsylvania, the court publishes the names and addresses of victims (and their children) who obtain protective orders (Safety Net, 2004).

Legal Issues and Legislative Solutions

Stalking has been legally designated a crime only since 1990. However, there have been descriptions of stalking behavior in film, fiction, and poetry during the past several hundred years (Lee, 1998). In the late 1980s and early 1990s, numerous high-profile cases involving celebrities began to catch the attention of the media and public policy leaders. Only then did such behavior begin to be described as stalking (Stalking Resource Center, 2003). California was the first state to pass an anti-stalking law in 1990 in response to the murder of actress Rebecca Schaeffer and five other Orange County women who were stalked and murdered by former intimate partners. By 1993, all 50 states had enacted stalking laws (U.S. Department of Justice, 1999) and all but four states (Idaho, Nebraska, New Jersey, Utah) and the District of Columbia currently have statutes that include stalking through electronic methods (Gregoire, 2004; WHOA, 2005). In several cases, however, state stalking laws have been interpreted to include stalking by video or GPS surveillance. In addition, a few states, such as Michigan and Nevada, prohibit a person from posting a message through electronic medium of communication without the victim's consent that substantially increases the risk of harm or violence to the victim (Medlin, 2002).

The web site Cyber-Stalking.net (2004) provides an overview of federal laws related to stalking by internet. In 1996, the U.S. Federal Interstate Stalking Law was passed, making it a federal crime to travel across state, tribal, or international lines to stalk someone or to stalk someone across state, tribal, or international lines using regular mail or "any facility of interstate or foreign commerce" (18 U.S.C § 2261A). In 2000, the law was amended to include threats made with electronic communication, such as e-mail or the internet (U.S. Department of Justice, 2001). In 2000, Congress also passed Amy Boyer's Law, (42 U.S.C. Section 1320 B–23 P.L. 106-553), which prohibits the sale or display of an individual's social security number to the public, including sales over the internet, without the person's expressed consent. Amy Boyer's Law is named after a young woman who was murdered after her stalker purchased her social security number over the internet and was able to then track her car license number and place of work. U.S. federal law provides specific protections against threatening electronic communications: 18 USC § 875(c) criminalizes interstate and foreign telephone or electronic communications containing a threat to abduct or injure another individual; 18 USC § 2510-2516 addresses wiretapping and provides protections against illegally tapping someone's telephone; and 47 USC § 223 of the Communication Decency Act prohibits interstate or foreign telecommunication that is used with the intent to annoy, abuse, threaten, or harass another. In addition, Title 42 of the Civil Rights Act may be utilized to address online victimization. This statute has been interpreted to prohibit sexual harassment in work environments. Conduct producing a hostile environment is specifically included in this statute. Thus, sexual harassment via e-mail may be prosecuted under this statute (McGrath and Casey, 2002).

In 1992, in an effort to create enforceable and constitutional anti-stalking laws, Congress passed legislation requiring the U.S. attorney general to develop model anti-stalking laws for distribution to the states (U.S. Department of Justice, 2001). As noted, however, there is still considerable variation in state stalking statutes. In 2004, the Stalking Resource Center launched a model initiative focused on analyzing the state stalking codes. The project seeks to develop common language that nationwide legislators can adopt to make existing stalking laws more inclusive of the use of technology to stalk and to further define specific legal aspects to make the requirement of intent clearer.

The Stalking Resource Center (2003) recommends that states review their laws to ensure that they prohibit and appropriately punish acts of stalking accomplished through technology and offers the following guide for those interested in revising their state's current stalking codes:

- Stalking laws should define the conduct that constitutes stalking as broadly as possible without being unconstitutionally vague.

- States should ask three questions:

  - 1. Will the language used in the law cover all conduct and communications that future advances in technology may generate?

  - 2. Does the law require or imply the need for direct physical contact between the perpetrator and the victim, or can electronic monitoring and surveillance be considered stalking?

  - 3. Does the law cover third-party contact initiated by the stalker?

- Law enforcement organizations should be encouraged to address the full range of technologies used as part of stalking and the co-occurrence of non-technology-related crimes when technology is misused in intimate partner stalking (Stalking Resource Center, 2003). In addition, law enforcement, prosecutors, and judges will need periodic training about the use of new technologies used in stalking and in the application and changes of related laws.

Education and Advocacy

Education about technology for domestic violence advocates and for the organizations with which they interact is essential to providing safety and services for survivors. Most domestic violence advocates have had little or no training related to the use of technology as a component of intimate partner violence. A concerted effort is needed to organize training opportunities in local communities. Training should focus on the technologies previously discussed and include domestic violence advocates, volunteers, and board members and law enforcement and legislative groups.

Domestic violence organizations should assess their own policies and procedures related to technology. First, screening for possible difficulties related to stalking or harassment with technology should become part of intake protocols. Education about technology should be incorporated into development of safety plans with survivors (Safety Net, 2004). In addition, agencies should review their data-collection and data-sharing policies to keep victim data out of the hands of stalkers, abusers, and members of the public. Finally, domestic violence agencies should review their communication, technology, and confidentiality policies to ensure that they include and address all forms of technology.

Advocacy and consciousness raising are needed with government agencies, community groups, and other entities that publish or share sensitive information about survivors and the general public, especially if these are published on the internet. This should include courthouse publications, voter records, and residence information. For example, in Texas, when a survivor learned that only law enforcement and court officers could have their property tax records restricted from internet publication, she urged her state legislator to address this problem. Her initiative changed the law in Texas for thousands of survivors (Safety Net, 2004). The Texas Council on Family Violence (2003) summarizes H.B. 2819: "Victims of family violence whose batterer has been convicted of a felony or Class A misdemeanor can now request that their home address information held by a tax appraisal district remain confidential." Finally, advocates should examine their state's stalking law and analyze the variables suggested by the Stalking Resource Center.

Need for Further Research

Both quantitative and qualitative studies are needed to improve our understanding of the use of technology in intimate partner violence. In her summary of research issues related to cyberstalking, Spence-Diehl (2003) includes the need for generalizable studies of incidence data, documentation of the types and frequency of cyberstalking behaviors, examination of the relationship between terrestrial and cyberstalking, development of cyberstalker profiles and histories, and outcome studies related to intervention strategies that support victims and eliminate or reduce cyberstalking. In addition, qualitative studies of the stories of survivors are needed to promote understanding of the day-to-day experiences of survivors, the coping mechanisms used, and the short-term and long-term impacts on survivors. A national collaborative effort is needed to collect stories and reports of technology misuse in intimate partner violence in a centralized location to provide generalizable data. Research is also needed to assess the outcomes of various strategies for informing and training domestic violence advocates to intervene in cases of stalking with technology. Finally, case studies are needed that provide guidelines for successful campaigns to change local and state policies related to maintaining the privacy of survivors' records and clarifying state stalking laws.

Resources for Addressing Technology in Intimate Partner Stalking

Resources for Advocates

The Safety Net Project (http://www.nnedv.org/projects/safetynet .html) at the National Network to End Domestic Violence: Provides information, training, and consultation to advocates, collaborative agencies and organizations, and the community on issues related to use of technology in intimate partner violence.

Stalking Resource Center at the National Center for Victims of Crime (http://www.ncvc.org/src): Their dual mission is to raise national awareness of stalking and to encourage the development and implementation of multidisciplinary responses to stalking in local communities across the country.

Resources for Victims of Intimate Partner Technology Stalking

National Domestic Violence Hotline (http://www.ndvh.org; 800-799-7233 or 800-787-3224 [TTY]): The 24-hr. hotline provides information and referrals related to domestic violence. Contains a database of more than 4,000 shelters and service providers across the United States, Puerto Rico, and the U.S. Virgin Islands.

Stranger-Related Stalking Resources

CyberAngels (http://www.cyberangels.org): A nonprofit group devoted to assisting victims of online harassment and stalking.

Women Halting Online Abuse (WHOA) (http://www.haltabuse .org): WHOA also educates the online community to develop web site resources, including creating a safe-site and unsafe-site list to enable internet users to make informed decisions and providing information about how users can protect themselves against online harassment.

Safety Ed International (http://www.safetyed.org): A nonprofit organization assisting the internet community and providing specific advice, resources, and information to victims being harassed or stalked online.

Privacy Rights Resources

Online Privacy Alliance (http://www.privacyalliance.com): A coalition of more than 80 global companies and associations whose purpose is to define privacy policy for the new electronic medium and foster an online environment that respects consumer privacy. Available at this web site are resources for consumers, model internet privacy policies, and news stories about recent online privacy violations and issues.

Electronic Privacy Information Center (http://www.epic.org/epic): A public interest research center in Washington, D.C., that focuses public attention on emerging civil liberties issues and seeks to protect privacy, the First Amendment, and constitutional values. Monitors court cases related to technology and cyberstalking.

Privacy Rights Clearinghouse (PRC) (http://www.privacyrights.org): A nonprofit consumer and advocacy program that teaches consumers how to protect their personal privacy. PRC's services include a hotline to report privacy abuses and to request information on ways to protect privacy and prevent identity theft.

Consumer Identity Theft Resource

Federal Trade Commission, Consumer Affairs Department (http://www.consumer.gov/idtheft): A resource site for consumer information from the federal government, including contact information for victims of identity theft or misuse of a social security number and fraudulent credit card accounts.

Network Solutions's WHOIS (http://www.networksolutions.com/cgi-bin/whois/whois): An internet company that provides searches in its registrar database to assist persons in determining the contents of a domain name registration record found in the header of a received e-mail. The result provides the contact information for the sender's internet service provider and can be used to track e-mail harassment.

Conclusion

As national organizations continue to educate and mobilize the advocacy community, they do so knowing that, along with its benefits, technology brings challenges. The same technology that provides victims and survivors of intimate violence with easy access to information, domestic violence resources, and social support also increases the prevalence of inaccurate information, loss of privacy, identity theft, disinhibited communication, online harassment, and stalking with technology. Ever-changing and increasingly inexpensive technologies make it easier than ever before for abusers to monitor and control their victims. Individuals and human service agencies must work to understand and protect against these dangers. Prevention and education about online and technology safety issues are necessary but not sufficient. In addition to staying informed about current technology, advocates must raise community awareness about the privacy needs of survivors, galvanize communities to work toward legal protections for victims of technology-based abuse, and advocate for legal consequences for those that perpetrate it.

References

Bahm, T. (2003). *Eliminating "cyber-confusion."* Retrieved January 15, 2005, from http://www.ncvc.org/src/main.aspx?dbName?Document Viewer&Document ID??33500.

Brewster, M. P. (2003). Power and control dynamics in prestalking and stalking situations. *Journal of Family Violence*, 18, 207–217.

Cell phone tech maintains privacy. (2004, January 19). *Wired News*. Retrieved July 20, 2004, from http://www.wired.com/news/wireless/0,1382,61965,00.html.

Cyber-Stalking.net. (2004). *Overview on U.S. federal statutes or laws pertaining to cyberstalking*. Retrieved February 7, 2004, from http://www.cyber-stalking.net/legal_usfederal.htm.

D'Ovidio, R., and Doyle, J. (2003). A study on cyberstalking: Understanding investigative hurdles. *FBI Law Enforcement Bulletin*, 72(3), 10–17.

Finn, J. (2004). A survey of online harassment at a university campus. *Journal of Interpersonal Violence*, 19, 468–483.

Finn, J., and Banach, M. (2000). Victimization online: The downside of seeking services for women on the Internet. *Cyberpsychology and Behavior*, 3, 776–785.

Fisher, B. S., Cullen, F. T., and Turner, M. G. (2000). *The sexual victimization of college women*. Washington, DC: National Institute of Justice, Bureau of Justice Statistics.

Fremouw, W. J., Westrup, D., and Pennypacker, J. (1997). Stalking on campus: The prevalence and strategies for coping with stalking. *Journal of Forensic Sciences*, 42(4), 666–669.

Givens, B. (2002). *Public records on the Internet: The privacy dilemma.* Retrieved July 20, 2004, from http://www.cfp2002.0rg/proceedings/proceedings/givens.pdf.

Greenfeld, L. A., and Rand, M. R. (1998). *Violence by intimates. Analysis of data on crimes by current or former spouses, boyfriends, and girlfriends.* Washington DC: U.S. Department of Justice.

Gregoire, T. M. (2004). *Cyberstalking: Dangers on the information superhighway.* Retrieved July 21, 2004, from http://www.ncvc.org/src/main.aspx?dbID?DB_Cyberstalking814.

H.E.S. v. J.C.S., 815 A.2d 405 (2003).

Kranz, A. (2001). *Helpful or harmful? How innovative communication technology affects survivors of intimate violence.* Retrieved July 19, 2004, from http://www.vaw.umn.edu/documents/5survivortech/ 5survivortech .html.

Lee, R. K. (1998). Romantic and electronic stalking in a college context. *William and Mary Journal of Women and the Law, 4*(2), 373–409.

Man charged in Caller ID killing. (1995, March 30). *Dallas Morning News*, p. A33.

McGarth, M. G., and Casey, E. (2002). Forensic psychiatry and the Internet: Practical perspectives on sexual predators and obsessional harassers in cyberspace. *Journal of the American Academy of Psychiatry and the Law, 30*, 81–94.

Medlin, A. (2002). *Stalking to cyberstalking, a problem caused by the Internet.* Retrieved February 7, 2004, from http://gsulaw.gsu.edu/lawand/papers/fa02/medlin.

Ogilvie, E. (2000). *The Internet and cyberstalking.* Sydney: Australian Institute of Criminology.

Orland, K. (2003, February 6). *Stalker victims should check for GPS.* Retrieved July 20, 2004, from http://www.cbsnews.com/stories/2003/02/06/tech/main539596.shtml.

Privacy Rights Clearinghouse. (2002). *Wireless communications: Voice and data privacy.* Retrieved July 18, 2004, from http://www.privacyrights .org/fs/fs2-wire.htm.

Rogers, L. E., Castleton, A., and Lloyd, S. A. (1996). Relational control and physical aggression in satisfying marital relationships. In D. D. Cahn and S. A. Lloyd (Eds.), *Family violence from a communication perspective* (pp. 218–239). Thousand Oaks, CA: Sage.

Safety Net. (2004). *Technology, safety, and privacy issues for victims of domestic violence*. Washington, DC: National Network to End Domestic Violence.

Southworth, C. (2002, May). *Safety on the Internet* (Violence Against Women on the Internet Online Course, Module 5). Retrieved February 19, 2005, from http://cyber.law.harvard.edu/vaw02/module5.html.

Spence-Diehl, E. (2003). Stalking and technology: The double-edged sword. *Journal of Technology and Human Services, 22*(1), 5–18.

Spitzberg, B. H., and Hoobler, G. (2002). Cyberstalking and the technologies of interpersonal terrorism. *New Media & Society*, 4, 71–92.

Stalking Resource Center. (2003). Stalking technology outpaces state laws. *Stalking Resource Center Newsletter, 3*(2), 1, 4–5. Retrieved February 19, 2005, from http://www.ncvc.org/src/AGP.Net/Components/DocumentViewer/Download.aspxnz?DocumentID?33500.

Texas Council on Family Violence. (2003). *Information confidentiality held by governmental bodies. Legal history of the domestic violence movement*. Retrieved April 12, 2007, from http://www.tcfv.org/tcfv-content/policy.php?itemid?17.

Tjaden, P., and Thoennes, N. (1998). *Stalking in America: Findings from the National Violence Against Women Survey*. Washington, DC: U.S. Department of Justice.

U.S. Department of Justice. (1999). *Cyberstalking: A new challenge for law enforcement and industry*. Retrieved February 19, 2005, from http://www.usdoj.gov/criminal/cybercrime/cyberstalking.htm.

U.S. Department of Justice. (2001). *Stalking and domestic violence: Report to congress*. Retrieved April 12, 2007, from http://www.ncjrs.gov/pdffiles1/ojp/186157.pdf.

Walker, L. E. A. (1984). *The battered woman syndrome*. New York: Springer.

Wendland, M. (2001, September 6). Belleville man accused of electronic voyeurism. *Detroit Free Press*. Retrieved July 20, 2004, from http://www.freep.com/money/tech/spy6_20010906.htm.

Westrup, D. (1998). Applying functional analysis to stalking behavior. In J. R. Meloy (Ed.), *The psychology of stalking: Clinical and forensic perspectives* (pp. 275–294). San Diego, CA: Academic Press.

Working to Halt Online Abuse. (2004). *Online harassment statistics.* Retrieved July 18, 2004, from http://www.haltabuse.org/resources/stats/index.shtml.

Working to Halt Online Abuse. (2005). *Cyberstalking laws.* Retrieved February 12, 2005, from http://www.haltabuse.org/resources/laws/index.shtml.

Section 20.3

Victims Who Have Disabilities: Uniquely Vulnerable to Stalkers

When Anita left her abusive husband Ed, she found that escaping his violence would not be easy. She moved her two children into an apartment and sought expert advice on how to start a new life. She obtained an order of protection, a divorce, and full custody of her children. As she struggled to free herself from Ed, he began stalking her. Anita finally moved to a new city and even changed her name. Yet one afternoon when she picked up her children, Ed was waiting outside the school. Alarmed and frustrated, she prepared to flee again.

Anita's plight is hardly unique. Abusers often become stalkers. And stalkers tenaciously pursue their victims. Yet Anita's story is somewhat unusual. In her case, the stalker had little trouble finding his ex-wife because she has a disability: she is deaf.[1] To locate Anita, Ed (who is also deaf) simply contacted the Social Security Administration to "inquire" whether the Security Disability Insurance (SSDI) checks his children receive as his dependents were reaching them. In answering Ed's question, the agency gave him Anita's new address.

Victims with Disabilities

Anita's difficulties in escaping her ex-husband suggest the complex challenges that stalking victims with disabilities face. Stalkers may target these victims because of their disabilities or exploit their disabilities in committing crimes. Victims face formidable burdens in protecting themselves, unique barriers to reporting, and difficulty accessing or receiving victim services.

Approximately 20 percent of noninstitutionalized Americans have a disability.[2] And people with disabilities suffer alarming rates of victimization. Women with disabilities experience the highest rate of personal violence—violence at the hands of spouses, partners, boyfriends, family members, caregivers, and strangers—of any group in our society today.[3] Of the 200 women with physical and cognitive disabilities who responded to a 2002 survey, 67 percent reported having experienced physical abuse, and 53 percent of the women reported having experienced sexual abuse.[4] Some researchers believe that 90 percent of people with developmental disabilities will at some point in their lives be the victims of sexual assault and that only three percent of these crimes will be reported.[5]

Vulnerability to Stalking

Given the level of physical violence experienced by people with disabilities, as well as the established link between intimate partner violence and stalking,[6] it is highly probable that people with disabilities experience significant levels of stalking. While the Stalking Resource Center (SRC) has found little research to establish the prevalence of stalking among people with disabilities, experience suggests that stalking is likely to occur in this population. In this section, SRC attempts to lay the groundwork for such research, to elicit feedback from providers who may have served such victims, and to explore the best ways to help them.

Offender Manipulation

People with disabilities are particularly vulnerable to stalking because they are sometimes perceived to be easier to control than other victims. "The balance of power in all abusive relationships shifts very subtly," says Debora L. Beck-Massey of the Domestic Violence Initiative for Women with Disabilities in Denver, Colorado, "so more and more of the control, decision making, and options slide toward the batterer's side." Abusers of people with disabilities often control victims' access to basic necessities such as food and transportation to increase their dependence.

If the relationships end, these abusers are particularly well equipped to stalk the victim. They have access to a significant amount of personal information, such as bank account numbers, passwords, and Social Security numbers, which they can use to take money from victims or to prevent them from accessing their funds. They are familiar with victims' work arrangements and any special transportation systems their victims use. These controlling behaviors, as part of an overall pattern of conduct, produce substantial emotional distress and are likely to cause fear in the victim.

Protection Problems

Stalking victims often have great difficulty protecting themselves and their families. They may have to change their entire lives—move to a different community, change jobs, alter their physical appearance, and even change names—all to avoid their offender's next move. "For stalking victims with disabilities," said Beck-Massey, "the very systems they rely on for support—for transportation, financial support, or services—may increase their vulnerabilities." Ed used the SSDI system to track Anita because she relied on SSDI support for her children. A victim with a disability living in government-subsidized housing may find it impossible to move quickly, even to escape a dangerous situation, because of six- to twelve-month waiting periods for apartments in such facilities.

Barriers to Reporting and Receiving Services

Stalking victims with disabilities confront the same barriers to reporting the crime (such as fear of not being believed) that most victims face.[7] In addition, victims with disabilities have to contend with physical or social isolation, impediments to communication or mobility, or physical or financial dependence on a caregiver who may also be the perpetrator.[8] For example, a victim who is housebound because of her disability may never sufficiently escape her caregiver to be able to report her victimization to law enforcement.

Victims are also vulnerable to stalkers' exploiting their disabilities to avoid criminal justice intervention. For example, a stalker may escape being investigated as a suspect by posing as a concerned friend checking up on a victim. Or, if a victim has a developmental disability and an investigating officer finds two differing versions of events—one from a woman who seemed confused and another from a coherent, ostensibly concerned "friend" of the victim—the officer might be easily convinced that the victim was not victimized at all. Stalkers can also pressure victims to drop charges by threatening them in ways that, absent the context of a disability, might seem less malignant. For example, by canceling a victim's food delivery or transportation to a crucial doctor's appointment, a stalker can remind the victim that he can control her life.

Stalkers can also exploit the victims' reliance on assistive technologies, such as text telephone (TTY) machines and e-mail. For example, a stalker who is able to hack into the victim's e-mail or gain access to her TTY machine can pose as the victim to interfere with communications with her victim advocate or the police department (for example, posing as the victim, the stalker requests that the police discontinue their investigation of the stalking case).

Identifying Needs and Providing Effective Services

For all stalking victims and victim advocates, recognizing the problem is half the battle. Criminal justice professionals and victim service providers must first know who in our communities may be at most risk for being victimized. Then, to improve their responses, they must identify the barriers to reporting crime and accessing services for these victims.

How to Work with Victims with Disabilities

- Consult disability agencies and victims with disabilities when devising your community's response to stalking.

- Collaborate with disability services agencies to provide training for criminal justice professionals and victim service providers on best practices for working with people with disabilities. Train disability rights workers to recognize and address stalking.

- Use targeted outreach and appropriate services (for example, use inclusive language and symbols in organization materials and provide the local telecommunications relay service (TRS) with a current list of victim service hotlines).

- Observe Americans with Disabilities Act (ADA) requirements. Compliance with the law helps victims with disabilities and protects government agencies and government-funded organizations from liability for discrimination.

Conclusion

Victim advocates, criminal justice agencies, and disability rights workers should take a closer look at the complex and challenging needs of stalking victims with disabilities. Researchers would benefit from studying the incidence of stalking among these victims, and victim service providers and criminal justice professionals could use the resulting knowledge to improve their response to victims with disabilities. The Stalking Resource Center would appreciate hearing from providers who have worked with such victims, and welcomes information on appropriate best practices, protocols, or policies. To share information with the SRC or to learn more about stalking, please contact at src@ncvc.org.

Endnotes

1. The Stalking Resource Center (SRC) recognizes the unique culture of the deaf community and the desire of its members to be independently identified. However, for the purposes of this brief article, the SRC adopts the Americans with Disabilities Act (ADA) definition of an individual with a disability as "a person who has a physical or mental impairment that substantially limits one or more major life activities,...who has a history or record of such an impairment, or ...who is perceived by others as having such an impairment." Examples included in the ADA definition include orthopedic, visual, speech, and hearing impairments, as well as many other conditions.

2. U.S. Census Bureau, "Disability Status: 2000," Census 2000 Brief (March 2003), http://www.census.gov/prod/2003pubs/c2kbr-17.pdf, (Accessed October 31, 2005).

3. W. Abramson et al., eds., "From the Editors," *Impact: Feature Issue on Violence Against Women with Developmental or Other Disabilities 13*, No. 3 (2000), http://ici.umn.edu/products/impact/133, (Accessed: October 31, 2005).

4. L.E. Powers and M. Oschwald, "Violence and Abuse Against People with Disabilities: Experiences, Barriers and Prevention Strategies," Center on Self-Determination, Oregon Institute on Disability and Development, Oregon Health and Science University, Citing: L.E. Powers, M.A. Curry, M. Oschwald, S. Maley, M. Saxton, and K. Eckels, "Barriers and Strategies in Addressing

Abuse: A Survey of Disabled Women's Experiences," *Journal of Rehabilitation 68*, No. 1 (2002): 4–13.

5. D. Sobsey and T. Doe, "Patterns of Sexual Abuse and Assault," *Sexuality and Disability 9*, No. 3 (1991): 243–259; and C. Tyiska, "Working with Victims of Crime with Disabilities," *Office for Victims of Crime Bulletin*, (Washington, DC: U.S. Department of Justice, 1998).

6. M.B. Mechanic et al., "Intimate Partner Violence and Stalking Behavior: Exploration of Patterns and Correlates in a Sample of Acutely Battered Women," *Violence and Victims 15*, No. 1 (2000): 55–72.

Chapter 21

Trafficking in Persons

Chapter Contents

Section 21.1

Scope and Nature of Modern-Day Slavery

This section includes text from "Trafficking in Persons: Facts and Figures," *In the Spotlight*, National Criminal Justice Reference Service, U.S. Department of Justice, updated May 28, 2008; and, excerpts from "Trafficking in Persons Report," U.S. Department of State, June 2008.

Facts and Figures about Trafficking in Persons

- As of May 2004, the U.S. Government estimates that 14,500 to 17,500 people are trafficked annually into the United States, and 600,000 to 800,000 are trafficked globally. This estimate covers men, women, and children trafficked across borders and recruited, harbored, transported, provided, or obtained for forced labor or sexual exploitation—severe forms of trafficking as defined in the Trafficking Victims Protection Act.

- Approximately 80 percent of the victims are female; 70 percent of those females are trafficked for the commercial sex industry.

- The largest number of people trafficked into the United States come from East Asia and the Pacific (5,000 to 7,000). The next highest numbers come from Latin America and from Europe and Eurasia, at between 3,500 and 5,500 victims from each.

- In June 2007, U.S. Immigration and Customs Enforcement (ICE) reported that they had made "more than 61 arrests under the child sex tourism provisions of the PROTECT Act" since Operation Predator was initiated in July 2003 (*Operation Predator Fact Sheet*, U.S. Department of Homeland Security, U.S. Immigration and Customs Enforcement, 2007).

Information from the 2008 Trafficking in Persons Report

The U.S. law that guides anti-human trafficking efforts, the Trafficking Victims Protection Act of 2000 (TVPA), as amended, states that the purpose of combating human trafficking is to punish traffickers, to protect victims, and to prevent trafficking from occurring. Freeing those trapped in slave-like conditions is the ultimate goal of the U.S. government's antihuman trafficking policy.

Human trafficking is a multidimensional threat. It deprives people of their human rights and freedoms, it increases global health risks, and it fuels the growth of organized crime.

Human trafficking has a devastating impact on individual victims, who often suffer physical and emotional abuse, rape, threats against self and family, and even death. But the impact of human trafficking goes beyond individual victims; it undermines the health, safety, and security of all nations it touches.

Trafficking Defined

The TVPA defines severe forms of trafficking as:

a. sex trafficking in which a commercial sex act is induced by force, fraud, or coercion, or in which the person induced to perform such an act has not attained 18 years of age; or

b. the recruitment, harboring, transportation, provision, or obtaining of a person for labor or services, through the use of force, fraud, or coercion for the purpose of subjection to involuntary servitude, peonage, debt bondage, or slavery.

A victim need not be physically transported from one location to another in order for the crime to fall within these definitions.

Modern-Day Slavery

The common denominator of trafficking scenarios is the use of force, fraud, or coercion to exploit a person for profit. A victim can be subjected to labor exploitation, sexual exploitation, or both. Labor exploitation includes traditional chattel slavery, forced labor, and debt bondage. Sexual exploitation typically includes abuse within the commercial sex industry. In other cases, victims are exploited in private homes by individuals who often demand sex as well as work. The use of force or coercion can be direct and violent or psychological.

A wide range of estimates exists on the scope and magnitude of modern-day slavery. The International Labor Organization (ILO)— the United Nations agency charged with addressing labor standards, employment, and social protection issues—estimates that there are 12.3 million people in forced labor, bonded labor, forced child labor, and sexual servitude at any given time; other estimates range from four million to 27 million.

Annually, according to U.S. government-sponsored research completed in 2006, approximately 800,000 people are trafficked across national borders, which does not include millions trafficked within their own countries. Approximately 80 percent of transnational victims are women and girls and up to 50 percent are minors. The majority of transnational victims are females trafficked into commercial sexual exploitation. These numbers do not include millions of female and male victims around the world who are trafficked within their own national borders—the majority for forced or bonded labor.

Human traffickers prey on the vulnerable. Their targets are often children and young women, and their ploys are creative and ruthless, designed to trick, coerce, and win the confidence of potential victims. Very often these ruses involve promises of a better life through employment, educational opportunities, or marriage.

The nationalities of trafficked people are as diverse as the world's cultures. Some leave developing countries, seeking to improve their lives through low-skilled jobs in more prosperous countries. Others fall victim to forced or bonded labor in their own countries. Women, eager for a better future, are susceptible to promises of jobs abroad as baby-sitters, housekeepers, waitresses, or models—jobs that traffickers turn into the nightmare of forced prostitution without exit. Some families give children to adults, often relatives, who promise education and opportunity—but sell the children into exploitative situations for money. But poverty alone does not explain this tragedy, which is driven by fraudulent recruiters, employers, and corrupt officials who seek to reap unlawful profits from others' desperation.

Forced Labor and Sexual Servitude: The Varying Forms of Human Trafficking

The hidden nature of trafficking in persons prevents a precise count of the number of victims around the world, but available research indicates that, when trafficking within a country's borders is included in the count, more people fall victim to labor forms of trafficking than sex trafficking. Although labor trafficking and sex trafficking are usually analyzed as separate trafficking in persons issues, victims of both forms of trafficking often share a common denominator—their trafficking ordeal started with a migration in search of economic alternatives.

The theme of migration is often heard in reporting on trafficking in persons and indeed the movement of victims is a common trait in many trafficking crimes. Yet servitude can also occur without the movement of a person. In analyzing trafficking in persons issues and designing effective responses, the focus should be on the exploitation and control of a person through force, fraud, or coercion—not on the movement of that person.

Major Forms of Trafficking in Persons

Forced Labor

Most instances of forced labor occur as unscrupulous employers take advantage of gaps in law enforcement to exploit vulnerable workers. These workers are made more vulnerable to forced labor practices because of unemployment, poverty, crime, discrimination, corruption, political conflict, and cultural acceptance of the practice. Immigrants are particularly vulnerable, but individuals are also forced into labor in their own countries. Female victims of forced or bonded labor, especially women and girls in domestic servitude, are often sexually exploited as well. Forced labor is a form of human trafficking that can be harder to identify and estimate than sex trafficking. It may not involve the same criminal networks profiting from transnational sex trafficking, but may instead involve individuals who subject anywhere from one to hundreds of workers to involuntary servitude, perhaps through forced or coerced household work or work at a factory.

Bonded Labor

One form of force or coercion is the use of a bond, or debt, to keep a person under subjugation. This is referred to in law and policy as bonded labor or debt bondage. It is criminalized under U.S. law and included as a form of exploitation related to trafficking in the United Nations Trafficking in Persons (UN TIP) Protocol. Many workers around the world fall victim to debt bondage when traffickers or recruiters unlawfully exploit an initial debt the worker assumed as part of the terms of employment, or when workers inherit debt in more traditional systems of bonded labor. Traditional bonded labor in South Asia enslaves huge numbers of people from generation to generation.

Debt Bondage and Involuntary Servitude Among Migrant Laborers

The vulnerability of migrant laborers to trafficking schemes is especially disturbing because this population is so sizable in some regions. Three potential contributors can be discerned: 1) abuse of contracts;

2) inadequate local laws governing the recruitment and employment of migrant laborers; and 3) the intentional imposition of exploitative and often illegal costs and debts on these laborers in the source country or state, often with the complicity and/or support of labor agencies and employers in the destination country or state.

Some abuses of contracts and hazardous conditions of employment do not in themselves constitute involuntary servitude, though use or threat of physical force or restraint to compel a worker to enter into or continue labor or service may convert a situation into one of forced labor. Costs imposed on laborers for the privilege of working abroad can place laborers in a situation highly vulnerable to debt bondage. However, these costs alone do not constitute debt bondage or involuntary servitude. When combined with exploitation by unscrupulous labor agents or employers in the destination country, these costs or debts, when excessive, can become a form of debt bondage.

Involuntary Domestic Servitude

Domestic workers may be trapped in servitude through the use of force or coercion, such as physical (including sexual) or emotional abuse. Children are particularly vulnerable. Domestic servitude is particularly difficult to detect because it occurs in private homes, which are often unregulated by public authorities. For example, there is great demand in some wealthier countries of Asia and the Middle East for domestic servants who sometimes fall victim to conditions of involuntary servitude.

Forced Child Labor

Most international organizations and national laws recognize that children may legally engage in light work. In contrast, the worst forms of child labor are being targeted for eradication by nations across the globe. The sale and trafficking of children and their entrapment in bonded and forced labor are clearly among the worst forms of child labor. Any child who is subject to involuntary servitude, debt bondage, peonage, or slavery through the use of force, fraud, or coercion is a victim of trafficking in persons regardless of the location of that exploitation.

Sex Trafficking and Prostitution

Sex trafficking comprises a significant portion of overall trafficking and the majority of transnational modern-day slavery. Sex trafficking would not exist without the demand for commercial sex flourishing around the world. The U.S. government adopted a strong position against prostitution in a December 2002 policy decision, which notes that prostitution is inherently harmful and dehumanizing and fuels trafficking in persons. Turning people into dehumanized commodities creates an enabling environment for human trafficking.

The United States government opposes prostitution and any related activities, including pimping, pandering, or maintaining brothels as contributing to the phenomenon of trafficking in persons, and maintains that these activities should not be regulated as a legitimate form of work for any human being. Those who patronize the commercial sex industry form a demand which traffickers seek to satisfy.

Children Exploited for Commercial Sex

Each year, more than two million children are exploited in the global commercial sex trade. Many of these children are trapped in prostitution. The commercial sexual exploitation of children is trafficking, regardless of circumstances. International covenants and protocols obligate criminalization of the commercial sexual exploitation of children. The use of children in the commercial sex trade is prohibited under both U.S. law and the U.N. TIP Protocol. There can be no exceptions, no cultural or socioeconomic rationalizations that prevent the rescue of children from sexual servitude. Terms such as "child sex worker" are unacceptable because they falsely sanitize the brutality of this exploitation.

Child Sex Tourism

Child sex tourism (CST) involves people who travel from their own country—often a country where child sexual exploitation is illegal or culturally abhorrent—to another country where they engage in commercial sex acts with children. CST is a shameful assault on the dignity of children and a form of violent child abuse. The commercial sexual exploitation of children has devastating consequences for minors, which may include long-lasting physical and psychological trauma, disease (including human immunodeficiency virus [HIV] and acquired immunodeficiency syndrome [AIDS]), drug addiction, unwanted pregnancy, malnutrition, social ostracism, and possibly death).

Tourists engaging in CST often travel to developing countries looking for anonymity and the availability of children being used in prostitution. The crime is typically fueled by weak law enforcement, corruption, the internet, ease of travel, and poverty. Sex offenders come from all socioeconomic backgrounds and may in some cases hold positions of trust. Cases of child sex tourism involving U.S. citizens have included a pediatrician, a retired Army sergeant, a dentist, and a university professor. Child pornography is frequently involved in these cases, and drugs may also be used to solicit or control the minors.

Section 21.2

Health Consequences of Trafficking in Persons

"Health Consequences of Trafficking in Persons,"
U.S. Department of State, August 8, 2007.

Trafficking in persons has serious public health implications, such as spreading the human immunodeficiency virus (HIV) and acquired immunodeficiency syndrome (AIDS) epidemic, besides being a human rights and national security issue.

Physical Trauma and Mental Health

By definition, human trafficking entails "force, fraud, or coercion" which typically includes confinement, and often, physical and psychological abuse. Research has demonstrated that violence and abuse are at the core of trafficking for prostitution. A study of women trafficked for prostitution into the European Union found that 95% of victims had been violently assaulted or coerced into a sexual act, and over 60% of victims reported fatigue, neurological symptoms, gastrointestinal problems, back pain, and gynecological infections.

A nine-country assessment first published in the *Journal of Trauma Practice* concluded that 73% of women used in prostitution were physically assaulted, 89% wanted to escape, 63% were raped, and 68% met the criteria for posttraumatic stress disorder. Additional psychological consequences common among prostituted women include dissociative and personality disorders, anxiety, and depression.

Another study (2001) revealed that 86% of women trafficked within their countries and 85% of women trafficked across international borders suffer from severe depression.

As with sex trafficking, those who are trafficked for labor also suffer physical and mental health problems, such as posttraumatic stress disorder due to physical assaults and beatings, and depression that elevates the risk of suicide. Victims of labor servitude have limited ability to determine the conditions in which they work, which may put them at higher risk of physical and mental health damage. There is a need for more data on the health consequences of trafficking for forced labor.

The Link Between HIV/AIDS and Trafficking in Persons

Approximately 42 million people worldwide are living with HIV/AIDS, and sex trafficking plays a major role in spreading the epidemic. In 2005, the Joint United Nations Programme on HIV/AIDS reported, "Across Asia, the [HIV] epidemics are propelled by combinations of injecting drug use and commercial sex." Thus, both prostitution and sex trafficking contribute to the spread of HIV/AIDS.

Globally, people in prostitution have a high incidence of HIV. For example, HIV prevalence among women trafficked from Nepal and prostituted in India is 38%. The rate of HIV infection exceeded 60% among girls prostituted prior to 15 years of age. In South Africa, the number reaches 70.4%. According to the World Congress Against Commercial Sexual Exploitation of Children, between "50 and 90 percent of children rescued from brothels in Southeast Asia are infected with HIV."

Experts believe that sex trafficking is contributing to the global dispersion of HIV subtypes and in the mutation of the HIV virus, as well as the development of drug-resistant strains of other sexually transmitted infections. In brothels in Indonesia, for example, 89% of prostituted women with gonorrhea were resistant to penicillin and 98% to tetracycline. The presence of some sexually transmitted infections (STI) greatly increases the risk of HIV transmission.

Sexual and Reproductive Health

Untreated sexually transmitted infections may lead to serious consequences for long-term health. One such implication, pelvic inflammatory disease, may result in infertility, ectopic pregnancy, chronic pelvic pain, and an increased risk of hysterectomy.

Research by Brian M. Willis and Barry Levy reveals that of the millions of women and girls forced into prostitution each year, approximately 45% are infected with the human papillomavirus (HPV). The National Cancer Institute has confirmed that HPV infection causes cervical cancer. Prostituted girls are left more susceptible to developing the disease since cervical cancer is associated with a high number of sexual partners and with young age at first intercourse.

It is common for sex trafficking to result in pregnancy, a situation that frequently leads to forced abortions, according to a 2003 European Union study on the health consequences of human trafficking. Trafficked women are particularly vulnerable to post-abortion risks, such as incomplete abortion, sepsis (infections of the bloodstream), hemorrhaging, and intra-abdominal injury. These complications reportedly account for most maternal deaths. The study also found that many women exploited for commercial sex are given insufficient time to recuperate, thereby increasing the risk of post-abortion infection. The Christian Medical and Dental Association points out that these abortions are probably carried out by unqualified individuals with little regard to sanitation, resulting in infection, mutilation, or infertility.

Part Three

Victims and Perpetrators

Chapter 22

Victims of Domestic Violence

Victims of domestic violence do not possess a set of universal characteristics or personality traits, but they do share the common experience of being abused by someone close to them. Anyone can become a victim of domestic violence. Victims of domestic violence can be women, men, adolescents, disabled persons, gays, or lesbians. They can be of any age and work in any profession. Normally, victims of domestic violence are not easily recognized because they are not usually covered in marks or bruises. If there are injuries, victims have often learned to conceal them to avoid detection, suspicion, and shame.

Unfortunately, an array of misconceptions about victims of domestic violence has led to harmful stereotypes about who they are and the realities of their abuse. Consequently, victims of domestic violence often feel stigmatized and misunderstood by the people in their lives. These people may be well-intended family members and friends or persons trained to help them, such as social workers, police officers, or doctors.

Barriers to Leaving an Abusive Relationship

The most commonly asked question about victims of domestic violence is: "Why do they stay?" Family, friends, coworkers, and community professionals who try to understand the reasons why a victim of

Text in this chapter is excerpted from "Child Protection in Families Experiencing Domestic Violence: Chapter 3," U.S. Department of Health and Human Services (HHS), updated December 10, 2007.

violence has not left the abusive partner often feel perplexed strated. Some victims of domestic violence do leave their violent partners while others may leave and return at different points throughout the abusive relationship. Leaving a violent relationship is a process, not an event, for many victims, who cannot simply "pick up and go" because they have many factors to consider. To understand the complex nature of terminating a violent relationship, it is essential to look at the barriers and risks faced by victims when they consider or attempt to leave. Individual, systemic, and societal barriers faced by victims of domestic violence include:

Fear: Perpetrators commonly make threats to find victims, inflict harm, or kill them if they end the relationship. This fear becomes a reality for many victims who are stalked by their partner after leaving. It also is common for abusers to seek or threaten to seek sole custody, make child abuse allegations, or kidnap the children. Historically, there has been a lack of protection and assistance from law enforcement, the judicial system, and social service agencies charged with responding to domestic violence. Inadequacies in the system and the failure of past efforts by victims of domestic violence seeking help have led many to believe that they will not be protected from the abuser and are safer at home. While much remains to be done, there is a growing trend of increased legal protection and community support for these victims.

Isolation: One effective tactic abusers use to establish control over victims is to isolate them from any support system other than the primary intimate relationship. As a result, some victims are unaware of services or people that can help. Many believe they are alone in dealing with the abuse. This isolation deepens when society labels them as "masochistic" or "weak" for enduring the abuse. Victims often separate themselves from friends and family because they are ashamed of the abuse or want to protect others from the abuser's violence.

Financial dependence: Some victims do not have access to any income and have been prevented from obtaining an education or employment. Victims who lack viable job skills or education, transportation, affordable daycare, safe housing, and health benefits face very limited options. Poverty and marginal economic support services can present enormous challenges to victims who seek safety and stability. Often, victims find themselves choosing between homelessness, living in impoverished and unsafe communities, or returning to their abusive partner.

Guilt and shame: Many victims believe the abuse is their fault. The perpetrator, family, friends, and society sometimes deepen this belief by accusing the victim of provoking the violence and casting blame for not preventing it. Victims of violence rarely want their family and friends to know they are abused by their partner and are fearful that people will criticize them for not leaving the relationship. Victims often feel responsible for changing their partner's abusive behavior or changing themselves in order for the abuse to stop. Guilt and shame may be felt especially by those who are not commonly recognized as victims of domestic violence. This may include men, gays, lesbians, and partners of individuals in visible or respected professions, such as the clergy and law enforcement.

Emotional and physical impairment: Abusers often use a series of psychological strategies to break down the victim's self-esteem and emotional strength. In order to survive, some victims begin to perceive reality through the abuser's paradigm, become emotionally dependent, and believe they are unable to function without their partner. The psychological and physical effects of domestic violence also can affect a victim's daily functioning and mental stability. This can make the process of leaving and planning for safety challenging for victims who may be depressed, physically injured, or suicidal. Victims who have a physical or developmental disability are extremely vulnerable because the disability can compound their emotional, financial, and physical dependence on their abusive partner.

Individual belief system: The personal, familial, religious, and cultural values of victims of domestic violence are frequently interwoven in their decisions to leave or remain in abusive relationships. For example, victims who hold strong convictions regarding the sanctity of marriage may not view divorce or separation as an option. Their religious beliefs may tell them divorce is "wrong." Some victims of domestic violence believe that their children still need to be with the offender and that divorce will be emotionally damaging to them.

Hope: Like most people, victims of domestic violence are invested in their intimate relationships and frequently strive to make them healthy and loving. Some victims hope the violence will end if they become the person their partner wants them to be. Others believe and have faith in their partner's promises to change. Perpetrators are not "all bad" and have positive, as well as, negative qualities. The abuser's "good side" can give victims reason to think their partner is capable of being nurturing, kind, and nonviolent.

Community services and societal values: For victims who are prepared to leave and want protection, there are a variety of institutional barriers that make escaping abuse difficult and frustrating. Communities that have inadequate resources and limited victim advocacy services and whose response to domestic abuse is fragmented, punitive, or ineffective can not provide realistic or safe solutions for victims and their children.

Cultural hurdles: The lack of culturally sensitive and appropriate services for victims of color and those who are non-English speaking pose additional barriers to leaving violent relationships. Minority populations include African-Americans, Hispanics, Asians, and other ethnic groups whose cultural values and customs can influence their beliefs about the role of men and women, interpersonal relationships, and intimate partner violence. For example, the Hispanic cultural value of "machismo" supports some Latino men's belief that they are superior to women and the "head of their household" in determining familial decisions. "Machismo" may cause some Hispanic men to believe that they have the right to use violent or abusive behavior to control their partners or children. In turn, Latina women and other family or community members may excuse violent or controlling behavior because they believe that husbands have ultimate authority over them and their children.

Examples of culturally competent services include offering written translation of domestic violence materials, providing translators in domestic violence programs, and implementing intervention strategies that incorporate cultural values, norms, and practices to effectively address the needs of victims and abusers. The lack of culturally competent services that fail to incorporate issues of culture and language can present obstacles for victims who want to escape abuse and for effective interventions with domestic violence perpetrators. Well-intended family, friends, and community members also can create additional pressures for the victim to "make things work."

The Impact of Domestic Violence on Victims

As with anyone who has been traumatized, victims demonstrate a wide range of effects from domestic violence. The perpetrator's abusive behavior can cause an array of health problems and physical injuries. Victims may require medical attention for immediate injuries, hospitalization for severe assaults, or chronic care for debilitating health problems resulting from the perpetrator's physical attacks. The direct physical effects of domestic violence can range from minor scratches or bruises to fractured bones or sexually transmitted diseases resulting from forced sexual activity and other practices. The indirect physical effects of domestic violence can range from recurring headaches or stomachaches to severe health problems due to withheld medical attention or medications.

Many victims of abuse make frequent visits to their physicians for health problems and for domestic violence-related injuries. Unfortunately, research shows that many victims will not disclose the abuse unless they are directly asked or screened for domestic violence by the physician. It is imperative, therefore, that health care providers directly inquire about possible domestic violence so victims receive proper treatment for injuries or illnesses and are offered further assistance for addressing the abuse.

The impact of domestic violence on victims can result in acute and chronic mental health problems. Some victims, however, have histories of psychiatric illnesses that may be exacerbated by the abuse; others may develop psychological problems as a direct result of the abuse. Following are some examples of emotional and behavioral effects of domestic violence include many common coping responses to trauma:

- Emotional withdrawal
- Denial or minimization of the abuse
- Impulsivity or aggressiveness
- Apprehension or fear
- Helplessness
- Anger
- Anxiety or hypervigilance
- Disturbance of eating or sleeping patterns
- Substance abuse
- Depression
- Suicide
- Posttraumatic stress disorder

Some of these effects also serve as coping mechanisms for victims. For example, some victims turn to alcohol to lessen the physical and emotional pain of the abuse. Unfortunately, these coping mechanisms can serve as barriers for victims who want help or want to leave their abusive relationships. Psychiatrists, psychologists, therapists, and counselors who provide screening, comprehensive assessment, and treatment for victims can serve as the catalyst that helps them address or escape the abuse.

Parenting and the Victim

Emerging research indicates that the harmful effects of domestic violence can negatively influence parenting behaviors. Parents who are suffering from abuse may experience higher stress levels, which in turn, can influence the nature of their relationship with and responses to their children. Victims who are preoccupied with avoiding physical attacks and coping with the violence confront additional challenges in their efforts to provide safety, support, and nurturance to their children. Unfortunately, some victims of domestic violence are emotionally or physically unavailable to their children due to injuries, emotional exhaustion, or depression.

Studies have found that victims of domestic violence are more likely to maltreat their children than those who are not abused by their partners. In some cases, victims who use physical force or inappropriate discipline techniques are trying to protect their children from potentially more severe forms of violence or discipline by the abuser. For example, a victim of domestic violence might slap the child when the abuser threatens harm if the child is not quiet. Seemingly, neglectful behaviors by the victim also may be a direct result of the domestic violence. This is illustrated when the abuser prevents the victim from taking the child to the doctor or to school because the adult victim's injuries would reveal the abusiveness.

The majority of victims of domestic violence are not bad, ineffective, or abusive parents, but researchers note that domestic violence is one of a multitude of stressors that can negatively influence parenting. However, many victims, despite ongoing abuse, are supportive, nurturing parents who mediate the impact of their children's exposure to domestic violence. Given the impact of violence on parenting behaviors, it is beneficial that victims receive services that alleviate their distress so they can support and benefit the children.

Strategies Victims Use to Protect Themselves and Their Children

Protective strategies that frequently are recommended by family, friends, and social services providers include contacting the police, obtaining a restraining order, or seeking refuge at a friend or relative's home or at a domestic violence shelter. It is ordinarily assumed that these suggestions are successful at keeping victims and their children safe from violence. It is crucial to remember, however, that while these strategies can be effective for some victims of domestic violence, they can be unrealistic and even dangerous options for other victims. For example, obtaining a restraining order can be useful in deterring some perpetrators, but it can cause other perpetrators to become increasingly abusive and threatening. Since these recommendations are concrete and observable, they tend to reassure people that the victim of domestic violence is actively taking steps to address the abuse and to be safe, even if they create additional risks. Furthermore, these options only address the physical violence in a victim's life. They do not address the economic or housing challenges the victim must overcome to survive, nor do they provide the emotional and psychological safety the victims need. Therefore, victims often weigh "perpetrator-generated" risks versus "life-generated" risks as they try to make decisions and find safety.

Typically, victims do not passively tolerate the violence in their lives. They often use very creative methods to avoid and deescalate their partner's abusive behavior. Some of these are successful and others are not. Victims develop their own unique set of protective strategies based on their past experience of what is effective at keeping them emotionally and physically protected from their partner's violence. In deciding which survival mechanism to use, victims engage in a methodical problem-solving process that involves analyzing: available and realistic safety options, the level of danger created by the abuser's violence, and the prior effectiveness and consequences of previously used strategies. After careful consideration, victims of domestic violence decide whether to use, adapt, replace, or discard certain approaches given the risks they believe it will pose to them and their children. Examples of additional protective strategies victims use to survive and protect themselves include the following:

- Complying, placating, or colluding with the perpetrator

- Minimizing, denying, or refusing to talk about the abuse for fear of making it worse

- Leaving or staying in the relationship so the violence does not escalate

- Fighting back or defying the abuser

- Sending the children to a neighbor or family member's home

- Engaging in manipulative behaviors, such as lying, as a way to survive

- Refusing or not following through with services to avoid angering the abuser

- Using or abusing substances as an "escape" or to numb physical pain

- Lying about the abuser's criminal activity or abuse of the children to avoid a possible attack

- Trying to improve the relationship or finding help for the perpetrator

Although these protective strategies act as coping and survival mechanisms for victims, they are frequently misinterpreted by laypersons and professionals who view the victim's behavior as uncooperative, ineffective, or neglectful. Because victims are very familiar with their partner's pattern of behavior, they can help the caseworker in developing a safety plan that is effective for both the victim and the children, especially when exploring options not previously considered.

Chapter 23

Nature and Scope of Violence against Women

- Women experience more intimate partner violence than do men:
  22.1 percent of surveyed women, compared with 7.4 percent of
  surveyed men, reported they were physically assaulted by a current or former spouse, cohabiting partner, boyfriend, girlfriend,
  or date in their lifetime; 1.9 percent of surveyed women and 3.4
  percent of surveyed men reported experiencing such violence in
  the previous 12 months. Approximately 1.3 million women and
  835,000 men are physically assaulted by an intimate partner
  annually in the United States.

- The National Violence Against Women Survey (NVAWS) found
  that 17.6 percent of surveyed women and three percent of surveyed men were raped at some point in their lifetime.

- Rape prevalence statistics by race and ethnicity illustrate no
  statistically significant differences between minority and non-
  minority women—19 percent of minority women and 17.9 percent of non-minority women reported a rape at some point in
  their lifetime. Examining rape prevalence statistics by specific
  racial and ethnic backgrounds, however, shows that American
  Indian/Alaska Native women are significantly more likely than
  women from all other backgrounds to have been raped at some
  point in their lifetime.

Excerpted from "Selected Research Results on Violence Against Women," U.S.
Department of Justice (DOJ), November 2007.

- Most victims, male and female, identified in the NVAWS were raped by just one person during their lifetime. Among female rape victims, 78.2 percent were raped by one person, 13.5 percent were raped by two people, and 8.3 percent were raped by three or more people. For male rape victims, 83.3 percent were raped by one person, 12.1 percent were raped by two people, and 4.6 percent were raped by three or more people.

- Women are significantly more likely than men to be injured during an assault: 31.5 percent of female rape victims, compared with 16.1 percent of male rape victims, reported being injured during their most recent rape; 39.0 percent of female physical assault victims, compared with 24.8 percent of male physical assault victims, reported being injured during their most recent physical assault.

- Stalking is more prevalent than previously thought: 8.1 percent of surveyed women and 2.2 percent of surveyed men reported being stalked at some time in their life; 1.0 percent of women surveyed and 0.4 percent of men surveyed reported being stalked in the 12 months preceding the survey. Approximately one million women and 371,000 men are stalked annually in the United States.

- Fifty-four percent of female victims and 71 percent of male victims were first raped before their 18th birthday—29.4 percent of female victims and 16.6 percent of male victims were 18 to 24 years old when they were first raped, and 16.6 percent of female victims and 12.3 percent of male victims were age 25 or older. Although most rape victims identified by NVAWS were under 18 when they were first raped, the survey found that more women were raped as adults than as children or adolescents.

- Intimate partner homicides make up 40–50 percent of all murders of women in the United States according to city or state specific databases. In 70–80 percent of intimate partner homicides, no matter which partner was killed, the man physically abused the woman before the murder.

- A survey of college women found that 2.8 percent of the sample had experienced either a completed rape (1.7 percent) or an attempted rape (1.1 percent). The study also found that this rate is approximately 11 times higher than that using a National Crime Victimization Survey (NCVS)-type survey.

- The majority of more than 36 studies reviewed indicate that approximately 30–60 percent of children whose mothers are being abused are themselves likely to be abused.

- Most domestic violence offenders with prior official criminal records have also been involved in nonviolent criminal behavior. Data from the Spousal Abuse Replication Program (SARP) illustrates a mix of offenders who escalated and deescalated the severity of their attacks over time.

Causes, Correlates, and Consequences of Violence against Women

- In the United States from 1976 to 1996, while legal advocacy and hotlines increased sharply, rates of homicides by intimate partners dropped about 30 percent.

- A study of intimate partner homicide found that for about one in five women, the fatal or life-threatening incident was the first physical violence they had experienced from their partner. This study also found that a woman's attempt to leave was the precipitating factor in 45 percent of the murders of a woman by a man.

- Women who had children by age 21 were twice as likely to be victims of domestic violence as women who were not mothers. Men who had fathered children by age 21 were more than three times as likely to be perpetrators of abuse as men who were not fathers.

- While alcohol is not the cause of violence against women, there appears to be a significant relationship between male perpetrator problem drinking and violence against intimate female partners. Findings also suggest that severe problem drinking of alcohol increases the risk for lethal and violent victimization of women in violent intimate partner relationships. More than two-thirds of the homicide and attempted homicide offenders used alcohol, drugs, or both during the incident; less than one-fourth of the victims did.

- A longitudinal cohort of sexually assaulted and not-sexually assaulted women found that 68 percent of physically abused women also report sexual assault. Furthermore, of the 148 sexual assault victims identified in the study: 27 percent of the women began drinking or increased their use of alcohol, illicit drugs, or nicotine; 20 percent became pregnant; and 15 percent contracted a sexually transmitted disease following the sexual assault. Eighty-eight percent of the victims' children were exposed to violence against their mothers, with 64 percent witnessing the abuse by age three. Only 30 percent of those children received counseling.

- Sexual assault or forced sex occurs in approximately 40–45 percent of battering relationships. Sexual assault is defined as sexual acts coerced by physical force or threat thereof or by power differential such as those that would exist between adults and children, employers and employees, or professors and students.

- Child sexual abuse before the age of 13 is not by itself a risk factor for adult sexual or domestic violence victimization, but girls who were victimized both before turning 12 and then again as adolescents between the ages of 13 and 17 were at much greater risk of both types of victimization as adults than any other women (Siegel and Williams, 2001, 2004). While this study was conducted among an urban sample of women (primarily black), similar results were found in a sample of college women. Women who experienced physical and sexual abuse in childhood and adolescence were most likely to suffer abuse in college. Moreover, college women who were physically or sexually abused as children but not as adolescents, were not more likely to experience abuse in college (White and Smith, 2004). Data from the NVAWS illustrate that women who were raped as minors were twice as likely to report being raped as adults—18.3 percent who were raped before age 18 also reported being raped after turning 18 compared to 8.7 percent who did not report being raped before age 18.

- Among families referred for child welfare investigations for child maltreatment, lifetime prevalence of domestic violence is 44.8 percent, past year prevalence is 29 percent, and caregiver depression is associated with increased prevalence.

- Family violence researchers agree that low income is a risk factor for partner violence. It is not only severe poverty and its associated stressors that increase the risk for partner violence; in addition, the higher income is, the lower are reported intimate violence rates (Carlson et al., 2003). Having a need for domestic violence services significantly impaired women in finding employment under welfare reform. Reductions in Aid to Families with Dependent Children (AFDC) benefits have also been associated with an increase in intimate partner homicide.

- Mental and emotional distress faced by women experiencing serious abuse is overwhelming. Almost half the women reporting serious domestic violence also meet the criteria for major depression; one-fourth for posttraumatic stress disorder (PTSD), and 28 percent had symptom scores as high as a group of persons entering outpatient treatment.

- Intimate partner violence is more severe and occurs more often in economically disadvantaged neighborhoods. Women living in disadvantaged communities are more than twice as likely to be victims of intimate violence compared to women living in more advantaged communities. Therefore, as African-Americans are more likely to live in disadvantaged communities and face more economic distress, they experience higher rates of intimate violence compared with whites. When comparing African-Americans and whites of similar income levels, the levels of intimate violence are similar.

- A longitudinal study of extremely poor women found that women with low self-esteem were more likely to be victimized by abusive partners. Although these women had a higher lifetime prevalence of intimate partner violence, most of their experiences with violence were episodic and limited over time. Intimate partner violence was predictive of subsequent drug, but not alcohol abuse, after controlling for factors of interest. Those women with a history of adult partner violence had almost three times the odds of using illegal drugs during the subsequent study years than women who had not experienced partner violence as adults.

- Homeless women are far more likely to experience violence of all sorts than American women in general, ranging from two to four times more likely, depending on the violence type. Approximately one homeless woman in four is homeless mainly because of her experiences with violence.

Chapter 24

Male Victims of Violence

Why It Matters

Men, as well as women, are victimized by violence. Sexual abuse and rape create substantial physical and psychological harm to male victims and perpetuate the cycle of violence.[1] Men and boys are less likely to report the violence and seek services due to the following challenges: the stigma of being a male victim, the perceived failure to conform to the macho stereotype, the fear of not being believed, the denial of victim status, and the lack of support from society, family members, and friends.[2]

Did you know?

- One out of fourteen men has been physically assaulted by a current or former spouse, live-in partner, boyfriend or girlfriend, or date at some point in their lives.[3]

- It is estimated that 835,000 men are physically assaulted by an intimate partner annually.[3]

- In terms of victimization, intimate partner violence against men is overwhelmingly committed in same-sex relationships rather than in heterosexual relationships.[4]

The Effects of Violence

- According to the National Center for Victims of Crime,[5] men experience many of the same psychological reactions to violence as women. These include the following:
  - Guilt, shame, and humiliation
  - Anger and anxiety
  - Depression
  - Withdrawal from relationships
- According to a study published by the American Medical Association, boys are less likely to report sexual abuse due to fear, anxiety associated with being perceived as gay, the desire to appear self-reliant, and the will to be independent. [6]
- In a male-perpetrated assault, the male victim is more likely to be strangled, beaten with closed fists, and threatened with guns or other weapons.[7]
- In a female-perpetrated assault, the male victim is more likely to be kicked, slapped, or have objects thrown at him.[7]
- Men who witnessed domestic violence as children are twice as likely to abuse their own partners and children than those who did not witness domestic violence.[8]

Perpetrators

- 86% of adult men who were physically assaulted were physically assaulted by a man.[3]
- 70% of adult men who were raped were raped by a man.[3]
- 56% of adult men who reported being physically assaulted were assaulted by a stranger.[3]

Intimate Partner Violence

- 16% of adult men who reported being raped and/or physically assaulted were assaulted by a current or former spouse, live-in partner, boyfriend or girlfriend, or date.[3]
- 40% of gay and bisexual men will experience abuse at the hands of an intimate partner.[9]

- In the National Violence Against Women Survey, approximately 23% of men reported being raped, physically assaulted, and/or stalked by a male intimate partner; 7% of men reported such violence by a wife or female cohabitant.[3]

- According to a Bureau of Justice Statistics 2004 report, 5.5% of male homicide victims were murdered by a spouse, ex-spouse, boyfriend, or girlfriend.[10]

- Women committing lethal acts of violence against their male partners are 7–10 times more likely than men to act in self-defense.[11]

- Because men are more likely to be financially independent and less likely to experience fear upon leaving a violent relationship, men are less likely to seek emergency shelter, and therefore do not take advantage of other domestic violence services that shelters provide.[7]

Sexual Abuse and Rape

- One in 33 men have been the victim of a completed or attempted rape.[3]

- 94% of the perpetrators of sexual abuse against boys are men.[12]

- One in six boys will be sexually abused by age 16.[13]

- 66% of men surveyed in the National Violence Against Women Survey said that they were physically assaulted as a child by an adult caretaker.[3]

- 21% of inmates in seven midwestern prisons had experienced at least one episode of pressured or forced sex during their incarceration.[14]

Types of Abuse[15]

- **Physical abuse** is the use of physical force against another in a way that injures that person or puts the victim at risk of being injured. Physical abuse ranges from physical restraint to murder and may include pushing, throwing, tripping, slapping, hitting, kicking, punching, grabbing, chocking, shaking, and so forth.

- **Emotional/psychological abuse** is any use of words, tone, action, or lack of action meant to control, hurt, or demean another person. Emotional abuse typically includes ridicule, intimidation, or coercion. Verbal abuse is included in this category.

- **Sexual abuse** is any forced or coerced sexual act or behavior motivated to acquire power and control over the partner. It includes forced sexual contact and contact that demeans, humiliates, or instigates feelings of shame or vulnerability, particularly in regards to the body, sexual performance, or sexuality.

- **Financial abuse** is the use or misuse of the financial or monetary resources of the partner or of the partnership without the partner's freely given consent. It can include preventing the partner from working or jeopardizing his or her employment so as to prevent them from gaining financial independence.

- **Identity abuse** is using personal characteristics to demean, manipulate, and control the partner.

- **Spiritual abuse** is using the victim's religious or spiritual beliefs to manipulate them. It can include preventing the victim from practicing their beliefs or ridiculing his or her beliefs.

Sources

1. Felson, R.B., and Pare, P.P. (2005) "The Reporting of Domestic Violence and Sexual Assault by Nonstrangers to the Police." *Journal of Marriage and Family, 67*(3), 597–610.

2. FORGE: For Ourselves: Reworking Gender Expression. Accessed July 2007 http://www.forge-forward.org.

3. Thoennes, N., and Tjaden, P. (2000) *Full Report of the Prevalence, Incidence, and Consequences of Violence Against Women*; Findings from the National Violence Against Women Survey. National Institute of Justice and Centers for Disease Control and Prevention.

4. Stephan S. Owen and Tod W. Burke, *An Exploration of the Prevalence of Domestic Violence in Same-Sex Relationships*, 95 Psychological Reports, Aug. 2004, at 129.

5. The National Center for Victims of Crime (1997) *Male Rape*. Accessed July 2007. http://www.ncvc.org.

6. Holmes, W.C., and Slap, G.B. (1998) "Sexual Abuse of Boys: Definitions, Prevalence, Sequelae, and Manage." *Journal of the American Medical Association*, 280(21), 1855–1862.

7.   Hamberger, L.K., and Guse, C. (2002) "Men's and Women's Use of Intimate Partner Violence in Clinical Samples." *Violence Against Women, 8*(11), 1301–1331.

8.   Strauss, M., et al. (1990). *Physical Violence in American Families: Risk Factors and Adaptations to Violence in 8,145 Families*. New Brunswick: Transaction Publishers.

9.   Greenwod, G.L. (2002) "Battering and Victimization among a Probability Based Sample of Men who have Sex with Men." *American Journal of Public Health*, 92, 1964–1969.

10. Fox, J.A., and Zawitz, M.W. (2004). *Homicide Trends in the U.S.: Trends by Gender*. Bureau of Justice Statistics: Accessed July 2007 http://www.ojp.usdoj.gov/bjs/homicide/gender.htm.

11. Saunders, D.G. (2002). "Are Physical Assaults by Wives and Girlfriends a Major Social Problem?" *Violence Against Women* 8(12), 1424–1448.

12. Snyder, H.N. (2000). "Sexual Assault of Young Children as Reported to Law Enforcement: Victim, Incident and Offender Characteristics." Bureau of Justice Statistics. Accessed July 2007 http://www.ojp.usdoj.gov/bjs/pub/pdf/saycrle.pdf.

13. Hopper, J. (2006). *Sexual Abuse of Males: Prevalence, Possible Lasting Effects, and Resources*. Accessed July 2007 http://www.jimhopper.com/male-ab.

14. Struckman-Johnson, C., and Struckman-Johnson, D. (2000) "Sexual Coercion Rates in Seven Midwestern Prisons for Men." *The Prison Journal*, 80(4), 379–390.

15. Gay Men's Domestic Violence Project. Types of Abuse. Accessed July 26, 2007 http://www.gmdvp.org/domestic_vio/gen_info/dynam3.htm.

16. HelpGuide. *Domestic Violence and Abuse*. Accessed July 2007 from www.helpguide.org/mental/domestic_violence_abuse_types_signs_causes_effects.htm.

For More Information

National Child Abuse Hotline
15757 N. 78th St.
Scottsdale, AZ 85260
Toll-Free: 800-4-A-CHILD (22-4453)

Toll-Free TDD: 800-222-4453
Phone: 480-922-8212
Fax: 480-922-7061
Website: http://www.region4wib.org/ChildhelpUSA.htm
E-mail: info@childhelpusa.org

National Domestic Violence Hotline
P.O. Box 161810
Austin, TX 78716
Toll-Free Hotline: 800-799-SAFE (7233)
Toll-Free TTY: 800-787-3224
Website: http://www.ndvh.org

National Sexual Assault Hotline
Rape, Abuse & Incest National Network (RAINN)
2000 L Street, NW, Suite 406
Washington, DC 20036
Toll-Free: 800-656-HOPE (4673)
Phone: 202-544-3064
Fax: 202-544-3556
Website: http://www.rainn.org
E-mail: info@rainn.org

Chapter 25

Domestic Violence among African Americans

Domestic Violence: Is It a Black Thing?

Activists in the growing movement to support battered African-American women agree on what's needed to stem domestic violence: more services that are culturally informed and integrated into victims' communities.

"Color blindness is not what you need if you're trying to serve diverse communities," says Oliver Williams, executive director of the Institute on Domestic Violence in the African-American Community at the University of Minnesota in Minneapolis. "The trend is toward an increase in community-based, faith-based, and grassroots services."

While the battered women's movement has long striven to serve all women, few projects can identify specific programs designed to reach out to diverse communities. That can be a barrier to safety for black women, who tend to reach out for help through informal networks in their communities, such as a church, rather than consulting a shelter or hotline, according to experts.

African-American women face a higher risk for experiencing domestic violence than other women, according to the most recent data from the Justice Department. In fact, they are more than twice as likely to die at the hands of a spouse or a boyfriend. They are also at greater risk of more severe violence, according to the Centers for

Disease Control in Atlanta and the Bureau of Justice Statistics (BJS) in Washington, DC.

"When you're talking about African-American women, you're talking about everything bad about family violence, and then some," says Tonya Lovelace, executive director of the Women of Color Network, a project of the National Resource Center on Domestic Violence based in Harrisburg, Pennsylvania. "The way that communities of color experience violence is affected by our history, and by other issues." Some behavior can be grouped by race, but differences can be deceiving, Williams said.

"Black women are more likely to leave than other women, but they are also more likely to return," he said. "A lot of the reasons may speak more to poverty and a lack of resources, because a woman may just not have a different place to go."

Organizations such as Atlanta's Black Church and Domestic Violence Institute, Williams' institute, and the National Resource Center on Domestic Violence's Women of Color Network are all engaged in training domestic violence groups and community service agencies in each others' work.

Much of the funding comes through the federal Violence Against Women Act, and much of the activity is coordinated and supported by the Violence Against Women Office at the U.S. Department of Justice. National groups such as the National Network to End Domestic Violence in Washington, DC, and the National Resource Center on Domestic Violence coordinate and facilitate the work.

While scholars and activists agree that higher rates of poverty among African-Americans probably shape some statistics about violence, they are quick to point out that higher incomes do not immunize against domestic violence.

An October 2006 article in *Essence* magazine, for example, details how Prince George's County, Maryland, the wealthiest predominantly black county in the nation, has a high rate of intimate partner homicide. According to the Maryland Network Against Domestic Violence, 48 people, mostly women, died there between 2001 and 2006 as a result of domestic violence, second only to Baltimore County which had 72 deaths.

One of the starkest realities for African-American women is their vulnerability to homicide. The risk of violence is higher for women in bigger cities, according to the BJS.

Homicide is the second leading cause of death for black women between the ages of 15 and 24, according to the Centers for Disease Control. Only young black men have a higher homicide rate, and only black men have a higher rate of intimate partner homicide than black women, BJS reported.

Barriers to seeking help are believed to contribute to the higher rate of homicide for both women and men because violence has escalated to a greater degree before a woman can reach safety, scholars and activists generally agree. The homicide rate for black men has dropped more than for black women in recent decades, according to federal statistics.

All the factors that contribute to greater violence probably explain the higher intimate partner homicide rate of black men, Lovelace said. "Black women get arrested more, we get convicted more, and we have had fewer places to go. The statistics don't account for self-defense," she said.

One of the biggest roadblocks to safety, says Tricia Bent-Goodley, a professor at Howard University, is the troubled, violent histories many black communities have with the police and social service agencies. That provides one more cultural barrier to seeking police intervention, even though African-American women report intimate partner violence to the police more often—in 66.4 percent of incidents—than other women.

In addition, black women face a greater likelihood of being arrested along with a perpetrator, and their children are more likely to end up in foster care when authorities are involved, Bent-Goodley said in a training webcast last year.

"If I'm being battered, the decision to pick up the phone to call for help is different for me," Lovelace said. "There are more black men incarcerated than there are in college, so that makes it a bigger burden, and I have to question whether he will be brutalized."

Chapter 26

Barriers That Prevent Asian and Pacific Islander Women from Seeking Help When Abused

Domestic violence is perpetuated by cultural beliefs and norms based on the devaluation of women. It is often legitimized, obscured, or denied by familial and social institutions.

Intimate partner violence is a pattern of behaviors that includes physical, sexual, verbal, emotional, economic, and/or psychological abuse used by adults or adolescents against (current or former) intimate partners, and sometimes against other family members. Domestic violence is also marked by a climate of fear in the home. It occurs in all communities regardless of race, class, faith, immigration status, education, gender identity, or sexual orientation. Asians and Pacific Islanders are no exception. This chapter has been compiled to raise awareness about what Asian and Pacific Islander (API) women are reporting and suffering, to conceptualize the available data, and to influence the development of culturally specific interventions. Only within the past two decades, have researchers and advocates begun to gather data on domestic violence within API communities in the United States. Their findings reveal how cultural, linguistic, socioeconomic, and political barriers prevent API women from seeking help. The magnitude of the problem is therefore considerably greater than studies indicate.

"Fact Sheet: Domestic Violence in Asian Communities," © 2005 Asian & Pacific Islander Institute on Domestic Violence/Asian & Pacific Islander American Health Forum (www.apiahf.org/apidvinstitute). Reprinted with permission.

Extent of the Problem

A compilation of community-based studies points to the high prevalence of domestic violence in Asian communities:

- 41–60% of respondents have reported experiencing domestic violence (physical and/or sexual) during their lifetime.[1]

In a telephone survey of a nationally representative sample of 8,000 women and 8,000 men from all ethnic backgrounds conducted from November 1995 to May 1996:[2]

- 12.8% of Asian and Pacific Islander women reported experiencing physical assault by an intimate partner at least once during their lifetime; 3.8% reported having been raped. The rate of physical assault was lower than those reported by whites (21.3%); African-Americans (26.3%); Hispanic, of any race, (21.2%); mixed race (27.0%); and American Indians and Alaskan Natives (30.7%). The low rate for Asian and Pacific Islander women may be attributed to underreporting.

The National Asian Women's Health Organization (NAWHO) interviewed 336 Asian American women aged 18–34 who reside the San Francisco and Los Angeles areas, via telephone (NAWHO study, hereinafter):[3]

- 16% of the respondents reported having experienced "pressure to have sex without their consent by an intimate partner."

- 27% experienced emotional abuse by an intimate partner.

Domestic Violence in Specific Asian Communities

Cambodian

In a study conducted by the Asian Task Force Against Domestic Violence in Boston, using a self-administered questionnaire at ethnic fairs (Asian Task Force study, hereinafter):[4]

- 44–47% of Cambodians interviewed said they knew a woman who experienced domestic violence.

Chinese

In a random telephone survey of 262 Chinese men and women in Los Angeles County:[5]

- 18.1% of respondents reported experiencing "minor physical violence" by a spouse or intimate partner within their lifetime, and 8% of respondents reported "severe physical violence" experienced during their lifetime. ["Minor to severe" categories were based on the researcher's classification criteria.]

- More acculturated respondents (as assessed by the researchers) were twice as likely to have been victims of severe physical violence. [Although the author states, "It is possible that traditional cultural values serve as a protective buffer against stressors engendered by immigration" (p. 263), higher rates among more acculturated respondents may be due to their increased likelihood to report abuse.]

Filipina

In a survey conducted by the Immigrant Women's Task Force of the Coalition for Immigrant and Refugee Rights and Services:[6]

- 20% of 54 undocumented Filipina women living in the San Francisco Bay Area reported having experienced some form of domestic violence, including physical, emotional, or sexual abuse, either in their country of origin or in the United States.

Japanese

In a face-to-face interview study of a random sample of 211 Japanese immigrant women and Japanese American women in Los Angeles County conducted in 1995 (Yoshihama study, hereinafter):

- 61% reported some form of physical, emotional, or sexual partner violence that they considered abusive—including culturally demeaning practices such as overturning a dining table, or throwing liquid at a woman—sometime prior to the interview.[7]

- 52% reported having experienced physical violence during their lifetime. When the probability that some women who have not been victimized at the time of the interview, but may be abused at a later date is calculated, 57% of women are estimated to experience a partner's physical violence by age 49.[8]

- No significant generational differences were found in the age-adjusted risk of experiencing intimate physical, sexual, or emotional violence.[9]

Korean

In a study of 256 Korean men from randomly selected Korean households in Chicago and in Queens (which then had the largest Korean population on the East Coast) in 1993:[10]

- 18% of the respondents reported committing at least one of the following acts of physical violence within the past year: throwing something, pushing, grabbing, shoving, or slapping their wife.

- 6.3% of the men committed what the researcher classified as "severe violence" (kicking, biting, hitting with a fist, threatening with a gun or knife, shooting, or stabbing).

- 33% of "male-dominated relationships" experienced at least one incident of domestic violence during the year, whereas only 12% of "egalitarian" relationships did. [Researchers classified couples into four types of relationships—egalitarian, divided power, male-dominated, and female-dominated—based on the respondents' answers about how the couple makes decisions.]

- Nearly 39% of husbands who were categorized as experiencing "high stress" perpetrated domestic violence during the past year, whereas one out of 66 husbands categorized as experiencing "low stress" did so. [This correlation does not necessarily mean that stress causes or leads to domestic violence. Women and non-abusive men are also exposed to high stress and do not resort to domestic violence.]

In a survey of a convenience sample of 214 Korean women and 121 Korean men in the San Francisco Bay Area conducted in 2000 by Shimtuh, a project serving Korean women in crisis (Shimtuh study, hereinafter):[11]

- 42% of the respondents said they knew of a Korean woman who experienced physical violence from a husband or boyfriend.

- About 50% of the respondents knew someone who suffered regular emotional abuse.

A 1986 study involving face-to-face interviews of a convenience sample of 150 Korean women living in Chicago found that:[12]

- 60% reported experiencing physical abuse by an intimate partner sometime in their lives.

- 36.7% reported sexual violence by an intimate partner some-time in their lives.

South Asian[13]

The Raj and Silverman study of 160 South Asian women (who were married or in a heterosexual relationship), recruited through community outreach methods such as flyers, snowball sampling, and referrals in Greater Boston, found that:[14]

- 40.8% of the participants reported that they had been physically and/or sexually abused in some way by their current male partners in their lifetime; 36.9% reported having been victimized in the past year.

- 65% of the women reporting physical abuse also reported sexual abuse, and almost a third (30.4%) of those reporting sexual abuse reported injuries, some requiring medical attention.

- No significant difference was found in the prevalence of domestic violence between arranged marriages [typically refers to marriages arranged by parents or relatives of each member of the couple] and non-arranged marriages.[15]

Vietnamese

In a study of 30 Vietnamese women recruited from a civic association that serves Vietnamese women in Boston:[16]

- 47% reported intimate physical violence sometime in their lifetime.

- 30% reported intimate physical violence in the past year.

Types of Abuse

Project AWARE (Asian Women Advocating Respect and Empowerment) in Washington, DC, conducted an anonymous survey in 2000–2001 to examine the experiences of abuse, service needs, and barriers to service among Asian women (Project AWARE study, hereinafter). Using a snowball method, a convenience sample of 178 Asian women was recruited:[17]

- 81.1% of the women reported experiencing at least one form of intimate partner violence (domination/controlling/psychological, physical, and/or sexual abuse as categorized by the researchers) in the past year.

- 67% "occasionally" experienced some form of domination/controlling/psychological abuse; 48% experienced it "frequently" in the past year.

- 32% experienced physical or sexual abuse at least "occasionally" during the past year.

- Of the 23 women who reported not having experienced intimate partner violence themselves, more than half (64%) said they knew of an Asian friend who had experienced intimate partner violence. Smaller proportions of respondents reported that their mothers (9%) and sisters (11%) had experienced intimate partner violence.

- 28.5% of the survey participants knew of a woman who was being abused by her in-laws.

Service Utilization

- Berkeley, California: Over 1,000 telephone requests per year were made to Narika, a Bay Area domestic violence help line for South Asian women in 1999 and 2000. Callers included victims of domestic violence, friends and family members calling on the victim's behalf, and other service agencies and providers requesting information and assistance.[18]

- San Francisco, California: Over 4,000 Asian women and children from across the country utilize a range of services provided by Asian Women's Shelter each year.[19] AWS turns away 75% of the battered women who call for shelter because of lack of shelter space.[20]

- Chicago, Illinois: In 2000, 28 API women used shelter services at Apna Ghar, a domestic violence program for South Asian women in Chicago; 106 received legal assistance, counseling, and case management services; and 253 API women called Apna Ghar's hotline. In 2001, the numbers were 31, 142, and 230 respectively.[21]

- New Jersey: 160 South Asian women received services between July 1996 and June 1997 from Manavi, a service program and shelter for South Asian women. The number of women receiving assistance increased to 252 (July 1997–June 1998) and 258 (July 1998–June 1999).[22]

- New York: Over 3,000 women who are abused by their partners (including being bitten, punched, stabbed, shot, threatened with knives or guns, or denied food and money) call the New York Asian Women's Center for help annually.[23]

- Austin, Texas: Saheli (a domestic violence program for South Asian women) received 388 calls in 2000 and assisted 68 cases, providing counseling, referral, and advocacy.[24]

Attitudes toward Domestic Violence

In a telephone survey of a national random sample of women and men conducted in 1992 by the Family Violence Prevention Fund of San Francisco where 18% of the respondents were Asian (156 Asian women, 161 Asian men):[25]

- Asian women tended to be less likely to categorize various interactions as domestic violence than women of other ethnic groups.

The Asian Task Force study found that:[26]

- Older Chinese respondents were more tolerant of the use of force and more likely to justify a husband's use of violence against his wife. Immigration status and level of education were not associated with the likelihood of justifying the husband's use of violence against his wife.

- The average score for all respondents on male privilege was 8.5 out of 24; for Vietnamese respondents it was 12 out of 24 (the highest score amongst the different ethnic groups in the study). The higher the score, the more an individual believes in male privilege. The average score of 8.5 is a low score indicating that overall, respondents do not believe that a husband has the right to discipline his wife, can expect to have sex with his wife whenever he wants it, is the ruler of his home, or that some wives deserve beatings.

- Cambodian participants of a focus group felt that "surviving the genocide in their native country has left people more vulnerable to stress and depression, which may contribute to domestic violence" in their community.

In a population-based study of a random sample of 211 women of Japanese descent living in Los Angeles in 1995:

- 71% of the respondents reported that their Japanese background influenced their experiences with their partner's violence. They identified the following aspects of their Japanese backgrounds as having influenced the way they responded to their partners' violence: conflict avoidance, the value of endurance, acceptance of male domination, the value of collective family welfare, and an aversion to seeking help.[27]

In a telephone survey of 31 randomly selected Chinese men and women in the San Gabriel Valley in Los Angeles County:[28]

- Respondents (men and women) overall did not agree with the use of domestic violence as an effective means of solving problems.

- Respondents (15 women and 16 men) tended to agree that physical and sexual aggression (slapping, pushing, throwing objects, and insisting a spouse have sex) was an indicator of violence between spouses. However, they were less likely to consider psychological aggression or financial abuse as indicators of violence between spouses.

- Respondents were more likely to implicate individual factors (for example: inability to control one's temper, inability to talk to one's spouse) and environmental factors (job pressure, acculturative stress, alcohol) as the causes of domestic violence, than structural factors (women working outside the home, breakdown of traditional family roles) and cultural factors (women's lower status in Chinese culture, belief that men are the heads of households).

In a study of 20 Vietnamese women (ten were known to be in physically abusive relationships and another ten were not known to be battered) conducted by Bui and Morash in 1999 (Bui and Morash study, hereinafter):[29]

- 70% of the women reported that their husbands believed that men should dominate women, while 90% of the women believed that men and women should have equal rights in the family.

In the NAWHO study of 336 Asian American women aged 18–34:[30]

- 18% of the respondents did not believe that rape occurs between people who are in a relationship.

Attitudes to Seeking Help or Intervention

In the Project AWARE study:[31]

- 45% of the Asian women surveyed reported that they or other Asian women they knew to be abused did "nothing" to protect themselves from abusive events. (The report's authors noted that "Doing nothing can serve as a strategy of resistance in an attempt [to] avoid or lessen abuse.")

- 34% sought help from their family, and 32% sought help from friends. Only 16% reported that they or the person they knew to be abused, called the police, and 9% actually obtained help from an agency.

- Although the majority of women (78%) who confided in someone about their experience of abuse felt better afterwards, 35% indicated that they felt ashamed.

In the Asian Task Force study:[32]

- 29% of Korean respondents said a woman being abused should not tell anyone about abuse; higher than the rates for Cambodian (22%), Chinese (18%), South Asian (5%), and Vietnamese (9%) respondents.

- 82% of South Asian respondents indicated that a battered woman should turn to a friend for help, whereas only 44% of Cambodian, 37% of Chinese, 41% of Korean, and 29% of Vietnamese respondents agreed with this statement.

- 74% of South Asian respondents supported a battered woman calling the police for help, whereas 47% of Cambodian, 52% of Chinese, 27% of Korean, and 49% of Vietnamese respondents agreed.

The Raj and Silverman study of 160 South Asian women found that:[33]

- 11% of South Asian women reporting intimate partner violence indicated receiving counseling support services for domestic abuse.

- Only 3.1% of the abused South Asian women in the study had ever obtained a restraining order against an abusive partner.

This rate is substantially lower than that reported in a study of women in Massachusetts, in which over 33% of women who reported intimate partner violence in the past five years had obtained a restraining order.

In the Yoshihama study of Japanese immigrant and Japanese American women:[34]

- U.S.-born respondents, compared to their Japan-born counterparts, were more likely (83% versus 43%) to seek help from friends; to confront their partners (86% versus 68%); and to find these methods more effective.

- Japan-born respondents were more likely to minimize the seriousness of the situation as a strategy to cope with abuse (90%) than U.S.-born respondents (58%); and rated this strategy as more helpful than did the U.S.-born respondents (3.1 versus 2.3 on a four-point scale).

- Although only 19% of women who had experienced partner violence (both U.S.-born and Japan-born respondents) used counseling, those who used counseling reported a high rate of satisfaction with it (3.3 out of 4 points).

In the Bui and Morash study:[35]

- Most women (90%) did not view family violence as a private matter and favored governmental intervention. (Despite this belief, few women called the police when they were abused due to language barriers and fears of husbands being arrested and subjected to racial discrimination.)

Abuse Witnessed or Experienced as a Child

In the Asian Task Force study:[36]

- 69% of the overall respondents reported being hit regularly as children. The proportion of respondents who were hit regularly by their parents as children varied slightly across ethnic groups: Cambodian (70%), Chinese (61%), Koreans (80%), South Asians (79%), and Vietnamese (72%).

- 27% of the Vietnamese respondents witnessed their fathers regularly hit their mothers; whereas 15% saw their mothers regularly hit their fathers.

250

- 30% of Korean respondents reported witnessing their fathers regularly hit their mothers, and 17% reported that their mothers regularly hit their fathers.

In the Yoshihama study of Japanese immigrant and Japanese American women in Los Angeles County:

- 13% of the respondents reported having experienced physical and/or sexual abuse during childhood.[37]

- 36.4% of the first generation respondents (those born in Japan and immigrated to the U.S. after age 13), and 13.2% of the 1st, 2nd, 3rd, and 4th generation respondents, reported that their father abused their mother.[38]

In the Shimtuh study in the San Francisco Bay Area:[39]

- 33% of the respondents (women and men) recalled their fathers hitting their mothers at least once.

Domestic Violence-Related Homicides

- 31% (16 out of 51 cases) of women killed in domestic violence-related deaths from 1993–1997 in California's Santa Clara County were Asian,[40] although Asians comprised only 17.5% of the county's population.

- 13% of women and children killed in domestic violence-related homicides in Massachusetts in 1991 were Asian, although Asians represented only 2.4% of the population in the state.[41]

- 6% of women killed by their abusers in Massachusetts in 1998 were Asian, a four-year low. During the same year requests for services to the Asian Task Force Against Domestic Violence increased by 36%.[42]

- 63 separate reports of murder and attempted murder of South Asian women in the U.S. and Canada between 1981–2000 were compiled from ethnic and local newspapers (not an exhaustive compilation). Although the majority of victims were women, the women's children and relatives were also killed in these domestic-violence related homicides, some of which were murder-suicides.[43]

- Seven domestic violence related homicides were reported in 2000 in Hawaii.[44] According to the Domestic Violence Clearinghouse and Legal Hotline, five of the seven women killed were of Filipina descent;[45] a disproportionately high rate given that Filipinos represent only 12.3% of the total population of Hawaii.[46]

References

1. This estimate is based on studies of women's experiences of domestic violence conducted among different Asian ethnic groups in the U.S.; cited in the *Fact Sheet on Domestic Violence in Asian Communities* compiled by the Asian and Pacific Islander Institute on Domestic Violence. The low end of the range is from a study by A. Raj and J. Silverman, Intimate partner violence against South-Asian women in Greater Boston *J Am Med Women's Assoc.* 2002; 57(2): 111–114. The high end of the range is from a study by M. Yoshihama, Domestic violence against women of Japanese descent in Los Angeles: Two methods of estimating prevalence. *Violence Against Women*. 1999; 5(8): 869–897.

2. Tjaden P, Thoennes N. *Extent, Nature, and Consequences of Intimate Partner Violence: Research Report.* Washington, DC: National Institute of Justice and the Centers for Disease Control and Prevention; July 2000. Available at: http://www.ncjrs .org/txtfiles1/nij/181867.txt, or 800-851-3420 (877-712-9279, TTY).

3. National Asian Women's Health Organization. *Silence, Not an Option!* San Francisco, CA: Author; 2002.

4. Yoshioka MR, Dang Q. *Asian Family Violence Report: A Study of the Cambodian, Chinese, Korean, South Asian, and Vietnamese Communities in Massachusetts.* Boston: Asian Task Force Against Domestic Violence, Inc.; 2000. Available at: www .atask.org.

5. Yick AG. Predictors of physical spousal/intimate violence in Chinese American families. *J Fam Violence*, 2000; 15(3): 249–267.

6. Hoagland C, Rosen K. *Dreams Lost, Dreams Found: Undocumented Women in the Land of Opportunity.* San Francisco, CA: Coalition for Immigrant and Refugee Rights and Services, Immigrant Women's Task Force; Spring 1990.

7. Yoshihama M. Domestic violence against women of Japanese descent in Los Angeles: Two methods of estimating prevalence. *Violence Against Women.* 1999; 5(8): 869–897.

8. Yoshihama M, Gillespie B. Age adjustment and recall bias in the analysis of domestic violence data: Methodological improvement through the application of survival analysis methods. *J Fam Violence.* 2002; 17(3): 199–221.

9. Yoshihama M, Horrocks J. Post–traumatic stress symptoms and victimization among Japanese American women. *J Consult Clin Psychol.* 2002; 70(2): 205–215.

10. Kim JY, Sung K. Conjugal violence in Korean American families: A residue of the cultural tradition. *J Fam Violence.* 2000; 15(4): 331–345.

11. Shimtuh, Korean American Domestic Violence Program. *Korean American Community of the Bay Area Domestic Violence Needs Assessment Report.* Oakland, CA: Author; 2000.

12. Song–Kim YI. Battered Korean Women in Urban United States. In: Furuto SM, Renuka B, Chung DK, Murase K, Ross-Sheriff F, eds. *Social Work Practice with Asian Americans: Sage Sourcebooks for the Human Services Series.* Vol. 20. Newbury Park, CA: Sage. 1992; 213–226.

13. This term refers to those who trace their origins to the countries or diasporal communities of Bangladesh, Bhutan, India, Nepal, Pakistan and Sri Lanka.

14. Raj A, Silverman J. Intimate partner violence against South-Asian women in Greater Boston. *J Am Med Women's Assoc.* 2002; 57(2): 111–114.

15. Raj A, Silverman J. Unpublished data.

16. Tran CG. *Domestic violence among Vietnamese refugee women: Prevalence, abuse characteristics, psychiatric symptoms, and psychosocial factors* [dissertation]. Boston, MA: Boston University; 1997.

17. McDonnell KA, Abdulla SE. *Project AWARE.* Washington, DC: Asian/Pacific Islander Domestic Violence Resource Project; 2001. Available at: www.DVRP.org

18. Narika. *Changing Voices.* Newsletter, 2001; 1(1). Available at: www.narika.org.

19. Asian Women's Shelter: Unpublished internal statistics.

20. Campbell DW, Masaki B, Torress S. Water on rock: Changing domestic violence perceptions in the African American, Asian American and Latino communities. In: Klein E, Campbell J, Soler E, Ghez M, eds. *Ending Domestic Violence: Changing Public Perceptions / Halting the Epidemic.* Thousand Oaks, CA: Sage; 1997; 64–87.

21. E-mail message from K. Sujata, Executive Director, Apna Ghar: March 18, 2002.

22. Dasgupta SD. Charting the course: An overview of domestic violence in the South Asian community in the United States. *J Soc Distress Homeless.* 2000; 9(3): 173–185.

23. Eng P. Domestic violence in Asian/Pacific Island communities: A public health issue. *Health Issues for Women of Color: A Cultural Diversity Perspective.* Thousand Oaks, CA: Sage; 1995:78–88.

24. E-mail message from Saheli: March 12, 2002.

25. Klein E, Campbell J, Soler E, Ghez M, eds. *Ending Domestic Violence: Changing Public Perceptions / Halting the Epidemic.* Thousand Oaks, CA: Sage; 1997: 79.

26. Yoshioka and Dang. *Asian Family Violence Report.*

27. Yoshihama M. Reinterpreting strength and safety in a socio-cultural context: Dynamics of domestic violence and experiences of women of Japanese descent. *Children Youth Services Rev.* 2000; 22: 207–229.

28. Yick AG, Agbayani–Siewert P. Perceptions of domestic violence in a Chinese American community. *J Interpersonal Violence.* 1997; 12(6): 832–846.

29. Bui HN, Morash M. Domestic violence in the Vietnamese immigrant community: An exploratory study. *Violence Against Women.* 1999; 5(7): 769–795.

30. National Asian Women's Health Organization. *Silence, Not an Option!*

31. McDonnell and Abdulla. *Project AWARE.*

32. Yoshioka and Dang. *Asian Family Violence Report.*

33. Raj and Silverman. Intimate partner violence against South-Asian women in Greater Boston.

34. Yoshihama M. Battered women's coping strategies and psychological distress: Differences by immigration status. *Am J Community Psychol.* 2002; 30(3): 429–452.

35. Bui and Morash. Domestic violence in the Vietnamese immigrant community.

36. Yoshioka and Dang. *Asian Family Violence Report.*

37. Yoshihama and Horrocks. Posttraumatic stress symptoms and victimization among Japanese American women.

38. Yoshihama M. Model minority demystified: Emotional costs of multiple victimizations in the lives of women of Japanese descent. *J Hum Behav in the Soc Environ.* 2001; 3(3/4): 201–224.

39. Shimtuh, Korean American Domestic Violence Program. *Korean American Community of the Bay Area Domestic Violence Needs Assessment Report.*

40. Santa Clara County Death Review Sub-Committee of the Domestic Violence Council, *Death Review Committee Final Report.* San Jose: Author; 1997.

41. Tong BQM. A haven without barriers: Task force is seeking a refuge for battered Asian women. *Boston Globe.* November 9, 1992; 17.

42. Malone H. Asian task force encouraged by drop in domestic abuse deaths, group will hold its sixth annual fundraiser today. *Boston Globe.* Sept. 25, 1999: B3.

43. Dasgupta SD. Data presented at the Asian and Pacific Islander Institute on Domestic Violence, National Summit 2002, San Francisco. Summit proceedings available from the Institute at apidvinstitute@apiahf.org.

44. Hawaii State Coalition Against Domestic Violence. *Domestic Violence Deaths in Hawaii, 2000.* Honolulu, HI: Author; 2001.

45. Domestic Violence Clearinghouse and Legal Hotline, Honolulu, HI. E–mail from Jennifer Rose: April 3, 2002.

46. The Department of Business, Economic Development and Tourism. *The State of Hawaii Data Book 2000*. Honolulu, HI: Author; 2000. Available at: http://www.hawaii.gov/dbedt/db00/index.html.

Chapter 27

Domestic Violence
in Tribal Communities

Why It Matters

Domestic violence is an issue for large numbers of Native American women both on tribal lands and outside of Indian country.[1] American Indian and Alaskan Native women are battered, raped, and stalked at far greater rates than any other group of women in the United States.[2] The U.S. Department of Justice estimates that Native American women are stalked at a rate at least twice that of any other group in the nation, and three out of four American Indian women have been victims of domestic violence.[3] This disproportionate amount of violence destroys the quality of the life of Native Americans and threatens the stability and security of their families, communities, and tribes.

Did You Know?

American Indians experience per capita rates of violence that are more than twice that of the U.S. resident population.[4]

• One out of three American Indian and Alaskan Native women are raped in their lifetime, compared to about one in five women in the nation as a whole.[5]

- 70% of American Indians who are the victims of violent crimes are victimized by a non-native individual.[6]

- One in five violent victimizations against American Indians involved an offender who was an intimate or member of the victim's family (between 1992 and 2001).[7]

- 25% of employed American Indian victims of violence said that the incident occurred in the workplace.[8]

- 17% of American Indian women—at least twice that of other groups—are stalked each year.[9]

- In one study of tribal jurisdictions between 1996 and 2001, 70% of orders of protection filed by prosecutors on behalf of American Indian women were violated.[10]

- 69% of American Indian children report exposure to violence in the home.[11]

Challenges

"Jurisdictional complexities, geographic isolation, and institutional resistance impede effective protection of women subjected to violence within Indian country."—Ninth Circuit Gender Bias Task Force report[12]

There are many challenges impeding efforts to decrease violence against Indian women:

- There is insufficient funding for domestic violence services in Native communities.[13]

- Victims fear that judicial, law enforcement, or medical personnel will not be sympathetic to them because of misperceptions

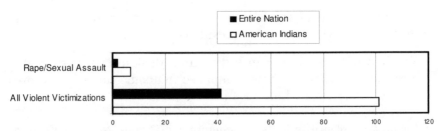

Figure 27.1. *Annual Average Rate of Violent Victimizations per 1,000 Individuals*

about Indian tribes, racial prejudices, or stereotypes of Indian people.[14]

• Tribal law enforcement agencies do not have jurisdiction over serious felonies committed by a non-tribal member against a tribal member, and native victims of non-tribal members must count on the Federal Bureau of Investigation (FBI) to arrest these perpetrators.[15]

• Orders of protection issued by a tribal court are often not given full faith and credit by state courts or even by courts of other tribes, so they are not enforced outside of tribal grounds.[16]

• Although 85% of domestic violence and sexual assault incidents against American Indians involved alcohol, funding restrictions prevent tribes from confronting alcohol abuse directly.[17]

• Many tribes cannot afford to provide shelters, forcing victims to leave the tribe for assistance and making it hard for them to continue work, attend school, and receive help from families.[18]

• In some tribes, law enforcement and victim services do not have any formal channels of communication.[19]

Violence Against Indian Women and Violence Against Women Act (VAWA)

The federal Services Training-Officers-Prosecutors (STOP) Violence Against Indian Women (VAIW) program was initiated in 1995 as part of the Violence Against Women Act (VAWA) to reduce violent crimes against American Indian women. It provides federal funds to Indian tribal governments to develop and strengthen the response of tribal justice systems to violent crimes committed against Indian women. The Office of Justice Programs originally set aside 2% of total annual STOP funding for Indian tribal governments and raised this amount to 4% in 2005—even though only approximately 1% to 2% of Americans are American Indian—in recognition of the seriousness of domestic violence in tribes.[20]

The 2005 reauthorization of VAWA continued to address violence against Indian women by strengthening tribal-based services, establishing a tribal registry to track perpetrators of violence against Indian women, establishing a Deputy Director for Tribal Affairs in the Office on Violence Against Women, and increasing tribal access to funding for domestic violence prevention.[21] For fiscal year (FY) 2007, no money was appropriated for research on violence against Indian women or tracking of violence against Indian women.

Although much work still needs to be done to reduce violence against American Indian women, since the initiation of the STOP VAIW program, tribal responses to domestic violence and sexual assault have improved. One study[22] showed the following:

- An over 400% increase in complaints filed by prosecutors on behalf of domestic violence victims.

- A 36% increase in arrests of offenders.

- An increase in restraining orders. Protection orders are now available in 93% of tribal court jurisdictions.

- 76 tribal grantees developed mandatory arrest policies.

- 39 tribes addressed collateral arrests in their codes, whereas 15 more indicate that dual arrests should not occur.

- Tribes improved channels of communication between law enforcement services and victim services.

- Improved training of law enforcement officers led to more perpetrator arrests and less mutual battery arrests.

- Tribes employed tribal members in limited prosecutorial roles.

- The use of domestic violence shelters increased.

- Tribes developed working relationships with surrounding state and tribal governments to ensure the full faith and credit of their protection orders is recognized.

Sources

[1] The National Congress of American Indians. "Fact Sheet: Violence Against Women in Indian Country." www.ncai.org.

[2, 3] Sacred Circle National Resource Center to End Violence Against Native Women, *VAWA 2005 Title IX-Tribal Provisions*. http://www.sacred-circle.com/Tribal%20Programs%20Title%20IX.htm.

[4, 7, 15, 16] Perry, Steven. Bureau of Justice Statistics, *A BJS Statistical Profile 1992–2001: American Indians and Crime*. http://www.usdoj.gov/otj/pdf/american_indians_and_crime.pdf.

[5, 6] The National Congress of American Indians. "Fact Sheet: Violence Against Women in Indian Country." www.ncai.org.

[8] Greenfeld, Lawrence A., and Steven K. Smith. 1999. *American Indians and Crime*. http://www.ojp.usdoj.gov/bjs/pub/pdf/aic.pdf.

[9] Sacred Circle National Resource Center to End Violence Against Native Women. *2005 Testimony*. http://www.sacred-circle.com/2005%20SC%20testimony.htm.

[10, 11] Luna-Firebaugh, Eileen M. (2006) "Violence Against American Indian Women and the Services-Training-Officers-Prosecutors Violence Against Indian Women (STOP VAIW) Program." *Violence Against Women Journal*. 12(2): 125–136.

[12, 13, 14] The National Congress of American Indians. "Fact Sheet: Violence Against Women in Indian Country." www.ncai.org.

[17] Luna-Firebaugh, Eileen M. (2006).

[18] Sacred Circle. *Cultural Competency and Native Women: A Guide for Non-Natives Who Advocate for Battered Women and Rape Victims*.

[19, 20, 22] *Luna-Firebaugh*, Eileen M. (2006)

[21] National Network to End Domestic Violence. "The Violence Against Women Act: Reauthorization 2005." http://www.endabuse.org/vawa/factsheets/Reauthorization.pdf.

For More Information

Clan Star, Inc.
64 Minnie Lane
P.O. Box 1630
Cherokee, NC 28719
Toll-Free: 888-636-4748
Phone: 828-497-5507
Fax: 828-497-5688
Website: http://www.clanstar.org

Mending the Sacred Hoop
202 E. Superior St.
Duluth, MN 55802
Toll-Free: 888-305-1650
Phone: 218-623-HOOP (4667)
Fax: 218-722-5775
Website: http://www.msh-ta.org

National Coalition Against Domestic Violence
P.O. Box 18749
Denver, CO, 80218-0749

Phone: 303-839-1852
Fax: 303-831-9251
TTY: 303-839-1681
Website: http://www.ncadv.org

Sacred Circle
National Resource Center to End Violence Against Native Women
722 St. Joseph St.
Rapid City, SD 57701
Toll-Free: 877-RED-ROAD (733-7623)
Phone: 605-341-2050
Fax: 605-341-2472
Website: http://www.sacred-circle.com
E-mail: scircle@sacred-circle.com

Walking the Healing Path
P.O. Box 447
Window Rock, AZ 86515
Phone: 505-409-4403, 505-612-9245, or 505-409-6200
Website: http://www.walkingthehealingpath.org

To Get Help

National Domestic Violence Hotline
P.O. Box 161810
Austin, TX 78716
Toll-Free Hotline: 800-799-SAFE (7233)
Toll-Free TTY: 800-787-3224
Website: http://www.ndvh.org

National Sexual Assault Hotline
Rape, Abuse & Incest National Network (RAINN)
2000 L Street, NW, Suite 406
Washington, DC 20036
Toll-Free: 800-656-HOPE (4673)
Phone: 202-544-3064
Fax: 202-544-3556
Website: http://www.rainn.org
E-mail: info@rainn.org

Chapter 28

Rural Victims of Violence

Why It Matters

According to the U.S. Census Bureau, 25% of Americans live in rural areas.[1] However, domestic violence and sexual assault services are primarily concentrated in urban and suburban areas. As a result, in many parts of the country it is not unusual for victims to drive several hours—or even fly—in order to obtain victim services.[2] Unique aspects of rural life, such as distance from cities and towns, the extremely close-knit nature of rural communities, scarcity of employment and educational opportunities, and delayed police and medical response times make it difficult for victims of domestic violence and sexual assault to report the abuse, leave abusive relationships, and seek services.[3]

Did You Know?

- Although absolute numbers of domestic violence and sexual assault are higher in urban areas, the rate of domestic violence and sexual assault victimization is higher in rural areas.[4]

- 27% of rural women experiencing domestic violence also experience sexual assault.[5]

- 34 million rural Americans live in areas with extreme shortages of medical and mental health professionals.[6]

- Rural victims of domestic violence and sexual assault are more likely than urban victims to be married to their abusers.[7]

Child and Elder Abuse

- While the number of children who have been physically or sexually abused is higher is urban areas, the child abuse rate is higher in rural areas.[8]

- Because many teachers, nurses, and child care providers in rural areas have long-standing personal relationships with perpetrators and their families, they may be less likely to label the abuse a crime and report it to the authorities.[9]

- One study found that elder abuse in rural areas is more likely to consist of physical abuse and deprivation because isolation allows greater opportunities for serious abuse to occur and remain unnoticed.[10]

Rural Perpetrators of Abuse

- One study found that 45% of rural perpetrators of domestic violence own firearms or other weapons.[11]

- Rural perpetrators of domestic violence and sexual assault are more likely than urban perpetrators to be socially networked with local law enforcement.[12]

- Perpetrators arrested for domestic violence in rural areas are twice as likely to abuse substances.[13]

- Rural domestic violence arrestees are more likely than urban perpetrators to be unemployed and less likely to have a high school diploma or have passed general educational development (GED) tests.[14]

Barriers to Seeking Services

- Many rural women hesitate to seek services because rural environments prevent anonymity. If a victim parks her car at a crisis center, clinic, or a police station, the entire community—including her abuser—will know very quickly.[15]

- Because most rural communities lack a public transportation system, batterers can manipulate transportation access, such as monitoring a car's odometer or disabling a vehicle, increasingly isolating victims.[16]

Barriers to Escaping Abuse

When attempting to escape an abusive relationship, rural women face unique challenges.

- Rural women overwhelmingly report that the greatest barriers to leaving their abusers include limited job opportunities, insufficient child care resources, and lack of available housing in their area.[17]

- For many rural families, finances are tied up in land and equipment. Therefore, a woman who considers terminating a relationship faces the reality that she and her partner will lose the family farm and their only means of income.[18]

- Rural women are significantly less likely than urban women to have credit in their own name, personal savings, individual checking accounts, or control over their own earnings.[19]

Protective Orders in Rural Areas

- In most cases, protective orders cannot be enforced until they are served on the perpetrator. However, one study found that 55% to 91% of protective orders in rural areas are not served.[20]

- Rural perpetrators violate protective orders three times more often than all other perpetrators.[21]

- Because many rural newspapers publish arrest logs and protective order requests, many rural victims of domestic violence do not seek protective orders out of fear that the entire community will find out.[22]

Services for Rural Victims[23]

The 2005 Violence Against Women Act (VAWA) reauthorized $55 million to strengthen existing domestic violence programs for victims in rural areas. The programs are designed to:

- fund cooperative efforts between law enforcement, prosecutors, and victim services;

- provide treatment, counseling and assistance to victims; and,

- work with rural communities to develop education and prevention strategies.

Funding for the Rural Grants program has led to the development of rural outreach services, the creation of domestic violence task forces and councils, enhanced coordination between law enforcement, prosecutors and victim services, and better enforcement of laws against domestic violence and sexual assault.

VAWA includes eligibility for rural areas in non-rural states and specifies dedicated funding to address sexual assault. Starting in fiscal year (FY) 2007, many more communities in need were able to apply for Rural Grant funds.

Funding of the Rural Grants program at the authorized level of $55 million will protect critical services to rural victims of violence and meet the overwhelming need for Rural Grand funds.

Sources

[1] United States Census Bureau. (1999). *1999 Statistical Abstract of the United States.* http://www.census.gov/Press-Release/www/1999/cb99–238.html.

[2, 4, 15] Lewis, S.H. (2003). *Unspoken Crimes: Sexual Assault in Rural America.* National Sexual Violence Resource Center: http://www.nsvrc.org/publications/ booklets/rural_txt.htm.

[3] Van Hightower, N.R. and Gorton, J. (2002). A Case Study of Community-Based Responses to Rural Women Battering. *Violence Against Women,* 8(7), 845–872.

[5, 17, 20, 21, 22] Logan, T.K., Shannon, L., and Walker, R. (2005). Protective Orders in Rural and Urban Areas: A Multiple Perspective Study. *Violence Against Women,* 11(7), 876–911.

[6, 7, 13, 14] Logan, T.K., Walker, R., and Leukefeld, C.G. (2001). Rural, Urban Influenced, and Urban Differences Among Domestic Violence Arrestees. *Journal of Interpersonal Violence,* 16(3), 266–283.

[8, 9] Menard, K.S. and Ruback, R.B. (2003). Prevalence and Processing of Child Sexual Abuse: A Multi-Data-Set Analysis of Urban and Rural Counties. *Law and Human Behavior,* 27(4), 385–402.

[10] Dimah, K.P. and Dimah, A. (2003). Elder Abuse and Neglect Among Rural and Urban Women. *Journal of Elder Abuse and Neglect,* 15(1), 75–93.

[11] DeKeseredy, W.S. and Joseph, C. (2006). Separation and/or Divorce Sexual Assault in Rural Ohio: Preliminary Results of an Exploratory Study. *Violence Against Women*, 12(3), 301–311.

[12, 16] Grossman, S.F., et al. (2005). Rural Versus Urban Victims of Violence: The Interplay of Race and Region. *Journal of Family Violence*, 20(2), 71–81.

[18] Women's Rural Advocacy Programs. (2006). *Problems of Rural Battered Women*. http://www.letswrap.com/dvinfo/rural.htm.

[19] Bosch, K. and Schumm, W.R. (2004). Accessibility to Resources: Helping Rural Women in Abusive Partner Relationships Become Free From Abuse. *Journal of Sex and Marital Therapy*, 30(5), 357–370.

[23] Campaign for Funding to End Domestic and Sexual Violence. 2007. *FY 2008 Appropriations Briefing Book*.

For More Information

National Coalition Against Domestic Violence
P.O. Box 18749
Denver, CO, 80218-0749
Phone: 303-839-1852
Fax: 303-831-9251
TTY: 303-839-1681
Website: http://www.ncadv.org

National Domestic Violence Hotline
P.O. Box 161810
Austin, TX 78716
Toll-Free Hotline: 800-799-SAFE (7233)
Toll-Free TTY: 800-787-3224
Website: http://www.ndvh.org

National Sexual Assault Hotline
Rape, Abuse & Incest National Network (RAINN)
2000 L Street, NW, Suite 406
Washington, DC 20036
Toll-Free: 800-656-HOPE (4673)
Phone: 202-544-3064
Fax: 202-544-3556
Website: http://www.rainn.org
E-mail: info@rainn.org

Rural Assistance Center
School of Medicine and Health Sciences, Rm. 4520
501 N. Columbia Rd., Stop 9037
Grand Forks, ND 58202-9037
Toll-Free: 800-270-1898
Fax: 800-270-1913
Website: http://www.raconline.org
E-mail: info@raconline.org

Chapter 29

Domestic Violence and Sexual Assault in the Military

Why It Matters

There are approximately 1.4 million active duty service members stationed in the U.S. and abroad.[1] Among this population are victims including men, women, and children who live daily with the realities of emotional, physical, and sexual abuse. Certain characteristics of military life such as constant relocation and a history of violence can make some families especially vulnerable to domestic violence.[2] Furthermore, many victims of domestic violence and sexual assault in the military community do not report incidents of abuse for fear that it will impact their partner's position.[1]

Did You Know?

- In one year there were more than 18,000 incidents of spousal abuse reported to the Department of Defense's Family Advocacy Program.[3]

- Domestic violence homicides in the military community from 1995–2001 include: 54 in the Navy or Marine Corps; 131 in the Army; and 32 in the Air Force.[4]

- Domestic violence victims in military communities are most likely to be women (66%)[5] and the civilian spouses of active duty personnel (62% of abusers are on active military duty).[6]

- Among active duty military women, 30% reported an adult lifetime prevalence of intimate partner abuse, while 22% reported intimate partner violence during military service.[7]

- Although data is hard to obtain, it is apparent that relatively few military personnel are prosecuted or administratively sanctioned on charges stemming from domestic violence.[8]

Institutional Barriers

- The only military personnel granted confidentiality in their communications are chaplains. Victim advocates, social workers, therapists, and physicians may not keep information confidential.[9]

- All military personnel (except chaplains) are required to report any suspected domestic violence regardless of circumstances.[10]

- In the military community, the person notified of the domestic violence allegation is the perpetrator's boss. Therefore, victims are reluctant to report incidents of abuse for fear of negative career consequences.[11]

Sexual Assault

- The prevalence of adult sexual assault among female veterans has been estimated as high as 41%.[12]

- 8% of female Persian Gulf War veterans in a survey reported being sexually abused during Desert Shield and Desert Storm.[13]

- 37% of women who reported a rape or attempted rape had been raped more than once; 14% of the victims reported having been gang raped.[14]

- Three-fourths of the female veterans who were raped did not report the incident to a ranking officer. One-third didn't know how to, and one-fifth believed that rape was to be expected in the military.[15]

Relevant Issues

- A high percentage of military personnel have prior histories of domestic violence in their families. Among Navy recruits, 54% of men and 40% of women have witnessed parental abuse prior to enlistment.[16]

- Constant relocation of military families from place to place, often with different culture and values, isolates victims by severing ties with family and loved ones.[17]

Protective Orders

- A military protective order (MPO) is issued by the command of a suspected abuser. A MPO may be verbal or written and may direct service members to stay away from victims or designated places; refrain from doing certain things; require the service member to move into government quarters; and provide support for family members. Enforcement of a MPO is the responsibility of the command issuing the order. Local law enforcement does not have the authority to arrest a service member for violation of a MPO.

- Disbarment orders govern the conduct of suspected civilian abusers and denies the civilian access to the military installation. Enforcement of disbarment orders is the responsibility of the command issuing the order. Apprehension and arrest are not mandated for military police or command. Local law enforcement may facilitate enforcement by responding to an incident and taking custody of the service member under a memorandum of understanding/agreement.

- Civilian protective orders must be enforced on military installations as required by The Armed Forces Domestic Security Act (P.L. 107–311).

Severity of Abuse

- The Department of Defense (DoD) divides the severity of abuse into three categories: severe physical abuse, moderate physical abuse, and mild physical abuse.

- The DoD severity definitions are inconsistent with the reality of domestic violence. For example, the DoD prerequisite to be categorized as "severe physical abuse" is "major physical injury requiring inpatient medical treatment or causing temporary or permanent disability or disfigurement." A strangulation case in the civilian community is considered very dangerous, whereas

271

at the DoD, it might be defined to be "mild" or "moderate abuse." As a result, 69% of domestic violence cases reported in one fiscal year were mild and only 6% were classified as severe.[14]

What You Can Do to Help

- Encourage partnerships between local victim advocacy agencies and military installations in your community.

- Volunteer with state, local, national, and international advocacy agencies that work to address domestic violence and sexual assault in the U.S. military.

- Write letters to the Department of Defense asking U.S. military leaders to change policies, adopt new laws, and provide funding to better service military families that experience violence.

- Lobby Congress to pass federal laws that protect victims' confidentiality and set aside DoD funds to address domestic violence and sexual assault in the military.

- Write letters to the editor and local media to draw attention to domestic violence and sexual assault in the U.S. military.

Sources

[1] Retrieved from www.military.com on July 13, 2007.

[2] "Defense Task Force on Domestic Violence, 2003 Third Year Report," U.S. Department of Defense, February 2003.

[3] Beals, Judith E., "The Military Response to Victims of Domestic Violence." Battered Women's Justice Project. http://www.bwjp.org/docurnents/BWJPMIL.pdf.

[4, 6] U.S. Department of Defense, Family Advocacy Program Report: "Child and Spouse Abuse Data," (FY97-01).

[5] U.S. Department of Defense, Family Advocacy Program Data, FY02.

[7] Campbell, Garza, et al., *Intimate Partner Violence and Abuse Among Active Duty Military Women*, Violence Against Women, 2003.

[8] Initial Report of the Defense Task Force on Domestic Violence, U.S. Department of Defense, 2001.

[9,10,11] Beals, Judith E., "The Military Response to Victims of Domestic Violence." Battered Women's Justice Project. http://www.bwjp.org/docurnents/BWJPMIL.pdf.

[12,14] Factors associated with women's risk of rape in the military. 2003. *Journal of Industrial Medicine.*

[13,15] Department of Defense. 2001. Initial Report of the Defense Task Force on Domestic Violence.

[16,17] "Defense Task Force on Domestic Violence, 2003 Third Year Report," U.S. Department of Defense, February 2003.

For More Information

U.S. Military's Sexual Assault Prevention and Response (SAPR)
Toll-Free Stateside Reporting: 800-342-9647
Toll-Free Overseas Reporting: 00-800-3429-6477
Phone: 703-697-7442 (Business)
Website: http://www.preventsexualassault.army.mil

To Get Help

National Domestic Violence Hotline
P.O. Box 161810
Austin, TX 78716
Toll-Free Hotline: 800-799-SAFE (7233)
Toll-Free TTY: 800-787-3224
Website: http://www.ndvh.org

National Sexual Assault Hotline
Rape, Abuse & Incest National Network (RAINN)
2000 L Street, NW, Suite 406
Washington, DC 20036
Toll-Free: 800-656-HOPE (4673)
Phone: 202-544-3064
Fax: 202-544-3556
Website: http://www.rainn.org
E-mail: info@rainn.org

Chapter 30

Domestic Violence Perpetrators

Chapter Contents

Section 30.1

Who Is a Perpetrator of Domestic Violence?

Excerpted from "Child Protection in Families Experiencing
Domestic Violence: Chapter 3," U.S. Department of Health and
Human Services (HHS), September 18, 2008.

As is the case with victims of domestic violence, abusers can be anyone and come from every age, sex, socioeconomic, racial, ethnic, occupational, educational, and religious group. They can be teenagers, college professors, farmers, counselors, electricians, police officers, doctors, clergy, judges, and popular celebrities. Perpetrators are not always angry and hostile, but can be charming, agreeable, and kind. Abusers differ in patterns of abuse and levels of dangerousness. While there is not an agreed upon universal psychological profile, perpetrators do share a behavioral profile that is described as "an ongoing pattern of coercive control involving various forms of intimidation, and psychological and physical abuse."

While many people think violent and abusive people are mentally ill, research shows that perpetrators do not share a set of personality characteristics or a psychiatric diagnosis that distinguishes them from people who are not abusive. There are some perpetrators who suffer from psychiatric problems, such as depression, posttraumatic stress disorder, or psychopathology. Yet, most do not have psychiatric illnesses, and caution is advised in attributing mental illness as a root cause of domestic violence. The Diagnostic and Statistical Manual of the American Psychological Association (DSM-IV) does not have a diagnostic category for perpetrators, but mental illness should be viewed as a factor that can influence the severity and nature of the abuse.

Examples of the most prevalent behavioral tactics by perpetrators include the following:

- **Abusing power and control:** The perpetrator's primary goal is to achieve power and control over their intimate partner. In order to do so, perpetrators often plan and utilize a pattern of coercive tactics aimed at instilling fear, shame, and helplessness in

276

the victim. Another part of this strategy is to change randomly the list of rules or expectations the victim must meet to avoid abuse. The abuser's incessant degradation, intimidation, and demands on their partner are effective in establishing fear and dependence. It is important to note that perpetrators may also engage in impulsive acts of domestic violence and that not all perpetrators act in such a planned or systematic way.

- **Having different public and private behavior:** Usually, people outside the immediate family are not aware of and do not witness the perpetrator's abusive behavior. Abusers who maintain an amiable public image accomplish the important task of deceiving others into thinking that he or she is a loving, normal person, and incapable of domestic violence. This allows perpetrators to escape accountability for their violence and reinforces the victims' fears that no one will believe them.

- **Projecting blame:** Abusers often engage in an insidious type of manipulation that involves blaming the victim for the violent behavior. Such perpetrators may accuse the victim of "pushing buttons" or provoking the abuse. By diverting attention to the victim's actions, the perpetrator avoids taking responsibility for the abusive behavior. In addition to projecting blame on the victim, abusers also may project blame on circumstances, such as making the excuse that alcohol or stress caused the violence.

- **Claiming loss of control or anger problems:** There is a common belief that domestic violence is a result of poor impulse control or anger management problems. Abusers routinely claim that they "just lost it," suggesting that the violence was an impulsive and rare event beyond control. Domestic violence is not typically a singular incident nor does it simply involve physical attacks. It is a deliberate set of tactics where physical violence is used to solidify the abuser's power in the relationship. In reality, only an estimated 5–10 percent of perpetrators have difficulty with controlling their aggression. Most abusers do not assault others outside the family, such as police officers, coworkers, or neighbors, but direct their abuse toward the victim or children. This distinction challenges claims that they cannot manage their anger.

- **Minimizing and denying the abuse:** Perpetrators rarely view themselves or their actions as violent or abusive. As a result, they often deny, justify, and minimize their behavior. For example, an abuser might forcibly push the victim down a flight of stairs and tell others that the victim tripped. Abusers also rationalize serious physical assaults, such as punching or choking, as self-defense. Abusers who refuse to admit they are harming their partner present enormous challenges to persons who are trying to intervene. Some perpetrators do acknowledge to the victim that the abusive behavior is wrong, but then plead for forgiveness or make promises of refraining from any future abuse. Even in situations such as this, the perpetrator commonly minimizes the severity or impact of the abuse.

It is equally important to acknowledge that abusers also possess positive qualities. There are abusers who are remorseful, accept responsibility for their violence, and eventually stop their abusive behavior. Perpetrators are not necessarily bad people, but their abusive behavior is unacceptable. Some perpetrators have childhood histories where they were physically or sexually abused, neglected, or exposed to domestic abuse. Some suffer from substance abuse and mental health problems. All of these factors can influence their psychological functioning and contribute to the complexity and severity of the abusive behavior. Perpetrators need support and intervention to end their violent behavior and any additional problems that compound their abusive behavior. Through specialized interventions, community services, and sanctions, some abusers can change and become nonviolent.

Indicators of Dangerousness

Different levels of violence and types of abuse are perpetrated by domestic violence offenders. Some abusers rarely use physical violence, while others assault their partners daily. There are perpetrators who are only abusive towards family members and others who are violent toward a variety of people. There are abusers who are more likely to inflict serious injury or become homicidal. Some frequently degrade the victim, while some rarely, if ever, implement that particular tactic.

It is critical that professionals and community service providers who intervene in domestic violence cases engage in thorough and continuous assessment of the perpetrator's level of dangerousness. Evaluating this dangerousness involves identifying risk indicators that reflect the capacity to continue perpetrating severe violence. Although domestic violence homicides or severe assaults cannot be predicted, there are several risk factors that help determine the likelihood that severe forms of violence may be imminent. The greater the number or the intensity of the following indicators, the more likely a severe or life-threatening attack will occur:

- Threats or thoughts of homicide and suicide
- Possession or access to weapons
- Use of weapons in a threatening or intimidating manner
- Extreme jealousy or obsession with the victim
- Physical attacks, verbal threats, and stalking during a separation or divorce
- Kidnapping or hostage taking
- Sexual assault or rape
- Prior abusive incidents that resulted in serious injury
- History of violence with previous partners and children
- Psychopathology or substance abuse

The listed factors pose a substantial risk to victims of domestic violence and possibly to their children. It also is important to ask for the victim's assessment of the abuser's dangerousness. Extremely dangerous perpetrators can be safety threats to people who are involved in the victim's life, individuals trying to help, or the children. It is crucial that community professionals who work with violent families incorporate these risk indicators into their assessments and interventions because failure to do so can seriously compromise the lives of everyone involved.

Section 30.2

Perpetrators and Parenting

Excerpted from "Child Protection in Families Experiencing
Domestic Violence: Chapter 3," U.S. Department of Health and
Human Services (HHS), September 18, 2008.

Can perpetrators be supportive parents when they are abusive towards the other parent? An emerging issue facing victims of domestic violence and child advocacy groups is the role and impact that perpetrators have in their children's lives. There are perpetrators who have positive interactions with their children, provide for their physical and financial needs, and are not abusive towards them. There also are perpetrators who neglect or physically harm their children. Although abusers vary tremendously in parenting styles, there are some behaviors common among perpetrators that can have harmful effects on children:

- **Authoritarianism:** Perpetrators can be rigid and demanding with their children. They often have high and unrealistic expectations and expect children to obey without question or resistance. This parenting style is intimidating for children and alters their sense of safety around the abuser. These perpetrators are more likely to use harsher forms of physical discipline, which can make the children increasingly vulnerable to becoming direct targets of violence.

- **Neglect, irresponsibility, and lack of involvement:** Some abusers are infrequently involved in the daily parenting activities of their children. They may view their children as hindrances and become easily annoyed with them. Furthermore, the perpetrator's preoccupation with controlling the partner and meeting his or her own emotional needs leaves little time to engage the children. Unfortunately, the perpetrator's physical and emotional unavailability can produce unrequited feelings of anticipation and fondness in the children who eagerly await attention.

- **Undermining the victim:** The perpetrator's coercive and violent behavior towards the victim sometimes sends children a message that it is acceptable for them to treat that parent in the same manner. More overt tactics that weaken the victim's influence over the children include the perpetrator disregarding the victim's parenting decisions, telling the children that the victim is an inadequate parent, and belittling the victim in the presence of the children. Being victimized by abuse can lead children to perceive the parent in a weaker, passive role with no real authority over their lives.

- **Self-centeredness:** Some perpetrators use their children to meet their own emotional needs. Perpetrators may expect their children to be immediately available only when they are interested and often overwhelm them with their problems. This can result in children feeling burdened and responsible for helping their parent while their own needs are neglected.

- **Manipulation:** To gain power in the home, perpetrators may manipulate their children into aligning against the victim. Abusers may make statements or exhibit behaviors that confuse the children regarding who is responsible for the violence and coerce them into believing that they are the preferable parent. Abusers also may directly or indirectly use their children to control and intimidate the victim. Perpetrators sometimes may threaten to abduct, seek sole custody of, or physically harm the children if the victim is not compliant. Sometimes these are threats exclusively and the abuser does not intend or really want to carry out the action, but the threats are typically perceived as being very real.

Children's Perceptions

Children's perception of the perpetrator's violence can play a significant role in the nature of their relationship. Children often feel anxious, scared, and angry when they witness abuse. At the same time, many children also feel affection, loyalty, and love for the abuser. It is common for children to experience ambivalent feelings towards the abuser and this can be difficult for them to resolve.

Domestic violence can influence the children's feelings toward the victim. Many children know the abuse is wrong and may even feel responsible for protecting the battered parent. Yet, they also experience confusion and resentment towards the victim for putting up with the abuse and are more likely to express their anger towards the victim rather than directly at the perpetrator.

Children need additional support as they struggle with their conflicting feelings towards the perpetrator. The responsibility of perpetrators as parents primarily focuses on preventing the recurrence of the violence. Some victims want their children to have a safe and positive relationship with the perpetrator, and some children crave that connection. Consequently, community service providers are confronted with the challenge of developing resources and strategies to help perpetrators become supportive and safe parents.

Examples of specific approaches that programs and service providers can use that will assist perpetrators in taking responsibility for the harm they pose to their children include the following:

- Educating abusers on the damaging effects of their behavior on their partners and children

- Providing intensive parenting skills programs that emphasize the needs of children affected by domestic abuse

- Offering safe exchange and supervised visitation programs

- Encouraging abusers to support their children attending groups for youths exposed to domestic violence

- Recruiting nonviolent fathers to mentor domestic violence perpetrators

Abuser's Role as Parent

A provocative issue for child protective services (CPS) caseworkers, service providers, and other community groups is determining the role abusers should have as parents or caretakers. Many voice legitimate concerns regarding the safety of the child victims.

There are special considerations and challenges in attempting to engage fathers who are abusive to their children or spouse, in activities that promote healthy involvement with the family. Some groups, such as some of those in the fatherhood movement, address this issue by helping fathers to increase their responsible involvement in their children's lives. Other groups, either through a prevention effort or an intervention treatment, seek to increase compassion, emotional awareness, and self-regulation skills in the belief that these skills remove the motivation for abusive behavior. Although juvenile court and protective order laws are designed to assign responsibility for child support and parental involvement, CPS caseworkers often face challenges in engaging fathers in the safety and care of their children. The difficulty with engaging some fathers in child protection efforts, however, stems from a cultural and gender bias of placing parenting responsibilities primarily on women. This is evidenced in child welfare systems where cases are tracked through the mother's name and subsequent case planning efforts are focused on her to make significant changes. Unfortunately, involving fathers or male caretakers typically does not occur unless they are willing participants or easily accessible in the CPS process. Thus, fathers can become essentially invisible in CPS efforts and unaccountable for the well-being of their children.

Unquestionably, balancing the protection of adult and child victims with the rights and responsibilities of perpetrators will require continuous dialogue and a movement towards collaboration. If communities are dedicated to ending domestic violence, they must strive to hear the voices of adults and children who suffer from abuse so that a collective agenda of building healthy, safe, and stable families can be accomplished.

Chapter 31

How Abusers
Stage Their Returns

While the smooth talk that it takes to get an abused spouse to take them back varies from person to person, there are five major strategies that seem to cover most of the wide range of tactics used by abusive partners:

The Honeymoon Syndrome

Also known as "Hearts and Flowers," this can include any bribe that will get you to return—and the sooner the better. Common bribes include promises to get therapy, promises not to be violent again (even after a long history), and even calculated doses of praise for you; saying things like "I know I don't deserve you, but if you'll take me back..."

Super Parent Syndrome

This is a very common ploy, especially if your partner has neglected the children in the past. An abuser might promise to start being a good parent, or might remind you how good they already are with the children. Many victims stay in abusive relationships because they believe that it's better for the children, but children are more aware than we give them credit for—and they know that abuse is occurring. In healthy parenting, children get to see both parents working together toward positive interactions for the whole family. When you stay with an abuser for the sake of the children, you are really slowly destroying one-half of their parenting system—yourself—thus robbing your children of the true and healthy "you" that should be in their futures and replacing it with the "you" that continues to be abused over time. Additionally, children depend on you to be able to do your job where they are concerned. This means they expect you to nourish them, protect them, and properly socialize them. Part of protecting them not only means directly protecting them, but also protecting their protector—you. Finally, a parent will always be a parent—even in the event of separation or divorce. A truly loving parent will continue to be a truly loving parent regardless of the shape and structure of the family. So before you cling to the promises of "super parent" abusers, consider carefully what's really in the long-term best interests of your children.

Revival Syndrome

"I have been going to church every Sunday since you left. I have accepted religion into my life." That's great, but so what? The real question is: has the violence stopped? Don't believe that just because someone spent an hour at church on a Sunday morning that violence and other abuse can't still be right around the corner. If you look at the massive amounts of literature directed at faith groups teaching them how to identify and respond to abusive relationships in their congregations, you'd quickly realize exactly how many god-fearing persons abuse, rape, beat, and murder their partners, even pastors. (Oprah did a show on domestic violence featuring a pastor who murdered his wife of 22 years because they argued over money and his unwillingness to get treatment for depression.)

Sobriety Syndrome

Whether it's drugs or alcohol, abusers have a higher incidence of substance use than the general population. Most substance-using abusers know that they have a substance abuse problem, or, they are aware that you believe they have a problem, even if they are in denial themselves. In the panic of facing losing their relationships, many will suddenly see the light and swear to you that they'll never touch it again. You'll want to hear it. You'll want to believe it. You'll want to support this effort. And you should, but don't just hear the words and breathe a sigh of relief. Actions speak louder than words and substance abuse and addiction is one of the hardest things to overcome by one-self. Withdrawal from chronic alcohol use, heroin, cigarettes, and even caffeine can cause vomiting, nausea, paranoia, and other unpleasant symptoms. When an abusive partner opens the door to getting sober, stick your foot in that door and help them to get more help—encourage them to talk to their doctor, to join a support group, to get substance abuse therapy, and so forth. Counseling, support, and therapy for substance abuse problems will address underlying problems and issues and help abusers to substitute healthier behaviors for their destructive coping mechanisms. Unless and until you see a substance using abuser actively participating in sobriety with outside help, don't fall for just the promise.

Counseling Syndrome

This is both a tactic to get you to stay and a tactic to maintain control and intimidation. You'll hear over and over again that abusers don't just stop their behavior without assistance to overcome issues and replace destructive behavior with healthy ones. Therapy is no exception. Friends, family, pastors, and even abusers might suggest couples counseling to you. Although they may have the best of intentions, couples counseling is not the solution to combat the behaviors of an abuser. Many abusers actually like the idea of couples counseling because it means that they don't have to take responsibility for their actions—instead, they get to drag you in as part of the problem. With your abuser sitting next to you in a counseling session, you are not emotionally free to say what you think without fear of repercussion, without the abuser twisting your words, and without them trying to coach you along as what to say or not to say. Safe, effective, and appropriate counseling for battering partners and abusers must be done without the victim present. Battering partners must take responsibility for their actions, must understand and admit that they have a problem, and be dedicated to the self-examination process to make positive long term changes possible. Couples counseling to combat domestic violence sounds like a great idea, but it is false advertising and can actually prolong and expand the emotional abuses that already exist.

Buy-Outs

The problem with all of these things is that in no case, no way, no how, does anything excuse or make up for the fact that a partner batters you. If you donate a million dollars to charity, it doesn't give you the right to go out and shoot someone. Similarly, don't fall into the trap of letting a partner buy their way out of violence in the relationship. Unless and until a battering partner owns up to their responsibility and gets some outside help to change their behavior, your relationship, your children, and your family are neither healthy nor safe.

Part Four

Domestic Violence Affects Children and Adolescents

Chapter 32

Complex Trauma in Children and Adolescents

The term complex trauma describes the dual problem of children's exposure to multiple traumatic events and the impact of this exposure on immediate and long-term outcomes. Typically, complex trauma exposure results when a child is abused or neglected, but it can also be caused by other kinds of events such as witnessing domestic violence, ethnic cleansing, or war. Many children involved in the child welfare system have experienced complex trauma. Often, the consequences of complex trauma exposure are devastating for a child. This is because complex trauma exposure typically interferes with the formation of a secure attachment bond between a child and her caregiver. Normally, the attachment between a child and caregiver is the primary source of safety and stability in a child's life. Lack of a secure attachment can result in a loss of core capacities for self-regulation and interpersonal relatedness. Children exposed to complex trauma often experience lifelong problems that place them at risk for additional trauma exposure and other difficulties, including psychiatric and addictive disorders, chronic medical illness, and legal, vocational, and family problems. These difficulties may extend from childhood through adolescence and into adulthood.

Cook, A., Spinazzola, J., Ford, J., Lanktree, C., Blaustein, M., Sprague, C., Cloitre, M., DeRosa, R., Hubbard, R., Kagan, R., Liautaud, J., Mallah, K., Olafson, E., and van der Kolk, B. Complex Trauma in Children and Adolescents. *Focal Point: Research, Policy and Practice in Children's Mental Health, Winter 2007.* © 2007 Research and Training Center on Family Support and Children's Mental Health–Portland State University (www.rtc.pdx.edu). Reprinted with permission.

The diagnosis of posttraumatic stress disorder (PTSD) does not capture the full range of developmental difficulties that traumatized children experience. Children exposed to maltreatment, family violence, or loss of their caregivers often meet diagnostic criteria for depression, attention-deficit/hyperactivity disorder (ADHD), oppositional defiant disorder (ODD), conduct disorder, anxiety disorders, eating disorders, sleep disorders, communication disorders, separation anxiety disorder, and/or reactive attachment disorder. Yet each of these diagnoses captures only a limited aspect of the traumatized child's complex self-regulatory and relational difficulties. A more comprehensive view of the impact of complex trauma can be gained by examining trauma's impact on a child's growth and development.

Impact on Development

A comprehensive review of the literature suggests seven primary domains of impairment observed in children exposed to complex trauma.

Attachment

Complex trauma is most likely to develop if an infant or child is exposed to danger that is unpredictable or uncontrollable, because the child's body must devote resources that are normally dedicated to growth and development instead to survival. The greatest source of danger and unpredictability is the absence of a caregiver who reliably and responsively protects and nurtures the child. The early caregiving relationship provides the primary context within which children learn about themselves, their emotions, and their relationships with others. A secure attachment supports a child's development in many essential areas, including his capacity for regulating physical and emotional states, his sense of safety (without which he will be reluctant to explore his environment), his early knowledge of how to exert an influence on the world, and his early capacity for communication.

When the child-caregiver relationship is the source of trauma, the attachment relationship is severely compromised. Caregiving that is erratic, rejecting, hostile, or abusive leaves a child feeling helpless and abandoned. In order to cope, the child attempts to exert some control, often by disconnecting from social relationships or by acting coercively towards others. Children exposed to unpredictable violence or repeated abandonment often learn to cope with threatening events and emotions by restricting their processing of what is happening around them. As a result, when they confront challenging situations, they cannot formulate a coherent, organized response. These children often have great difficulty regulating their emotions, managing stress, developing concern for others, and using language to solve problems. Over the long term, the child is placed at high risk for ongoing physical and social difficulties due to:

- increased susceptibility to stress (for example, difficulty focusing attention and controlling arousal),

- inability to regulate emotions without outside help or support (feeling and acting overwhelmed by intense emotions), and

- inappropriate help-seeking (such as, excessive help-seeking and dependency or social isolation and disengagement).

Biology

Toddlers or preschool-aged children with complex trauma histories are at risk for failing to develop brain capacities necessary for regulating emotions in response to stress. Trauma interferes with the integration of left and right hemisphere brain functioning, such that a child cannot access rational thought in the face of overwhelming emotion. Abused and neglected children are then prone to react with extreme helplessness, confusion, withdrawal, or rage when stressed.

In middle childhood and adolescence, the most rapidly developing brain areas are those that are crucial for success in forming interpersonal relationships and solving problems. Traumatic stressors or deficits in self-regulatory abilities impede this development, and can lead to difficulties in emotional regulation, behavior, consciousness, cognition, and identity formation.

It is important to note that supportive and sustaining relationships with adults—or, for adolescents, with peers—can protect children and adolescents from many of the consequences of traumatic stress. When interpersonal support is available, and when stressors are predictable, escapable, or controllable, children and adolescents can become highly resilient in the face of stress.

Affect Regulation

Exposure to complex trauma can lead to severe problems with affect regulation. Affect regulation begins with the accurate identification of internal emotional experiences. This requires the ability to differentiate among states of arousal, interpret these states, and apply appropriate labels (happy, frightened). When children are provided with inconsistent models of affect and behavior (for example, a smiling expression paired with rejecting behavior) or with inconsistent responses to affective display (child distress is met inconsistently with anger, rejection, nurturance, or neutrality), no coherent framework is provided through which to interpret experience.

Following the identification of an emotional state, a child must be able to express emotions safely and to adjust or regulate internal experience. Complexly traumatized children show impairment in both of these skills. Because they have difficulty in both self-regulating and self-soothing, these children may display dissociation, chronic numbing of emotional experience, dysphoria (a mood of general dissatisfaction, restlessness, depression, and anxiety), avoidance of emotional situations (including positive experiences), and maladaptive coping strategies (for example, substance abuse).

The existence of a strong relationship between early childhood trauma and subsequent depression is well-established. Recent twin studies, considered one of the highest forms of clinical scientific evidence because they can control for genetic and family factors, have conclusively documented that early childhood trauma, especially sexual abuse, dramatically increases risk for major depression, as well as many other negative outcomes. Not only does childhood trauma appear to increase the risk for major depression, it also appears to predispose toward earlier onset of depression, as well as longer duration, and poorer response to standard treatments.

Dissociation

Dissociation is one of the key features of complex trauma in children. In essence, dissociation is the failure to take in or integrate information and experiences. Thus, thoughts and emotions are disconnected, physical sensations are outside conscious awareness, and repetitive behavior takes place without conscious choice, planning, or self-awareness. Although dissociation begins as a protective mechanism in the face of overwhelming trauma, it can develop into a problematic disorder. Chronic trauma exposure may lead to an over-reliance on dissociation as a coping mechanism that, in turn, can exacerbate difficulties with behavioral management, affect regulation, and self-concept.

Behavioral Regulation

Complex childhood trauma is associated with both under-controlled and over-controlled behavior patterns. As early as the second year of life, abused children may demonstrate rigidly controlled behavior patterns, including compulsive compliance with adult requests, resistance to changes in routine, inflexible bathroom rituals, and rigid control of food intake. Childhood victimization also has been shown to be associated with the development of aggressive behavior and oppositional defiant disorder.

An alternative way of understanding the behavioral patterns of chronically traumatized children is that they represent children's defensive adaptations to overwhelming stress. Children may reenact behavioral aspects of their trauma (through aggression, self-injurious, or sexualized behaviors) as automatic behavioral reactions to trauma reminders or as attempts to gain mastery or control over their experiences. In the absence of more advanced coping strategies, traumatized children may use drugs or alcohol in order to avoid experiencing intolerable levels of emotional arousal. Similarly, in the absence of knowledge of how to form healthy interpersonal relationships, sexually abused children may engage in sexual behaviors in order to achieve acceptance and intimacy.

Cognition

Prospective studies have shown that children of abusive and neglectful parents demonstrate impaired cognitive functioning by late infancy when compared with non-abused children. The sensory and emotional deprivation associated with neglect appears to be particularly detrimental to cognitive development; neglected infants and toddlers demonstrate delays in expressive and receptive language development, as well as deficits in overall intelligence quotient (IQ). By early childhood, maltreated children demonstrate less flexibility and creativity in problem-solving tasks than same-age peers. Children and adolescents with a diagnosis of PTSD secondary to abuse or witnessing violence demonstrate deficits in attention, abstract reasoning, and problem solving.

By early elementary school, maltreated children are more frequently referred for special education services. A history of maltreatment is associated with lower grades and poorer scores on standardized tests and other indices of academic achievement. Maltreated children have three times the dropout rate of the general population. These findings have been demonstrated across a variety of trauma exposures (for example, physical abuse, sexual abuse, neglect, and exposure to domestic violence) and cannot be accounted for by the effects of other psychosocial stressors such as poverty.

Self-Concept

The early caregiver relationship has a profound effect on a child's development of a coherent sense of self. Responsive, sensitive caretaking and positive early life experiences allow a child to develop a model of self as generally worthy and competent. In contrast, repetitive experiences of harm and/or rejection by significant others and the associated failure to develop age-appropriate competencies are likely to lead to a sense of self as ineffective, helpless, deficient, and unlovable. Children who perceive themselves as powerless or incompetent and who expect others to reject and despise them are more likely to blame themselves for negative experiences and have problems eliciting and responding to social support.

By 18 months, maltreated toddlers already are more likely to respond to self-recognition with neutral or negative affect than nontraumatized children. In preschool, traumatized children are more resistant to talking about internal states, particularly those they perceive as negative. Traumatized children have problems estimating their own competence. Early exaggerations of competence in preschool shift to significantly lowered estimates of self-competence by late elementary school. By adulthood, they tend to suffer from a high degree of self-blame.

Family Context

The family, particularly the child's mother, plays a crucial role in determining how the child adapts to experiencing trauma. In the aftermath of trauma, family support and parents' emotional functioning strongly mitigate the development of PTSD symptoms and enhance a child's capacity to resolve the symptoms.

There are three main elements in caregivers' supportive responses to their children's trauma:

1. Believing and validating the child's experience.

2. Tolerating the child's affect.

3. Managing the caregiver's own emotional response.

When a caregiver denies the child's experiences, the child is forced to act as if the trauma did not occur. The child also learns he or she cannot trust the primary caregiver and does not learn to use language to deal with adversity. It is important to note that it is not caregiver distress per se that is necessarily detrimental to the child. Instead, when the caregiver's distress overrides or diverts attention away from the needs of the child, the child may be adversely affected. Children may respond to their caregiver's distress by avoiding or suppressing their own feelings or behaviors, by avoiding the caregiver altogether, or by acting in the role of a parent and attempting to reduce the distress of the caregiver.

Caregivers who have had impaired relationships with attachment figures in their own lives are especially vulnerable to problems in raising their own children. Caregivers with histories of childhood complex trauma may avoid experiencing their own emotions, which may make it difficult for them to respond appropriately to their child's emotional state. Parents and guardians may see a child's behavioral responses to trauma as a personal threat or provocation, rather than as a reenactment of what happened to the child or a behavioral representation of what the child cannot express verbally. The victimized child's simultaneous need for and fear of closeness also can trigger a caregiver's own memories of loss, rejection, or abuse, and thus diminish parenting abilities.

Ethnocultural Issues

Children's risk of exposure to complex trauma, as well as child and family responses to exposure, can also be affected by where they live and by their ethnocultural heritage and traditions. For example, war and genocide are prevalent in some parts of the world, and inner cities are frequently plagued with high levels of violence and racial tension. Children, parents, teachers, religious leaders, and the media from different cultural, national, linguistic, spiritual, and ethnic backgrounds define key trauma-related constructs in many different ways and with different expressions. For example, flashbacks may be "visions," hyperarousal may be "un ataque de nervios," and dissociation may be "spirit possession." These factors become important when considering how to treat the child.

Resilience Factors

While exposure to complex trauma has a potentially devastating impact on the developing child, there is also the possibility that a victimized child may function well in certain domains while exhibiting distress in others. Areas of competence also can shift as children are faced with new stressors and developmental challenges. Several factors have been shown to be linked to children's resilience in the face of stress: positive attachment and connections to emotionally supportive and competent adults within the family or community, development of cognitive and self-regulation abilities, and positive beliefs about oneself and motivation to act effectively in one's environment. Additional individual factors associated with resilience include an easygoing disposition, positive temperament, and sociable demeanor; internal locus of control and external attributions for blame; effective coping strategies; a high degree of mastery and autonomy; special talents; creativity; and spirituality.

The greatest threats to resilience appear to follow the breakdown of protective systems. This results in damage to brain development and associated cognitive and self-regulatory capacities, compromised caregiver-child relationships, and loss of motivation to interact with one's environment.

Assessment and Treatment

Regardless of the type of trauma that leads to a referral for services, the first step in care is a comprehensive assessment. A comprehensive assessment of complex trauma includes information from a number of sources, including the child's or adolescent's own disclosures, collateral reports from caregivers and other providers, the therapist's observations, and standardized assessment measures that have been completed by the child, caregiver, and, if possible, by the child's teacher. Assessments should be culturally sensitive and language-appropriate. Court evaluations, where required, must be conducted in a forensically sound and clinically rigorous manner.

The National Child Traumatic Stress Network is a partnership of organizations and individuals committed to raising the standard of care for traumatized children nationwide. The Complex Trauma Workgroup of the National Child Traumatic Stress Network has identified six core components of complex trauma intervention:

1. Safety: Creating a home, school, and community environment in which the child feels safe and cared for.

2. Self-regulation: Enhancing a child's capacity to modulate arousal and restore equilibrium following dysregulation of affect, behavior, physiology, cognition, interpersonal relatedness, and self-attribution.

3. Self-reflective information processing: Helping the child construct self-narratives, reflect on past and present experience, and develop skills in planning and decision making.

4. Traumatic experiences integration: Enabling the child to transform or resolve traumatic reminders and memories using such therapeutic strategies as meaning-making, traumatic memory containment or processing, remembrance and mourning of the traumatic loss, symptom management and development of coping skills, and cultivation of present-oriented thinking and behavior.

5. Relational engagement: Teaching the child to form appropriate attachments and to apply this knowledge to current interpersonal relationships, including the therapeutic alliance, with emphasis on development of such critical interpersonal skills as assertiveness, cooperation, perspective-taking, boundaries and limit-setting, reciprocity, social empathy, and the capacity for physical and emotional intimacy.

6. Positive affect enhancement: Enhancing a child's sense of self-worth, esteem, and positive self-appraisal through the cultivation of personal creativity, imagination, future orientation, achievement, competence, mastery-seeking, community-building, and the capacity to experience pleasure.

In light of the many individual and contextual differences in the lives of children and adolescents affected by complex trauma, good treatment requires the flexible adaptation of treatment strategies in response to such factors as patient age and developmental stage, gender, culture and ethnicity, socioeconomic status, and religious or community affiliation. However, in general, it is recommended that treatment proceed through a series of phases that focus on different goals. This can help avoid overloading children—who may well already have cognitive difficulties—with too much information at one time. A phase-based approach begins with a focus on providing safety, typically followed by teaching self-regulation. As children's capacity to identify, modulate and express their emotions stabilizes, treatment focus increasingly incorporates self-reflective information processing, relational engagement, and positive affect enhancement. These additional components play a critical role in helping children to develop in positive, healthy ways, and to avoid future trauma and victimization.

While it may be beneficial for some children affected by complex trauma to process their traumatic memories, this typically can only be successfully undertaken after a substantial period of stabilization in which internal and external resources have been established. Notably, several of the leading interventions for child complex trauma do not include revisiting traumatic memories but instead foster integration of traumatic experiences through a focus on recognizing and coping with present triggers within a trauma framework.

Best practice with this population typically involves adoption of a systems approach to intervention, which might involve working with child protective services, the court system, the schools, and social service agencies. Finally, there is a consensus that interventions should build strengths as well as reduce symptoms. In this way, treatment for children and adolescents also serves to protect against poor outcomes in adulthood.

References

This article has been adapted from the following sources:

Cook, A., Spinazzola, J., Ford, J., Lanktree, C., Blaustein, M.; Cloitre, M, DeRosa, R., Hubbard, R., Kagan, R., Liautaud, J., Mallah, K., Olafson, E., and van der Kolk, B. (2005). Complex trauma in children and adolescents. *Psychiatric Annals*, 35, 390–398.

Cook, A., Blaustein, M., Spinazzola, J, and van der Kolk, B. (Eds.). *Complex trauma in children and adolescents*. National Child Traumatic Stress Network. Available at http://www.nctsnet.org/nccts/nav.do?pid=typ_ct.

Chapter 33

Child Maltreatment and Domestic Violence

Over the past few decades, there has been a growing awareness of the co-occurrence of domestic violence and child maltreatment. Studies report that there are approximately between 750,000 and 2.3 million victims of domestic violence each year. Many of these victims are abused several times, so the number of domestic violence incidents is even greater. According to a national study by the U.S. Department of Health and Human Services (HHS), approximately 903,000 children were identified by child protective services (CPS) as victims of abuse or neglect in 2001. Increasingly, service providers and researchers have recognized that some of these adult and child victims are from the same families. Research suggests that in an estimated 30 to 60 percent of the families where either domestic violence or child maltreatment is identified, it is likely that both forms of abuse exist. Studies show that for victims who experience severe forms of domestic violence, their children also are in danger of suffering serious physical harm. In a national survey of over 6,000 American families, researchers found that 50 percent of men who frequently assaulted their wives also abused their children. Other studies demonstrate that perpetrators of domestic violence who were abused as children are more likely to physically harm their children.

Excerpted from "Child Protection in Families Experiencing Domestic Violence: Chapter 2," Child Welfare Information Gateway, U.S. Department of Health and Human Services (HHS), updated September 18, 2008.

Rates of Domestic Violence

Using the National Crime Victimization Survey (NCVS), a household counted as experiencing domestic violence was counted only once, regardless of the number of times that a victim experienced violence and regardless of the number of victims in the household during the year. The following statistics represent reported cases.

Table 33.1. Rates and Characteristics of Domestic Violence

Characteristic of the household	Percent of households that experienced domestic violence
Caucasian	0.4%
African-American	0.5%
Hispanic	0.5%
Other	0.5%
Urban	0.5%
Suburban	0.4%
Rural	0.4%
Northeast	0.3%
Midwest	0.7%
South	0.4%
West	0.5%
Household Size	
1 person	0.4%
2 to 3 persons	0.4%
4 to 5 persons	0.5%
6 or more persons	1.0%

The Co-Occurrence of Child Maltreatment and Domestic Violence

An estimated 3.3 to 10 million children a year are at risk for witnessing or being exposed to domestic violence, which can produce a range of emotional, psychological, and behavioral problems for children. This estimate is derived from an earlier landmark study that found approximately three million American households experienced at least one incident of serious violence each year. The broad range of this estimate highlights the fact that the exact number of domestic violence incidents is unknown, and there sometimes is incongruence or a lack of agreement about exactly what constitutes domestic violence.

One study estimates that as many as ten million teenagers are exposed to parental violence each year. This estimate comes from a survey in which adults were asked "whether, during their teenage years, their father had hit their mother and how often" and vice versa for the mother. The survey found that about one in eight, 12.6 percent of the sample, recalled such an incident. In these cases, 50 percent remembered their father hitting the mother, 19 percent recalled their mother hitting the father, and 31 percent recalled the parents hitting each other.

These estimates are based on research that identified maltreated children who accompanied victims of domestic violence to shelters and identified adult victims via CPS caseloads. Additionally, research examining the relationship between victims and their own use of violence indicate that they are more likely to perpetrate physical violence against their children than caretakers who are not abused by a partner or spouse. Children who witness domestic violence and are victimized by abuse exhibit more emotional and psychological problems than children who only witness domestic violence.

Current data regarding the co-occurrence between domestic violence and child maltreatment compel child welfare and programs that address domestic violence to re-evaluate their existing philosophies, policies, and practice approaches towards families experiencing both forms of violence. The overlap of these issues may be particularly critical in identifying cases with a high risk of violence, such as the relationship between domestic violence and child fatalities in CPS cases. A review of CPS cases in two states identified domestic violence in approximately 41 to 43 percent of cases resulting in the critical injury or death of a child. A number of protocols and practice guidelines have surfaced over the past decade to provide child welfare and service providers with specific assessment and intervention procedures aimed at enhancing the safety of children and victims of domestic violence.

Children's Exposure to Domestic Violence

Children who live in homes where a parent or caretaker is experiencing abuse are commonly referred to as child witnesses or children who are witnessing domestic violence. The term "children's exposure" to domestic violence, however, provides a more inclusive definition because it encompasses the multiple ways children experience domestic abuse. Although caretakers frequently believe they are protecting their children from witnessing their abuse, children living in these homes report differently. Researchers have found that 80 to 90 percent of children in homes where domestic violence occurs can provide detailed accounts of the violence in their homes. Research studies have proliferated regarding children's exposure to domestic violence, the problems associated with witnessing, and the protective factors that influence their responses to the violence. Children's exposure to domestic violence typically falls into three primary categories:

- Hearing a violent event

- Being directly involved as an eyewitness, intervening, or being used as a part of a violent event (for example, being used as a shield against abusive actions)

- Experiencing the aftermath of a violent event

Children's exposure to domestic violence also may include being used as a spy to interrogate the adult victim, being forced to watch or participate in the abuse of the victim, and being used as a pawn by the abuser to coerce the victim into returning to the violent relationship. Some children are physically injured as a direct result of the domestic violence. Some perpetrators intentionally physically, emotionally, or sexually abuse their children in an effort to intimidate and control their partner. While this is clearly child maltreatment, other cases may not be so clear. Children often are harmed accidentally during violent attacks on the adult victim. An object thrown or weapon used against the battered partner can hit the child. Assaults on younger children can occur while the adult victim is holding the child, and injury or harm to older children can happen when they intervene in violent episodes. In addition to being exposed to the abusive behavior, many children are further victimized by coercion to remain silent about the abuse, maintaining the family secret.

The Effects of Domestic Violence on Children

Children who live with domestic violence face numerous risks, such as the risk of exposure to traumatic events, the risk of neglect, the risk of being directly abused, and the risk of losing one or both of their parents. All of these can lead to negative outcomes for children and clearly have an impact on them. Research studies consistently have found the presence of three categories of childhood problems associated with exposure to domestic violence:

- **Behavioral, social, and emotional problems:** higher levels of aggression, anger, hostility, oppositional behavior, and disobedience; fear, anxiety, withdrawal, and depression; poor peer, sibling, and social relationships; low self-esteem.

- **Cognitive and attitudinal problems:** lower cognitive functioning, poor school performance, lack of conflict resolution skills, limited problem-solving skills, acceptance of violent behaviors and attitudes, belief in rigid gender stereotypes and male privilege.

- **Long-term problems:** higher levels of adult depression and trauma symptoms, increased tolerance for and use of violence in adult relationships.

Children also display specific problems unique to their physical, psychological, and social development. For example, infants exposed to violence may have difficulty developing attachments with their caregivers and in extreme cases suffer from failure to thrive. It should be noted that there also are limitations and uncertainties to the research since some of the children in such studies do not show elevated problem levels even under similar circumstances. Preschool children may regress developmentally or suffer from eating and sleep disturbances. School-aged children may struggle with peer relationships, academic performance, and emotional stability. Adolescents are at a higher risk for either perpetrating or becoming victims of teen dating violence. Reports from adults who repeatedly witnessed domestic violence as children show that many suffer from trauma-related symptoms, depression, and low self-esteem.

Possible Symptoms in Children Exposed to Domestic Violence

- Sleeplessness, fears of going to sleep, nightmares, dreams of danger
- Physical symptoms such as headaches or stomachaches
- Hypervigilance to danger or being hurt
- Fighting with others, hurting other children or animals
- Temper tantrums or defiant behavior

- Withdrawal from people or typical activities
- Listlessness, depression, low energy
- Feelings of loneliness and isolation
- Current or subsequent substance abuse
- Suicide attempts or engaging in dangerous behavior
- Poor school performance
- Difficulties concentrating and paying attention
- Fears of being separated from the non-abusing parent
- Feeling that his or her best is not good enough
- Taking on adult or parental responsibilities
- Excessive worrying
- Bed-wetting or regression to earlier developmental stages
- Dissociation
- Identifying with or mirroring behaviors of the abuser

Children's Protective Factors in Response to Domestic Violence

Studies documenting the types of problems associated with children who are exposed to domestic violence reveal a wide variation in their responses to the violence. Children's risk levels and reactions to domestic violence exist on a continuum where some children demonstrate enormous resiliency while others show signs of significant maladaptive adjustment. Protective factors such as social competence, intelligence, high self-esteem, outgoing temperament, strong sibling and peer relationships, and a supportive relationship with an adult, are thought to be important variables that help protect children from the adverse effects of exposure to domestic violence. In addition, research shows that the impact of domestic violence on children can be moderated by certain factors, including the following:

- **The nature of the violence:** Children, who witness frequent and severe forms of violence, perceive the violence as their fault. Because they fail to observe their caretakers resolving conflict, these children may undergo more distress than children who witness fewer incidences of physical violence. The frequency with which they witness positive interactions between their caregivers also affects them.

- **Coping strategies and skills:** Children with poor coping skills are more likely to experience problems than children with strong coping skills and supportive social networks. Children who utilize problem-solving strategies targeted directly at the source of disagreement demonstrate fewer maladaptive symptoms. Emotion-focused strategies, however, are less desirable because they often target internal responses to a stressful situation, which can result in less effective coping methods (for example, children fantasizing that their parents are getting along).

- **The age of the child:** Younger children appear to exhibit higher levels of emotional and psychological distress than older children. Age-related differences might result from older children's more fully developed cognitive abilities to understand the violence and select various coping strategies to alleviate upsetting emotions.

- **The time since exposure:** Children are observed to have heightened levels of anxiety and fear immediately after a recent violent event. Fewer observable effects are seen in children the longer time has past after they have witnessed the violence.

- **Gender:** In general, boys exhibit more externalized behaviors (aggression or acting out) while girls exhibit more internalized behaviors (withdrawal or depression). In addition, boys identify more with the male abuser and girls identify more with the female victim; both may continue these roles throughout life if the issues are not addressed.

- **The presence of child abuse:** Children who witness domestic abuse and are physically abused demonstrate increased levels of emotional and psychological maladjustment than children who only witness violence and are not abused.

Professionals Responding to Child Maltreatment and Domestic Violence: In Search of Common Ground

Although adult and child victims often are found in the same families, child protection and domestic violence programs have historically responded separately to victims. The divergent responses are largely due to the differences in each system's historical development, philosophy, mandate, policies, and practices. As a result, these differences have led to variations in desired outcomes and practice methods for child welfare caseworkers and service providers who lack a mutual understanding of one another's mission and approach when addressing the co-occurrence of child maltreatment and domestic violence.

Several key debates stemming from these differences have limited collaboration between the two fields. For CPS caseworkers, whose legal mandate is the protection of the abused child, responding to domestic violence has been widely regarded as a peripheral issue. Alternatively, service providers have primarily focused on pursuing safety and empowerment for adult victims. The differing opinion about whose safety is paramount has led to misconceptions and critical accusations by both systems. Child welfare advocates have charged service providers with discounting the safety needs of children by focusing primarily on the adult victim who also may be neglectful or abusive towards the children. Conversely, some service providers accuse child welfare caseworkers of "revictimizing" victims of domestic violence by placing responsibility and blame on adult victims for the violent behaviors of perpetrators or charging the adult victim with failing to protect the child. Furthermore, interactions with the perpetrator are markedly distinct for each system. CPS's growing emphasis on a family-centered approach may sometimes compel caseworkers to engage perpetrators, who are either biological parents or caretakers of the children, in efforts aimed at creating healthy and stable families. In contrast, service providers often view separation from perpetrators as a desirable intervention until the safety of all family members is assured.

Despite their differences, child welfare advocates and service providers share areas of common ground that can bridge the gap between them:

- Both want to end domestic violence and child maltreatment
- Both want children to be safe
- Both want adult victims to be protected—for their own safety and so their children are not harmed by the violence
- Both believe in supporting a parent's strengths
- Both prefer that children not be involved in CPS, if avoidable

Additionally, men historically have not been actively involved with CPS or domestic violence agencies in working to make the necessary behavior modifications that will facilitate change on these issues.

Chapter 34

Numbers and Trends in Child Maltreatment

Child Maltreatment 2006

All 50 states, the District of Columbia, and the U.S. territories have mandatory child abuse and neglect reporting laws that require certain professionals and institutions to report suspected maltreatment to a child protective services (CPS) agency. Examples of these mandatory reporters include health care providers and facilities, mental health care providers, teachers and other school staff, social workers, police officers, foster care providers, and daycare providers. The initial report of suspected child abuse or neglect is called a referral. Approximately one-third of referrals are screened out each year and do not receive further attention from CPS. The remaining referrals are screened in and an investigation or assessment is conducted by the CPS agency to determine the likelihood that maltreatment has occurred or that the child is at risk of maltreatment. After conducting interviews with family members, the alleged victim, and other people familiar with the family, the CPS agency makes a determination or finding concerning whether the child is a victim of abuse or neglect or is at risk of abuse or neglect. This determination often is called a disposition. Each state establishes specific dispositions and terminology.

This chapter includes text from "Child Maltreatment 2006: Summary," Administration for Children and Families, U.S. Department of Health and Human Services (HHS), April 3, 2008.

Each state has its own definitions of child abuse and neglect based on minimum standards set by federal law. Federal legislation provides a foundation for states by identifying a minimum set of acts or behaviors that define child abuse and neglect. The federal *Child Abuse Prevention and Treatment Act* (CAPTA), (42 U.S.C.A. §5106g), as amended by the *Keeping Children and Families Safe Act of 2003*, defines child abuse and neglect as:

- any recent act or failure to act on the part of a parent or caretaker which results in death, serious physical or emotional harm, sexual abuse or exploitation; or

- an act or failure to act which presents an imminent risk of serious harm.

Within the minimum standards set by CAPTA, each state is responsible for providing its own definitions of child abuse and neglect. Most states recognize four major types of maltreatment: neglect, physical abuse, sexual abuse, and emotional abuse. Although any of the forms of child maltreatment may be found separately, they also can occur in combination.

What is the National Child Abuse and Neglect Data System (NCANDS)?

NCANDS is a federally sponsored effort that collects and analyzes annual data on child abuse and neglect. The data are submitted voluntarily by the states, the District of Columbia, and the Commonwealth of Puerto Rico. The first report from NCANDS was based on data for 1990; the report for 2006 data is the 17th issuance of this annual report.

What data are collected?

NCANDS collects case-level data on all children who received an investigation or assessment by a CPS agency. States that are unable to provide case-level data submit aggregated counts of key indicators.

Case-level data include information on the characteristics of referrals of abuse or neglect that are made to CPS agencies, the children referred, the types of maltreatment that are alleged, the dispositions (or findings) of the investigations, the risk factors of the child and the caregivers, the services that are provided, and the perpetrators.

How many children were reported and received an investigation or assessment for abuse and neglect?

During federal fiscal year 2006, an estimated 3.3 million referrals, involving the alleged maltreatment of approximately 6.0 million children, were made to CPS agencies. An estimated 3.6 million children received an investigation or assessment.

- Approximately 60 percent (61.7%) of referrals were screened in for investigation or assessment by CPS agencies.

- Approximately 30 percent of the investigations or assessments determined at least one child who was found to be a victim of abuse or neglect with the following report dispositions: 25.2 percent substantiated, 3.0 percent indicated, and 0.4 percent alternative response victim.

- More than 70 percent of the investigations or assessments determined that the child was not a victim of maltreatment with the following dispositions: 60.4 percent unsubstantiated, 5.9 percent alternative response non-victim, 3.2 percent "other," 1.7 percent closed with no finding, and 0.1 percent intentionally false.

Who reported child maltreatment?

For 2006, 56.3% of alleged child abuse or neglect reports were made by professionals. The term professional means that the person had contact with the alleged child maltreatment victim as part of the report source's job. This term includes teachers, police officers, lawyers, and social services staff. The remaining reports were made by nonprofessionals, including friends, neighbors, sports coaches, and relatives.

- The three largest percentages of report sources were from such professionals as teachers (16.5%), lawyers or police officers (15.8%), and social services staff (10.0%).

Who were the child victims?

During 2006, an estimated 905,000 children were determined to be victims of abuse or neglect. Among the children confirmed as victims by CPS agencies in 2006:

- children in the age group of birth to one year had the highest rate of victimization at 24.4 per 1,000 children of the same age group in the national population;

- 51.5% of the child victims were girls and 48.2 percent were boys; and

- 48.9% of all victims were white; 22.8% were African-American; and 18.4 percent were Hispanic.

What were the most common types of maltreatment?

As in prior years, neglect was the most common form of child maltreatment. CPS investigations determined that:

- 64.1% of victims suffered neglect,

- 16.0% of the victims suffered physical abuse,

- 8.8% of the victims suffered sexual abuse, and

- 6.6% of the victims suffered from emotional maltreatment.

How many children died from abuse or neglect?

Child fatalities are the most tragic consequence of maltreatment. Yet, each year children die from abuse and neglect. During 2006:

- an estimated 1,530 children died due to child abuse or neglect;

- the overall rate of child fatalities was 2.04 deaths per 100,000 children;

- 41.1% of child fatalities were attributed to neglect; physical abuse also was a major contributor to child fatalities;

- 78.0% of the children who died due to child abuse and neglect were younger than four years old;

- infant boys (younger than one year) had the highest rate of fatalities, at 18.5 deaths per 100,000 boys of the same age in the national population; and

- infant girls had a rate of 14.7 deaths per 100,000 girls of the same age.

Who abused and neglected children?

In 2006, 79.4% of perpetrators of child maltreatment were parents, and another 6.7 percent were other relatives of the victim. Women comprised a larger percentage of all perpetrators than men, 57.9 percent compared to 42.1 percent. More than 75 percent (77.5%) of all perpetrators were younger than age 40.

- Of the perpetrators who maltreated children, 7.0% committed sexual abuse, while 60.4 percent committed neglect.

- Of the perpetrators who were parents, 91.5% were the biological parent of the victim.

Who received services?

During an investigation, CPS agencies provide services to children and their families, both in the home and in foster care.

- Of the children who received post-investigation services, 58.9% were victims and 30.3 percent were non-victims.

- Of the children who were placed in foster care, 21.5% were victims and 4.4 percent were non-victims.

Chapter 35

Effects of Childhood Stress on Health across the Lifespan

Stress is an inevitable part of life. Human beings experience stress early, even before they are born. A certain amount of stress is normal and necessary for survival. Stress helps children develop the skills they need to cope with and adapt to new and potentially threatening situations throughout life. Support from parents or other concerned caregivers is necessary for children to learn how to respond to stress in a physically and emotionally healthy manner.

The beneficial aspects of stress diminish when it is severe enough to overwhelm a child's ability to cope effectively. Intensive and prolonged stress can lead to a variety of short- and long-term negative health effects. It can disrupt early brain development and compromise functioning of the nervous and immune systems. In addition, childhood stress can lead to health problems later in life including alcoholism, depression, eating disorders, heart disease, cancer, and other chronic diseases.

The purpose of this chapter is to summarize the research on childhood stress and its implications for adult health and well-being. Of particular interest is the stress caused by child abuse, neglect, and repeated exposure to intimate partner violence (IPV).

Text in this chapter is excerpted from Middlebrooks JS, Audage NC. *The Effects of Childhood Stress on Health across the Lifespan.* Atlanta (GA): Centers for Disease Control and Prevention, National Center for Injury Prevention and Control; 2008. The complete report is available at http://www.cdc.gov/ncipc/pub-res/pdf/Childhood_Stress.pdf.

Types of Stress

Following are descriptions of the three types of stress that The National Scientific Council on the Developing Child has identified based on available research:

Positive stress results from adverse experiences that are short-lived. Children may encounter positive stress when they attend a new daycare, get a shot, meet new people, or have a toy taken away from them. This type of stress causes minor physiological changes including an increase in heart rate and changes in hormone levels. With the support of caring adults, children can learn how to manage and overcome positive stress. This type of stress is considered normal and coping with it is an important part of the development process.

Tolerable stress refers to adverse experiences that are more intense but still relatively short-lived. Examples include the death of a loved one, a natural disaster, a frightening accident, and family disruptions such as separation or divorce. If a child has the support of a caring adult, tolerable stress can usually be overcome. In many cases, tolerable stress can become positive stress and benefit the child developmentally. However, if the child lacks adequate support, tolerable stress can become toxic and lead to long-term negative health effects.

Toxic stress results from intense adverse experiences that may be sustained over a long period of time—weeks, months, or even years. An example of toxic stress is child maltreatment which includes abuse and neglect. Children are unable to effectively manage this type of stress by themselves. As a result, the stress response system gets activated for a prolonged amount of time. This can lead to permanent changes in the development of the brain. The negative effects of toxic stress can be lessened with the support of caring adults. Appropriate support and intervention can help in returning the stress response system back to its normal baseline.

The Effects of Toxic Stress on Brain Development in Early Childhood

The ability to manage stress is controlled by brain circuits and hormone systems that are activated early in life. When a child feels threatened, hormones are released and they circulate throughout the body. Prolonged exposure to stress hormones can impact the brain and impair functioning in a variety of ways.

- Toxic stress can impair the connection of brain circuits and, in the extreme, result in the development of a smaller brain.

- Brain circuits are especially vulnerable as they are developing during early childhood. Toxic stress can disrupt the development of these circuits. This can cause an individual to develop a low threshold for stress, thereby becoming overly reactive to adverse experiences throughout life.

- High levels of stress hormones, including cortisol, can suppress the body's immune response. This can leave an individual vulnerable to a variety of infections and chronic health problems.

- Sustained high levels of cortisol can damage the hippocampus, an area of the brain responsible for learning and memory. These cognitive deficits can continue into adulthood.

The Effects of Toxic Stress on Adult Health and Well-Being

Research findings demonstrate that childhood stress can impact adult health. The Adverse Childhood Experiences (ACE) Study is particularly noteworthy because it demonstrates a link between specific 1) violence-related stressors, including child abuse, neglect, and repeated exposure to intimate partner violence, and 2) risky behaviors and health problems in adulthood.

The ACE Study

The ACE Study, a collaboration between the Centers for Disease Control and Prevention (CDC) and Kaiser Permanente Health Appraisal Clinic in San Diego, uses a retrospective approach to examine the link between childhood stressors and adult health. Over 17,000 adults participated in the research, making it one of the largest studies of its kind. Each participant completed a questionnaire that asked for detailed information on their past history of abuse, neglect, and family dysfunction as well as their current behaviors and health status. Researchers were particularly interested in participants' exposure to the following ten adverse childhood experiences:

- Abuse
  - Emotional
  - Physical
  - Sexual

- Neglect
  - Emotional
  - Physical
- Household Dysfunction
  - Mother treated violently
  - Household substance abuse
  - Household mental illness
  - Parental separation or divorce
  - Incarcerated household member

General ACE Study Findings

The ACE Study findings have been published in more than 30 scientific articles. The following are some of the general findings of the study: Childhood abuse, neglect, and exposure to other adverse experiences are common (table 35.1). Almost two-thirds of study participants

Table 35.1. Prevalence of Individual Adverse Childhood Experiences

ACE Category	Women (N = 9,367)	Men (N = 7,970)	Total (N = 17,337)
Abuse			
Emotional Abuse	13.1%	7.6%	10.6%
Physical Abuse	27.0%	29.9%	28.3%
Sexual Abuse	24.7%	16.0%	20.7%
Neglect			
Emotional Neglect*	16.7%	12.4%	14.8%
Physical Neglect*	9.2%	10.7%	9.9%
Household Dysfunction			
Mother Treated Violently	13.7%	11.5%	12.7%
Household Substance Abuse	29.5%	23.8%	26.9%
Household Mental Illness	23.3%	14.8%	19.4%
Parental Separation or Divorce	24.5%	21.8%	23.3%
Incarcerated Household Member	5.2%	4.1%	4.7%

* Collected during the second survey wave only (N=8,667).

reported at least one ACE, and more than one in five reported three or more (table 35.2).

The short- and long-term outcomes of ACE include a multitude of health and behavioral problems. As the number of ACE a person experiences increases, the risk for the following health outcomes also increases:

- alcoholism and alcohol abuse
- chronic obstructive pulmonary disease
- depression
- fetal death
- illicit drug use
- ischemic heart disease
- liver disease
- risk for intimate partner violence
- multiple sexual partners
- sexually transmitted diseases
- smoking
- suicide attempts
- unintended pregnancies

ACE are also related to risky health behaviors in childhood and adolescence, including pregnancies, suicide attempts, early initiation of smoking, sexual activity, and illicit drug use.

As the number of ACE increases, the number of co-occurring health conditions increases.

Table 35.2. ACE Score

Number of Adverse Childhood Experiences (ACE Score)	Women	Men	Total
0	34.5%	38.0%	36.1%
1	24.5%	27.9%	26.0%
2	15.5%	16.4%	15.9%
3	10.3%	8.6%	9.5%
4 or more	15.2%	9.2%	12.5%

Violence-Related ACE Study Findings

Findings from the ACE Study confirm what we already know—that too many people in the United States are exposed at an early age to violence and other childhood stressors. The study also provides strong evidence that being exposed to certain childhood experiences, including being subjected to abuse or neglect or witnessing intimate partner violence (IPV), can lead to a wide array of negative behaviors and poor health outcomes. In addition, the ACE Study has found associations between experiencing ACE and two violent outcomes: suicide attempts and the risk of perpetrating or experiencing IPV.

Following is a summary of some of the ACE Study findings relevant to violence. Some findings relate to participants' past history of abuse, neglect, and IPV exposure, while others involve the link between ACE and adult behaviors and health status.

Child Maltreatment and Its Impact on Health and Behavior

- 25% of women and 16% of men reported experiencing child sexual abuse.

- Participants who were sexually abused as children were more likely to experience multiple other ACE.

- The ACE score increased as the child sexual abuse severity, duration, and frequency increased and the age at first occurrence decreased.

- Women and men who experienced child sexual abuse were more than twice as likely to report suicide attempts.

- A strong relationship was found between frequent physical abuse, sexual abuse, and witnessing of IPV as a child and a male's risk of involvement with a teenage pregnancy.

- Women who reported experiencing four or more types of abuse during their childhood were 1.5 times more likely to have an unintended pregnancy at or before the age of twenty.

- Men and women who reported being sexually abused were more at risk of marrying an alcoholic and having current marital problems.

Witnessing Intimate Partner Violence (IPV) as a Child and Its Impact on Health and Behavior

- Study participants who witnessed IPV were two to six times more likely to experience another ACE.

320

- As the frequency of witnessing IPV increased, the chance of reported alcoholism, illicit drug use, IV drug use, and depression also increased.

- Exposure to physical abuse, sexual abuse, and IPV in childhood resulted in women being 3.5 times more likely to report IPV victimization.

- Exposure to physical abuse, sexual abuse, and IPV in childhood resulted in men being 3.8 times more likely to report IPV perpetration.

The Link between ACE and Suicide Attempts

- 3.8% of study participants reported having attempted suicide at least once.

- Experiencing one ACE increased the risk of attempted suicide two to five times.

- As the ACE score increased so did the likelihood of attempting suicide.

- The relationship between ACE and the risk of attempted suicide appears to be influenced by alcoholism, depression, and illicit drug use.

ACE and Associated Health Behaviors

Associations were found between ACE and many negative health behaviors. Following is a partial list.

- Participants with higher ACE scores were at greater risk of alcoholism.

- Those with higher ACE scores were more likely to marry an alcoholic.

- Study participants with higher ACE scores were more likely to initiate drug use and experience addiction.

- Those with higher ACE scores were more likely to have 30 or more sexual partners, engage in sexual intercourse earlier, and feel more at risk of contracting acquired immunodeficiency syndrome (AIDS).

- Higher ACE scores in participants were linked to a higher probability of both lifetime and recent depressive disorders.

Chapter 36

Teen Dating Abuse

Chapter Contents

Section 36.1

Dating Violence Defined

Dating Violence: What Is It?

Dating violence is controlling, abusive, and aggressive behavior in a romantic relationship. It can happen in straight or gay relationships. It can include verbal, emotional, physical, or sexual abuse, or a combination.

Controlling behavior may include the following:

- Not letting you hang out with your friends
- Calling or paging you frequently to find out where you are, whom you're with, and what you're doing
- Telling you what to wear
- Having to be with you all the time

Verbal and emotional abuse may include the following:

- Calling you names
- Jealousy
- Belittling you (cutting you down)
- Threatening to hurt you, someone in your family, or himself or herself if you don't do what he or she wants

Physical abuse may include these actions:

- Shoving
- Punching
- Slapping
- Pinching
- Hitting
- Kicking
- Hair pulling
- Strangling

Sexual abuse may include the following:

- Unwanted touching and kissing
- Forcing you to have sex
- Not letting you use birth control
- Forcing you to do other sexual things

Anyone can be a victim of dating violence. Both boys and girls are victims, but boys and girls abuse their partners in different ways. Girls are more likely to yell, threaten to hurt themselves, pinch, slap, scratch, or kick. Boys injure girls more and are more likely to punch their partner and force them to participate in unwanted sexual activity. Some teen victims experience violence occasionally. Others are abused more often, sometimes daily.

If You Are a Victim of Dating Violence, You Might...

- Think it's your fault
- Feel angry, sad, lonely, depressed, or confused
- Feel helpless to stop the abuse
- Feel threatened or humiliated
- Feel anxious
- Not know what might happen next
- Feel like you can't talk to family and friends
- Be afraid of getting hurt more seriously
- Feel protective of your boyfriend or girlfriend

You're Not Alone

- One in five teens in a serious relationship reports having been hit, slapped, or pushed by a partner.[1]
- 50–80% of teens have reported knowing others who were involved in violent relationships.[2]
- Teens identifying as gay, lesbian, and bisexual are as likely to experience violence in same-sex dating relationships as youths involved in opposite sex dating.[3]
- Many studies indicate that, as a dating relationship becomes more serious, the potential for and nature of violent behavior escalates.[4]

- Young women, ages 16 to 24 years, experience the highest rates of relationship violence.[5]

Get Help

Being a victim of dating violence is not your fault. Nothing you say, wear, or do gives anyone the right to hurt you.

- If you think you are in an abusive relationship, get help immediately. Don't keep your concerns to yourself.

- Talk to someone you trust like a parent, teacher, school principal, counselor, or nurse.

- If you choose to tell, you should know that some adults are mandated reporters. This means they are legally required to report neglect or abuse to someone else, such as the police or child protective services. You can ask people if they are mandated reporters and then decide what you want to do. Some examples of mandated reporters are teachers, counselors, doctors, social workers, and in some cases, even coaches or activity leaders. If you want help deciding whom to talk to, call the National Crime Victim Helpline at 1-800-FYI-CALL or an anonymous crisis line in your area. You might also want to talk to a trusted family member, a friend's parent, an adult neighbor or friend, an older sibling or cousin, or other experienced person who you trust.

Help Yourself

Think about ways you can be safer. This means thinking about what to do, where to go for help, and who to call ahead of time.

- Where can you go for help?
- Who can you call?
- Who will help you?
- How will you escape a violent situation?

Here are other precautions you can take:

- Let friends or family know when you are afraid or need help.
- When you go out, say where you are going and when you'll be back.
- In an emergency, call 911 or your local police department.

- Memorize important phone numbers, such as the people to contact or places to go in an emergency.
- Keep spare change, calling cards, or a cell phone handy for immediate access to communication.
- Go out in a group or with other couples.
- Have money available for transportation if you need to take a taxi, bus, or subway to escape.

Help Someone Else

If you know someone who might be in an abusive relationship, you can help.

- Tell the person that you are worried.
- Be a good listener.
- Offer your friendship and support.
- Ask how you can help.
- Encourage your friend to seek help.
- Educate yourself about dating violence and healthy relationships.
- Avoid any confrontations with the abuser. This could be dangerous for you and your friend.

References

1. Liz Claiborne Inc., "Study on Teen Dating Abuse," (Teenage Research Unlimited, 2005), http://www.loveisnotabuse.com (accessed March 1, 2007).

2. Ibid.

3. L.L. Kupper et al., "Prevalence of Partner Violence in Same-Sex Romantic and Sexual Relationships in a National Sample of Adolescents," *Journal of Adolescent Health 35* (2004): 124–131.

4. *Teen Dating Violence Resource Manual*, (Denver: National Coalition Against Domestic Violence, 1997), 17.

5. C. M. Rennison and S. Welchans, "BJS Special Report: Intimate Partner Violence," (Washington, DC: Bureau of Justice Statistics, 2000).

Section 36.2

Dating Violence among U.S. High School Students

This section includes text from "Physical Dating Violence Among High School Students–United States, 2003," *MMWR Weekly 55*(19) pp. 532–535, Centers for Disease Control and Prevention (CDC), May 19, 2006. The full report is available at http://www.cdc.gov/mmwr/preview/mmwrhtml/ mm5519a3.htm.

Dating violence is defined as physical, sexual, or psychological violence within a dating relationship. In a study of dating violence victimization among students in grades 7–12 during 1994–1995, the 18-month prevalence of victimization from physical and psychological dating violence was estimated at 12% and 20%, respectively. In addition to the risk for injury and death, victims of dating violence are more likely to engage in risky sexual behavior, unhealthy dieting behaviors, substance use, and suicidal ideation/attempts. Dating violence victimization can be a precursor for intimate partner violence (IPV) victimization in adulthood, most notably among women. Among adult women in the United States, an estimated 5.3 million IPV incidents occur each year, resulting in approximately two million injuries and 1,300 deaths. By using data from the 2003 Youth Risk Behavior Survey (YRBS), the Centers for Disease Control and Prevention (CDC) analyzed the prevalence of physical dating violence (PDV) victimization among high school students and its association with five risk behaviors. The results indicated that 8.9% of students (8.9% of males and 8.8% of females) reported PDV victimization during the 12 months preceding the survey and that students reporting PDV victimization were more likely to engage in four of the five risk behaviors (sexual intercourse, attempted suicide, episodic heavy drinking, and physical fighting). Primary prevention programs are needed to educate high school students about healthy dating relationship behaviors, and secondary prevention programs should address risk behaviors associated with dating violence victimization.

The Youth Risk Behavior Surveillance System measures the prevalence of health risk behaviors among high school students through

Table 36.1. Prevalence of physical dating violence victimization* among high school students, by sex and selected characteristics– United States, 2003

Characteristic	Total (%)	Male (%)	Female (%)
Overall	8.9	8.9	8.9
Grade level			
9	8.1	7.8	8.6
10	8.8	9.3	8.2
11	8.1	7.9	8.2
12	10.1	10.1	10.2
Race/Ethnicity			
White, non-Hispanic	7.0	6.6	7.5
Black, non-Hispanic	13.9	13.7	14.0
Hispanic	9.3	9.2	9.2
Geographic region **			
Northeast	10.6	10.8	10.4
Midwest	7.5	8.3	6.5
South	9.6	9.3	9.9
West	6.9	6.1	7.8
Self-reported grades			
Mostly A's	6.1	6.6	5.7
Mostly B's	7.7	7.4	8.0
Mostly C's	11.2	10.4	12.3
Mostly D's or F's	13.7	13.0	14.9

*Defined as a response of yes to a single question: "During the past 12 months, did your boyfriend or girlfriend ever hit, slap, or physically hurt you on purpose?"

Northeast: Connecticut, Maine, Massachusetts, New Hampshire, New Jersey, New York, Pennsylvania, Rhode Island, and Vermont. **Midwest:** Illinois, Indiana, Iowa, Kansas, Michigan, Minnesota, Missouri, Nebraska, North Dakota, Ohio, South Dakota, and Wisconsin. **South:** Alabama, Arkansas, Delaware, District of Columbia, Florida, Georgia, Kentucky, Louisiana, Maryland, Mississippi, North Carolina, Oklahoma, South Carolina, Tennessee, Texas, Virginia, and West Virginia. **West:** Alaska, Arizona, California, Colorado, Hawaii, Idaho, Montana, Nevada, New Mexico, Oregon, Utah, Washington, and Wyoming.

biennial national, state, and local surveys. The 2003 national survey obtained cross-sectional data representative of public- and private-school students in grades 9–12 in the 50 states and the District of Columbia. The overall response rate was 67%. Data from 15,214 students in 158 schools were available for analysis; 14,956 (98.3%) students answered the dating violence question. Students completed an anonymous, self-administered questionnaire that included a question about dating violence victimization.

PDV victimization was defined as a response of "yes" to a single question: "During the past 12 months, did your boyfriend or girlfriend ever hit, slap, or physically hurt you on purpose?" Students were not asked whether they had had a boyfriend or girlfriend during the 12 months preceding the survey; therefore, a response of "no" might have included students who had not been dating.

Table 36.2. Association* between physical dating violence victimization[t] and reported risk behaviors among high school students, by sex–United States, 2003

Risk Behavior[a]	Total AOR**	Male AOR**	Female AOR**
Currently sexually active	2.6	3.3	2.0
Attempted suicide	3.3	3.8	3.1
Current cigarette use	1.1	1.1	1.1
Episodic heavy drinking	1.3	1.2	1.4
Physical fighting	1.7	1.7	1.8

*Models include all risk behaviors and control variables (for example, sex, grade level, race/ethnicity, and self-reported grades).

[t] Defined as a response of yes to a single question: "During the past 12 months, did your boyfriend or girlfriend ever hit, slap, or physically hurt you on purpose?"

[a] **Currently sexually active:** 34.3% of all students reported having sexual intercourse with at least one person during the three months preceding the survey. **Attempted suicide:** 8.5% reported actually attempting suicide at least one time during the 12 months preceding the survey. **Current cigarette use:** 21.9% reporting smoking cigarettes on one or more of the thirty days preceding the survey. **Episodic heavy drinking:** 28.3% reported having five or more alcoholic drinks in a row on at on one or more of the 30 days preceding the survey. **Physical fighting:** 33.0% reported being in a physical fight at least one time during the twelve months preceding the survey.

**Adjusted odds ratio.

The findings in this report suggest that PDV victimization affects a substantial number of high school students, with approximately one in eleven reporting PDV victimization during the 12 months preceding the survey, a ratio equating to nearly 1.5 million high school students nationwide. Prevalence of PDV victimization was similar and associated with risk behaviors for both male and female high school students, and no significant increases in PDV victimization were observed by grade level.

Medical and mental health-care providers and others consulted by teens (for example, school counselors) should be aware of the prevalence of dating violence and the potential for associated risk behaviors among teens who report dating violence. Appropriate intervention (such as, referral for counseling) to reduce the likelihood of further victimization is more likely if providers ask about dating violence when speaking with teens. The findings in this report and the resulting recommendations are consistent with recommendations by others that dating violence intervention and prevention can benefit from addressing dating violence in the context of other risk behaviors.

Section 36.3

Date Rape

When people think of rape, they might think of a stranger jumping out of a shadowy place and sexually attacking someone. But it's not only strangers who rape. In fact, about half of all people who are raped know the person who attacked them. Girls and women are most often raped, but guys can also be raped.

Most friendships, acquaintances, and dates never lead to violence, of course. But, sadly, sometimes it happens. When forced sex occurs between two people who already know each other, it is known as date rape or acquaintance rape.

Even if the two people know each other well, and even if they were intimate or had sex before, no one has the right to force a sexual act on another person against his or her will.

Although it involves forced sex, rape is not about sex or passion. Rape has nothing to do with love. Rape is an act of aggression and violence.

You may hear some people say that those who have been raped were somehow "asking for it" because of the clothes they wore or the way they acted. That's wrong: The person who is raped is not to blame. Rape is always the fault of the rapist. And that's also the case when two people are dating—or even in an intimate relationship. One person never owes the other person sex. If sex is forced against someone's will, that's rape.

Healthy relationships involve respect—including respect for the feelings of others. Someone who really cares about you will respect your wishes and not force or pressure you to have sex.

Alcohol and Drugs

Alcohol is often involved in date rapes. Drinking can loosen inhibitions, dull common sense, and—for some people—allow aggressive tendencies to surface.

Drugs may also play a role. You may have heard about "date rape" drugs like Rohypnol (roofies), gamma-hydroxybutyrate (GHB), and ketamine. Drugs like these can easily be mixed in drinks to make a person black out and forget things that happen. Both girls and guys who have been given these drugs report feeling paralyzed, having blurred vision, and lack of memory.

Mixing these drugs with alcohol is highly dangerous and can kill.

Protecting Yourself

The best defense against date rape is to try to prevent it whenever possible. Here are some things both girls and guys can do:

- Avoid secluded places (this may even mean your room or your partner's) until you trust your partner.

- Don't spend time alone with someone who makes you feel uneasy or uncomfortable. This means following your instincts and removing yourself from situations that you don't feel good about.

- Stay sober and aware. If you're with someone you don't know very well, be aware of what's going on around you and try to stay in control. Also, be aware of your date's ability to consent to sexual activity—you may become guilty of committing rape if the other person is not in a condition to respond or react.

- Know what you want. Be clear about what kind of relationship you want with another person. If you are not sure, then ask the other person to respect your feelings and to give you time. Don't allow yourself to be subject to peer pressure or encouraged to do something that you don't want to do.

- Go out with a group of friends and watch out for each other.

- Don't be afraid to ask for help if you feel threatened.

- Take self-defense courses. These can build confidence and teach valuable physical techniques a person can use to get away from an attacker.

Getting Help

Unfortunately, even if someone takes every precaution, date rape can still happen. If you're raped, here are some things that you can do:

- If you're injured, go straight to the emergency room—most medical centers and hospital emergency departments have doctors and counselors who have been trained to take care of someone who has been raped.

- Call or find a friend, family member, or someone you feel safe with and tell them what happened.

- If you want to report the rape, call the police right away. Preserve all the physical evidence. Don't change clothes or wash.

- Write down as much as you can remember about the event.

- If you aren't sure what to do, call a rape crisis center. If you don't know the number, your local phone book will have hotline numbers.

Don't be afraid to ask questions and get information. You'll have lots of questions as you go through the process—such as whether to report the rape, who to tell, and the kinds of reactions you may get from others.

Rape isn't just physically damaging—it can be emotionally traumatic as well. It may be hard to think or talk about something as personal as being raped by someone you know. But talking with a trained rape crisis counselor or other mental health professional can give you the right emotional attention, care, and support to begin the healing process. Working things through can help prevent lingering problems later on.

Chapter 37

Juveniles as Abusers

Chapter Contents

Section 37.1

Juvenile Perpetrators of Domestic Violence

"Spotlight on: Juvenile Perpetrators of Domestic Violence,"
by Jennifer Henderson. © 2001 National District Attorneys Association
(www.ndaa.org). Reprinted with permission.

Recent years have witnessed a groundswell of interest in domestic violence. Public service announcements, education campaigns, and popular media have attracted considerable attention. Statistics and research findings are abundant in the professional literature. Despite the resources and attention that are committed to this issue, however, comparatively little is directed to juveniles as the perpetrators of domestic violence.

For purposes of this chapter, domestic violence is defined to include two types of offenses: teen dating violence and family violence. Much of what we have learned about the dynamics of domestic violence, as well as effective interventions and prevention strategies, apply equally to cases involving adult and juvenile offenders. This chapter reviews several key principles having particular application to the juvenile perpetrator, and offers specific strategies to address issues unique to these forms of domestic violence committed by juveniles.

Dynamics of Domestic Violence

The Power and Control Wheel, developed by the Domestic Abuse Intervention Project in Duluth, Minnesota is a useful tool for understanding how certain behaviors contribute to the cyclical nature of domestic violence and the environment of fear it engenders.[2] It is a conceptual way of looking at some of the tactics perpetrators use and how they work together. Battering is not an isolated or accidental behavior. Although this framework was designed with adult perpetrators in mind, juvenile perpetrators use these same behaviors, with some variations that are described, and prosecutors must respond accordingly.

336

Teen Dating Violence

Violent relationships often begin in adolescence. Studies suggest that between 25 and 40 percent of teens have been assaulted by dates.[3] According to the 1997 Massachusetts Youth Risk Behavior Survey, 20 percent of high school girls and seven percent of high school boys had been victims of teen dating violence.[4] Abuse frequently escalates during pregnancy;[5] more than 70 percent of pregnant or parenting teenagers are beaten by their boyfriends.[6] Violent relationships in adolescence can have serious ramifications for victims: many will continue to be abused in their adult relationships[7] and are at higher risk for substance abuse, eating disorders, risky sexual behavior, and suicide.[8]

Between one-fourth and one-third of adolescent abusers reported instrumental uses of violence, for example, to "intimidate, frighten, or force the other person to give me something."[9] Intimidation, coercion, and threats are behaviors that are found in the Power and Control Wheel. Isolation from one's social circle is another abusive behavior that may be especially effective in teen dating relationships where the peer plays such a pivotal role. Insults and other forms of emotional abuse are likewise powerful acts commonly found in violent teen relationships.

The school environment has unique characteristics that may inhibit victims from reporting abuse. Victims may attend classes with the perpetrators and experience intense pressure to recant. Ostracism from the social group is a particularly powerful form of retribution among adolescents.

Family Violence

Juveniles commit family violence when they commit an act against a parent, caretaker, or sibling "intended to cause physical, psychological, or financial damage to gain power and control."[10] One source estimates that as many as 18 percent of all violent crimes committed by juveniles could be classified as family violence.[11]

Because control is the motivating factor, the behaviors of juveniles who perpetrate family violence are indicative of abuse, not some stereotypical teenage rebellion. Like their adult counterparts, juvenile abusers "victimize the people they see as vulnerable."[12]

Intrafamilial victims of juvenile abusers are extremely reluctant to come forward, for many reasons. Parents, in particular, have a natural instinct to protect their children and may choose to endure abuse directed toward them or other family members rather than see a child get in trouble with the juvenile justice system. Parents are also inhibited by shame, secrecy, and fears of retribution, whether by the juvenile or by the courts, which may order other children removed from their care.

Like other victims of domestic violence, family members simply want the abusive behavior to stop, ideally without formal justice system intervention. Once an incident is reported, victims may attempt to discourage responding officers from doing anything more than counseling the juvenile. Investigators and prosecutors who can identify abusive behaviors by juveniles as indicative of a pattern of family violence are better situated to fashion appropriate dispositions and to prevent future violence. Prosecutors should charge these crimes under their state's domestic violence statute, if applicable, or other appropriate offense category.

Prevention, Programs, and Solutions

The social, physical, and psychological consequences of domestic violence perpetrated by juveniles can be devastating, both for victims and for the perpetrators themselves, since abusive behaviors are likely to continue into adulthood. Prevention, education, and early intervention are key components of a comprehensive strategy to eradicate this serious problem.

Prevention and education programs typically are located in schools. In Massachusetts, for example, the State Department of Education has established Updated Guidelines for Schools on Addressing Teen Dating Violence. These guidelines encompass a written policy chart detailing certain behaviors, their consequences, and the persons involved. They also include a restraining order checklist, teen safety plan, and a model for implementation. In 2000, 50 schools in Massachusetts received funds to implement these guidelines.[13] Other programs, such as the Teen Dating Violence Prevention Program (TDVP) in Houston, also provide education to teens through partnerships with area shelters, local universities, or other women's programs. The TDVP is curriculum based, ranging from one hour presentations to a semester long program.

Many police departments around the country have established protocols for investigating domestic violence. These protocols should be reviewed to assure their applicability to juvenile offenders. In San Diego, for example, the language throughout the Domestic Violence Protocol does not exclude juvenile perpetrators. The protocol also has a section specifically pertaining to teen dating violence.

Santa Clara County, California, established a Juvenile Delinquency Domestic and Family Violence Court to encourage a coordinated community response to these problems. The Court mobilizes a wide range of specialized probation services, including comprehensive investigation, intensive supervision, age-appropriate violence prevention and batterers intervention programs, victim advocacy, referral and support services, and domestic and family violence prevention education programming.[14]

Batterers treatment programs for juvenile offenders should mirror their counterparts that serve adult perpetrators. These programs share six basic principles:[15]

1. Each person is responsible for his own behavior. The victim cannot cause the violence or eliminate it.

2. Provocation does not justify violence.

3. Violence is a choice—a dysfunctional, destructive choice with negative consequences.

4. Nonviolent choices exist as appropriate alternatives.

5. Violence is learned. Perpetrators can also learn to be nonviolent.

6. Violence impacts the whole family. Children learn that violence is an acceptable choice.

In addition to batterers treatment, juvenile offenders may benefit from other interventions, such as anger management, drug/alcohol therapy, family counseling, or individual therapy. Prosecutors must recognize, however, that none of the other interventions can substitute for treatment that is explicitly designed to confront and eliminate battering behaviors.

The Prosecutor's Role

Prosecutors can and should play an integral role in developing and implementing protocols for investigating and prosecuting domestic violence cases involving juvenile perpetrators. Working with local law enforcement on protocols, as was the case in the San Diego example, ensures all parties understand the applicable laws, opens lines of communication, and creates the opportunity for both police and the prosecutor to work together toward the common goal of addressing this violence and preventing future violence.

Prosecutors can be vigilant to charge juvenile domestic violence offenses for what they are. By documenting dating violence or family violence in all reports, case files, and court proceedings, prosecutors underscore the seriousness of this violence and lay the foundation for appropriate case disposition.

Like their counterparts in adult criminal court, juvenile court prosecutors often must contend with reluctant or recanting victims, or indeed, no victims at all. Often the hearsay rules and exceptions, as well as other rules of evidence, such as Rule 404(b), can be used to build a strong case in chief without a cooperative victim. Prosecutors should also maximize their use of photographs, medical information, and other witnesses.

In preparing dispositional recommendations, prosecutors should consider the wide range of treatment alternatives described. Frequently, these options are offered among an offender's probationary requirements. Some jurisdictions have first-time offense deferred sentencing statutes that allow dismissal of charges upon the successful completion of a probationary period and probation requirements.[16] Even where this option is not available, probation can be an effective way to hold juvenile offenders accountable for their behavior.

Prosecutors also have opportunities to educate the public and other personnel in the juvenile justice system. The dynamics of juvenile domestic violence can be discussed in the context of jury *voir dire* (if a jury trial is available for juveniles) or arguments and questioning of witnesses during a bench trial. Countywide trainings, in-service training, and community gatherings offer additional opportunities to reach judges, other court workers, police officers, treatment professionals, and the general public.

Conclusion

Dating violence and family violence committed by juveniles are serious crimes and serious harbingers of future violent behavior. By recognizing these behaviors among adolescents, treating them seriously within the juvenile justice system, and marshaling age-appropriate resources for juvenile offenders, prosecutors stand a far better chance of halting the trajectory of violence.

References

1. Staff Attorney, American Prosecutors Research Institute (APRI), National Juvenile Justice Prosecution Center.

2. The Power and Control Wheel can be found at www.duluth-model.org/daipmain.htm.

3. Houston Area Women's Center, Teen Dating Violence Website, hereafter, HAWC, www.hawc.org/topics/teen/facts.html.

4. Massachusetts Department of Education's Updated Guidelines for Schools on Addressing Teen Dating Violence, www.doe .mass.edu/lss.tdv/tdv1.html.

5. HAWC; See also Helping Victims of Teen Dating Violence, Connecticut Clearinghouse Fact Sheet, hereafter Connecticut Fact Sheet, www.ctclearinghouse.org/fteendt.htm and the American Bar Association Commission on Domestic Violence Statistics, www.abanet.org/domviol.stats.html.

6. Id., citing the Bureau of Justice Statistics that "95% of the reported incidents of assaults in relationships are committed by males."

7. National Crime Prevention Council, "Crime Prevention Program Ideas: Combating Teen Dating Violence."

8. Silverman, Jay G., Raj, Anita, Mucci, Lorelei A., Hathaway, Jeanne E., Dating Violence Against Adolescent Girls and Associated Substance Use, Unhealthy Weight Control, Sexual Risk Behavior, Pregnancy, and Suicidality, *Journal of the American Medical Association*, vol. 286, no. 5, August 1, 2001.

9. The American Bar Association Commission on Domestic Violence Statistics, citing Brustin, S., Legal Response to Teen Dating Violence, *Family Law Quarterly*, vol. 29, no. 2, 335 (Summer 1995).

10. Cottrell, Barbara, *Parent Abuse: The Abuse of Parents by Their Teenage Children*, page 3.

11. Snyder, Howard N., Juvenile Arrests 1998, *Juvenile Justice Bulletin OJJDP*, December 1999, page 5.

12. Cottrell, *Parent Abuse*, page 10.

13. Massachusetts Department of Education's Updated Guidelines for Schools on Addressing Teen Dating Violence, Background section, www.doe.mass.edu/lss.tdv/tdv1.html.

14. Available at http://www.santaclaracounty.org/ probation.Juvenile.html.

15. Center on Crime, Community, and Culture, citing Tolman and Edleson, *Intervention for Men Who Batter: A Review of Research* (1995).

16. See Michigan Compiled Laws 769.4a.

Note: This information is offered for educational purposes only and is not legal advice.

Section 37.2

Reported Domestic Assaults by Juvenile Offenders

This section is excerpted from "Domestic Assaults by Juvenile Offenders," by Howard N. Snyder and Carl McCurley, *Juvenile Justice Bulletin*, November 2008, U.S. Department of Justice. The complete report is available at http://www.ncjrs.gov/pdffiles1/ojjdp/219180.pdf.

According to data from the Federal Bureau of Investigation (FBI), National Incident-Based Reporting System (NIBRS), 48% of all sexual, aggravated, and simple assaults reported to law enforcement in 2004 were committed by offenders having a domestic relationship with the victim (for example, the victim and offender are connected by a family or romantic relationship). Most (91%) domestic assault offenders were adults—meaning that one of every twelve offenders who came to the attention of law enforcement for domestic assault offenses was younger than 18. From the perspective of law enforcement, 53% of adults and 24% of juveniles who committed an assault were in a domestic relationship with their victims. Offenders were more likely to be arrested in domestic assault incidents than in acquaintance or stranger assault incidents.

These findings and those that follow come from an analysis of NIBRS files that describe incidents reported to law enforcement agencies in 30 states in 2004. Agencies provide the FBI with demographic information on victims, their offender(s), and any arrestees. In addition, characteristics of the crime are reported, such as the type of offense, whether a weapon was used, the degree of injury to victims, and each victim's relationship to each offender. This enables the identification of sexual, aggravated, and simple assaults for which a domestic relationship existed between the victim and offender.

Other findings include the following:

- Females were 67% of the victims of juvenile domestic assault offenders.

- Half (51%) of juvenile domestic assault offenders victimized a parent and one-quarter (24%) victimized a sibling.

- The weapon most commonly used in domestic assaults by juveniles was a knife.

- About two-thirds (69%) of all juvenile domestic assault offenders victimized persons older than 18; however, the great majority (98%) of juvenile domestic sexual assault offenders victimized other juveniles.

- One-third (35%) of juvenile domestic assault offenders were female.

- Most (84%) juvenile domestic assault offenders acted alone.

- Most (88%) juvenile domestic assault offenders committed their crime in a residence.

- Juvenile offenders were less likely to be arrested in sexual assaults than in aggravated assaults and simple assaults reported to law enforcement. The same was true for adults.

Domestic Violence Is Defined in Many Ways

To some, domestic violence is limited to violence between spouses. To others, it includes crimes against other household and/or family members. Still others extend the definition to include persons in a dating or intimate relationship. This report uses an inclusive definition of domestic relationships that encompasses parents, children, siblings, other family members (such as cousins, grandparents), and intimate partners (current and former spouses and current boy/girl-friends, including homosexual relationships). Assault of intimate partners is only a small part of juvenile domestic assault, accounting for 3% of juvenile assault offenders, as opposed to 39% of adult assault offenders. Definitions of domestic violence that focus solely on intimate partners to the exclusion of parents, siblings, and other family members overlook most of the assaults that juvenile offenders perpetrated against persons linked to them by close relationships.

Although abuse within families takes many forms, such as emotional abuse, economic abuse, and stalking, the focus of this report is on physical assault or the threat of assault. For this chapter, assaults include sexual assaults (forcible rape, forcible sodomy, sexual assault with an object, and forcible fondling), aggravated assault, and simple assault (including intimidation).

One-Fourth of Juvenile Assaults Were Domestic Violence

In 2004, almost half (48%) of all assaults reported to law enforcement agencies can be classified as domestic violence using the inclusive definition. Twenty-four percent (24%) of assaults by juvenile offenders were committed against domestic victims, compared with 53% of assaults by adult offenders. The domestic proportion of assaults increased steadily with offender age, from 16% of offenders younger than age 12, to 25% for offenders ages 12–17, to 44% of offenders ages 18–24, to 57% of offenders age 25 or older.

One of Every 12 Domestic Assault Offenders Is a Juvenile

In the 2004 NIBRS data, juveniles were one-sixth (17%) of all assault offenders reported to law enforcement, and one-twelfth (9%) of domestic assault offenders. The juvenile proportion of domestic assault offenders was greater for sexual assaults (24%) than for other assaults (8%).

One-Third of Juvenile Domestic Assault Offenders Were Female

Overall, 31% of all juveniles who committed an assault were female. A juvenile female was the offender in 35% of juvenile domestic assaults, compared with 31% of juvenile assaults of acquaintances and 21% of juvenile assaults of strangers. The type of domestic assault committed by juveniles that was most likely to involve a female offender was the assault of a parent—41% of these juvenile offenders were female. In comparison, a female was most likely to be the offender in assaults by adults when the victim was the offender's child—35% of these adult offenders were female.

Two-Thirds of Juvenile Domestic Assault Offenders Victimized Females

In general, females were the victims in the majority (60%) of assaults. Assault victims of adult offenders, however, were more likely to be female than were victims of juvenile offenders. Half (50%) of all victims of assaults that juvenile offenders committed were female, compared with 62% of the assault victims of adult offenders.

- Except for assaults within romantic relationships, juvenile female offenders were far more likely to assault females than were juvenile male offenders.

Table 37.1. Juvenile Percentage of Offenders

Offense	Domestic assaults	All assaults
Total	9%	17%
All sex assaults	24	26
Forcible rape	18	18
Forcible sodomy	39	40
Assault w/ an object	25	27
Forcible fondling	25	31
Aggravated assault	8	15
Simple assault	8	17

Table 37.2. Female Percentage of Offenders

Offense	Juvenile offenders	Adult offenders
Assaults	31%	25%
Domestic violence	35	23
Parent	41	29
Child	35	35
Intimate partner	29	20
Sibling	27	29
Other family	29	30
Acquaintance	31	29
Stranger	21	19

345

- In domestic assaults against siblings, both juvenile male and juvenile female offenders were more likely to assault their sisters than their brothers (66% and 54%, respectively).

- Of all the boyfriends and girlfriends who are victims of juvenile offenders, 73% were female. This female percentage was greater for adult offenders (82%), and for the victims of adult offenders who were classified as spouses (79%).

Domestic assaults were far more likely to have female victims (74%) than were assaults of acquaintances (51%) or those of strangers (32%). This was true if the offender was a juvenile or an adult. Two-thirds (67%) of domestic assault victims of juvenile offenders were female, as were three-fourths (75%) of the domestic assault victims of adult offenders. Seventy-three percent (73%) of parents assaulted by a juvenile child were female, compared with 64% of parents assaulted by an adult child. In comparison, 46% of acquaintances and 32% of strangers assaulted by juveniles were female, as were 52% of acquaintances and 32% of strangers assaulted by adults.

In general, most assaults (63%) by juvenile males were against male victims and most assaults (78%) by juvenile females were against female victims. However, this pattern of same-gender victimization was not seen in domestic assaults. For both juvenile male and juvenile female offenders, the domestic violence victims were primarily female (66% and 70%, respectively). When the domestic assault was against a parent, the parent was most likely the mother for both juvenile male (68%) and juvenile female offenders (81%).

Victim/Offender Relationships

- A parent was the victim in half of all domestic assaults that juvenile offenders committed.

- One-fourth (24%) of the domestic assault victims of juvenile offenders were the offenders' siblings.

- An aggravated assault by an adult offender was more than twice as likely to be a domestic assault as was an aggravated assault by a juvenile offender (42% versus 20%).

- Three of every ten forcible rapes by both juvenile and adult offenders were crimes of domestic violence. The victims of domestic forcible rapes by juvenile offenders were equally likely to be siblings as boyfriends/girlfriends; for adult offenders, these victims were about as equally likely to be the offender's child as a boyfriend/girlfriend.

- Nearly eight of every ten domestic aggravated and domestic simple assault victims of juvenile offenders were parents or siblings. In contrast, seven of every ten domestic aggravated and domestic simple assault victims of adult offenders were boyfriends/girlfriends or other intimate partners.

Victims of Domestic Assaults by Juveniles Were Least Likely to Be Physically Injured

Domestic assaults by juvenile offenders were the least likely to result in victim injury: domestic (43%), versus acquaintance (50%), and stranger (52%). Domestic assaults reported to law enforcement with juvenile offenders were far less likely to involve an injured victim than domestic assaults that adult offenders committed (43% versus 56%).

Juvenile Female Assault Offenders Were More Likely Than Males to Victimize Their Parents

In 2004, 31% of all juvenile offenders in assault incidents were female. This percentage increased to 35% when the focus is only domestic assaults. Of all juvenile assault offenders, 16% of female and 10% of male offenders assaulted their parents. When limiting the crimes to domestic assaults, a greater proportion of female (60%) than male juvenile offenders (46%) assaulted their parents. In contrast, a greater proportion of the domestic assaults by male juvenile offenders than female juvenile offenders victimized siblings (27% versus 19%).

White Juvenile Assault Offenders Were More Likely Than Black Offenders to Have Victimized Their Parents

Relatively equal proportions of white and black adult assault offenders were domestic assault offenders (52% and 54%); in contrast, a much larger proportion of white than black juvenile assault offenders were reported to law enforcement for a domestic assault (28% versus 17%). For all offenders younger than 13, domestic assaults accounted for 10% of the assaults by black offenders and 21% of the assaults by white offenders. For juveniles ages 12–17, domestic assaults accounted for 19% of black and 30% of white juvenile assault offenders.

- Parents were the victims in a larger proportion of domestic assaults by white juvenile offenders (54%) than black (44%). Similar proportions of white and black juvenile domestic assault offenders victimized siblings (23% versus 25%).

Domestic Assault Victims Differed for Older Juveniles and Younger Adults

Half (51%) of the victims of older juvenile domestic assault offenders (ages 13–17) were parents, compared with 10% of the victims of young adult offenders (ages 18–24). In contrast, 11% of the victims of older juveniles and 51% of the victims of young adults were boyfriends/girlfriends. The domestic victims of older juveniles were more likely to be siblings than were the victims of young adults (23% versus 9%).

- Of all assault offenders who assaulted their own parents, 49% were between the ages of seven and 17, with almost two-thirds of all these offenders ages 15–17.

- For juvenile offenders, the ages of domestic victims of aggravated and simple assaults peaked in the late teens and late thirties, reflecting assaults on siblings and parents.

- For juvenile offenders, 70% of domestic victims of aggravated assault were adults, as were 78% of domestic victims of simple assaults.

Section 37.3

Sibling Violence Is a Predictor of Dating Violence

A study of 371 unmarried students with siblings at a Tampa, Florida community college finds that sibling violence can have long-term negative consequences, and that perpetrating sibling violence predicts perpetrating dating violence. Published in the March/April 2004 issue of the *American Journal of Health Behavior*, the study notes, "surprisingly, parent-to-child violence was a significant predictor of sibling violence, but parent-to-parent violence was not."

The authors charge that society has been slow to recognize youth violence, and that violence between siblings is rarely acknowledged, even though it may occur in 60 percent of American families with more than one child living at home. Author Virginia Noland of the University of Florida writes, "the findings suggest that sibling violence is not harmless and may be an important influence later in violence between intimate partners."

Participants included men and women age 16 to 30 who have siblings and who responded to a written questionnaire about conflict behaviors occurring between ages of ten and 14, which is when sibling violence peaks. "After the older sibling reaches 14, they tend to gravitate to their peer group and spend less and less time with their brothers and sisters," Noland said.

Seventy-eight percent of respondents reported being pushed or shoved by a sibling, while 77 percent said they had pushed or shoved their sibling. At the more extreme level, ten percent of men and eight percent of women said a sibling had used a knife or gun against them. The highest level of sibling violence was found between two brothers and the least between two sisters.

In addition to Noland, the authors are: Karen D. Liller, Ph.D.; Robert J. McDermott, Ph.D., FAAHB; Martha L. Coulter, Dr.PH.; and Anne

E. Seraphine, Ph.D. They note, "the presence of violent behavior, whether observed or experienced directly, can affect relationships later in life." They recommend further research into violence in blended households, single-parent families, and homes with paramours.

Part Five

Elder Abuse

Chapter 38

Facts about Late-Life Domestic Violence

Elder abuse is a growing problem. While we don't know all of the details about why abuse occurs or how to stop its spread, we do know that help is available for victims. Concerned people can spot the warning signs of a possible problem and make a call for help if an elder is in need of assistance.

What is elder abuse?

Elder abuse is a term referring to any knowing, intentional, or negligent act by a caregiver or any other person that causes harm or a serious risk of harm to a vulnerable adult. Elder abuse can affect people of all ethnic backgrounds and social status and can affect both men and women. The specificity of laws varies from state to state, but broadly defined, abuse may be:

- **Physical abuse:** Inflicting, or threatening to inflict, physical pain or injury on a vulnerable elder, or depriving them of a basic need.

- **Emotional abuse:** Inflicting mental pain, anguish, or distress on an elder person through verbal or nonverbal acts.

- **Sexual abuse:** Non-consensual sexual contact of any kind.

Text in this chapter is excerpted from "Frequently Asked Questions," National Center on Elder Abuse, Administration on Aging, September 19, 2008.

353

- **Exploitation:** Illegal taking, misuse, or concealment of funds, property, or assets of a vulnerable elder.

- **Neglect:** Refusal or failure by those responsible to provide food, shelter, health care or protection for a vulnerable elder.

- **Abandonment:** Desertion of a vulnerable elder by anyone who has assumed the responsibility for care or custody of that person.

What makes an older adult vulnerable to abuse?

Social isolation and mental impairment (such as dementia or Alzheimer disease) are two factors that may make an older person more vulnerable to abuse. But, in some situations, studies show that living with someone else (a caregiver or a friend) may increase the chances for abuse to occur. A history of domestic violence may also make a senior more susceptible to abuse.

Who are the abusers of older people?

Abusers of older adults are both women and men. Family members are more often the abusers than any other group. For several years, data showed that adult children were the most common abusers of family members; recent information indicates spouses are the most common perpetrators when state data concerning elders and vulnerable adults is combined.

The bottom line is that elder abuse is a family issue. As far as the types of abuse are concerned, neglect is the most common type of abuse identified.

Are there criminal penalties for the abusers?

Although there are variations across the country, in most states there are several laws that address criminal penalties for various types of elder abuse. Laws vary state to state. Some states have increased penalties for those who victimize older adults. Increasingly, across the country, law enforcement officers and prosecutors are trained on elder abuse and ways to use criminal and civil laws to bring abusers to justice.

How many people are suffering from elder abuse?

It is difficult to say how many older Americans are abused, neglected, or exploited, in large part because surveillance is limited and the problem remains greatly hidden. Findings from the often cited National Elder Abuse Incidence Study suggest that more than 500,000 Americans aged 60 and over were victims of domestic abuse in 1996.

This study also found that only 16 percent of the abusive situations are referred for help—84 percent remain hidden. While a couple of studies estimate that between 3–5 percent of the elderly population have been abused, the Senate Special Committee on Aging estimates that there may be as many as five million victims every year. One consistent finding, over a ten-year study period, is that reports have increased each year.

Who do I call if I suspect elder abuse?

Call the police or 9-1-1 immediately if someone you know is in immediate, life-threatening danger.

Each one of us has a responsibility to keep vulnerable elders safe from harm. The laws in most states require helping professions in the front lines—such as doctors and home health providers—to report suspected abuse or neglect. These professionals are called mandated reporters. Under the laws of eight states, "any person" is required to report a suspicion of mistreatment.

If the danger is not immediate, but you suspect that abuse has occurred or is occurring, please tell someone. Relay your concerns to the local adult protective services, long-term care ombudsman, or police.

If you have been the victim of abuse, exploitation, or neglect, you are not alone. Many people care and can help. Please tell your doctor, a friend, or a family member you trust, or call Eldercare Locator help line immediately.

What should I expect if I call someone for help?

When making the call, be ready to give the elder's name, address, contact information, and details about why you are concerned. You may be asked a series of questions to gain more insight into the nature of the situation.

- Are there any known medical problems (including confusion or memory loss)?

- What kinds of family or social supports are there?

- Have you seen or heard incidents of yelling, hitting, or other abusive behavior?

How can elder abuse be prevented?

Educating seniors, professionals, caregivers, and the public on abuse is critical to prevention. On an individual level, some simple but vital steps reduce the risk:

* Take care of your health.

* Seek professional help for drug, alcohol, and depression concerns, and urge family members to get help for these problems.

* Attend support groups for spouses and learn about domestic violence services.

* Plan for your own future. With a power of attorney or a living will, health care decisions can be addressed to avoid confusion and family problems, should you become incapacitated. Seek independent advice from someone you trust before signing any documents.

* Stay active in the community and connected with friends and family. This will decrease social isolation, which has been connected to elder abuse.

* Know your rights. If you engage the services of a paid or family caregiver, you have the right to voice your preferences and concerns. If you live in a nursing home or board and care home, call your Long-Term Care Ombudsman. The Ombudsman is your advocate and has the power to intervene.

All states have adult protective and long-term care ombudsman programs, family care supports, and home and community care services that can help older adults with activities of daily living. Call the Eldercare Locator at 800-677-1116 for information and referrals on services in your area.

How can I help stop elder abuse?

Knowing the warning signs of abuse is a first step toward protecting elders. Some specific tips: Become a community sentinel by keeping a watchful eye out for loved ones, friends, or neighbors who may be vulnerable. Speak up if you have concerns. That means even if you are not sure. You have a right to question. Be involved. Volunteer with older adults in your community. Support initiatives to increase and strengthen adult protective services in your state.

For More Information

National Center on Elder Abuse
c/o Center for Community Research and Services
University of Delaware
297 Graham Hall
Newark, DE 19716
Phone: 302-831-3525
Fax: 302-831-4225
Website: http://www.ncea.aoa.gov
E-mail: ncea-info@aoa.hhs.gov

Eldercare Locator
Toll-Free Voice/TTY: 800-677-1116
Website: http://www.eldercare.gov
E-mail: eldercarelocator@infospherix.com

Chapter 39

Major Types of Elder Abuse

Elder abuse is a growing problem. While we don't know all of the details about why abuse occurs or how to stop its spread, we do know that help is available for victims. Concerned people can spot the warning signs of a possible problem, and make a call for help if an elder is in need of assistance.

Physical abuse is defined as the use of physical force that may result in bodily injury, physical pain, or impairment. Physical abuse may include but is not limited to such acts of violence as striking (with or without an object), hitting, beating, pushing, shoving, shaking, slapping, kicking, pinching, and burning. In addition, inappropriate use of drugs and physical restraints, force-feeding, and physical punishment of any kind also are examples of physical abuse.

Signs and symptoms of physical abuse include but are not limited to:

- bruises, black eyes, welts, lacerations, and rope marks;
- bone fractures, broken bones, and skull fractures;
- open wounds, cuts, punctures, untreated injuries in various stages of healing;
- sprains, dislocations, and internal injuries/bleeding;

"Major Types of Elder Abuse," National Center on Elder Abuse, Administration on Aging, September 28, 2007.

- broken eyeglasses/frames, physical signs of being subjected to punishment, and signs of being restrained;
- laboratory findings of medication overdose or under utilization of prescribed drugs;
- an elder's report of being hit, slapped, kicked, or mistreated;
- an elder's sudden change in behavior; and
- the caregiver's refusal to allow visitors to see an elder alone.

Sexual abuse is defined as non-consensual sexual contact of any kind with an elderly person. Sexual contact with any person incapable of giving consent is also considered sexual abuse. It includes, but is not limited to, unwanted touching, all types of sexual assault or battery, such as rape, sodomy, coerced nudity, and sexually explicit photographing.

Signs and symptoms of sexual abuse include but are not limited to:

- bruises around the breasts or genital area;
- unexplained venereal disease or genital infections;
- unexplained vaginal or anal bleeding;
- torn, stained, or bloody underclothing; and
- an elder's report of being sexually assaulted or raped.

Emotional or psychological abuse is defined as the infliction of anguish, pain, or distress through verbal or nonverbal acts. Emotional/psychological abuse includes but is not limited to verbal assaults, insults, threats, intimidation, humiliation, and harassment. In addition, treating an older person like an infant; isolating an elderly person from his or her family, friends, or regular activities; giving an older person the silent treatment; and enforced social isolation are examples of emotional or psychological abuse.

Signs and symptoms of emotional or psychological abuse include but are not limited to:

- being emotionally upset or agitated;
- being extremely withdrawn and non communicative or non responsive;
- unusual behavior usually attributed to dementia (for example, sucking, biting, rocking); and
- an elder's report of being verbally or emotionally mistreated.

Neglect is defined as the refusal or failure to fulfill any part of a person's obligations or duties to an elder. Neglect may also include failure of a person who has fiduciary responsibilities to provide care for an elder (for example, pay for necessary home care services) or the failure on the part of an in-home service provider to provide necessary care.

Neglect typically means the refusal or failure to provide an elderly person with such life necessities as food, water, clothing, shelter, personal hygiene, medicine, comfort, personal safety, and other essentials included in an implied or agreed-upon responsibility to an elder.

Signs and symptoms of neglect include but are not limited to:

- dehydration, malnutrition, untreated bed sores, and poor personal hygiene;

- unattended or untreated health problems;

- hazardous or unsafe living condition or arrangements (for example: improper wiring, no heat, or no running water);

- unsanitary and unclean living conditions (such as dirt, fleas, lice on person, soiled bedding, fecal/urine smell, inadequate clothing); and

- an elder's report of being mistreated.

Abandonment is defined as the desertion of an elderly person by an individual who has assumed responsibility for providing care for an elder, or by a person with physical custody of an elder.

Signs and symptoms of abandonment include but are not limited to:

- the desertion of an elder at a hospital, a nursing facility, or other similar institution;

- the desertion of an elder at a shopping center or other public location; and

- an elder's own report of being abandoned.

Financial or material exploitation is defined as the illegal or improper use of an elder's funds, property, or assets. Examples include, but are not limited to, cashing an elderly person's checks without authorization or permission; forging an older person's signature; misusing or stealing an older person's money or possessions; coercing or deceiving an older person into signing any document (for example, contracts or will); and the improper use of conservatorship, guardianship, or power of attorney.

Signs and symptoms of financial or material exploitation include but are not limited to:

- sudden changes in bank account or banking practice, including an unexplained withdrawal of large sums of money by a person accompanying the elder;

- the inclusion of additional names on an elder's bank signature card;

- unauthorized withdrawal of the elder's funds using the elder's automatic teller machine (ATM) card;

- abrupt changes in a will or other financial documents;

- unexplained disappearance of funds or valuable possessions;

- substandard care being provided or bills unpaid despite the availability of adequate financial resources;

- discovery of an elder's signature being forged for financial transactions or for the titles of his or her possessions;

- sudden appearance of previously uninvolved relatives claiming their rights to an elder's affairs and possessions;

- unexplained sudden transfer of assets to a family member or someone outside the family;

- the provision of services that are not necessary; and

- an elder's report of financial exploitation.

Self-neglect is characterized as the behavior of an elderly person that threatens his or her own health or safety. Self-neglect generally manifests itself in an older person as a refusal or failure to provide himself or herself with adequate food, water, clothing, shelter, personal hygiene, medication (when indicated), and safety precautions.

The definition of self-neglect excludes a situation in which a mentally competent older person, who understands the consequences of his or her decisions, makes a conscious and voluntary decision to engage in acts that threaten his or her health or safety as a matter of personal choice.

Signs and symptoms of self-neglect include but are not limited to:

- dehydration, malnutrition, untreated or improperly attended medical conditions, and poor personal hygiene;

- hazardous or unsafe living conditions or arrangements (for example: improper wiring, no indoor plumbing, no heat, no running water);

- unsanitary or unclean living quarters (for example: animal or insect infestation, no functioning toilet, fecal or urine smell);

- inappropriate or inadequate clothing, lack of the necessary medical aids (eyeglasses, hearing aids, dentures); and

- grossly inadequate housing or homelessness.

Chapter 40

Reports of Abuse in Older Adults

This chapter contains results from a national survey on elder abuse conducted by the National Center on Elder Abuse (NCEA). Information presented here represents Fiscal Year (FY) 2003 data from Adult Protective Services (APS) in all fifty states, the District of Columbia, and Guam. The report primarily summarizes data concerning reports of abuse for individuals 60 years of age and older.

The purpose of the *2004 Survey of Adult Protective Services* was to gather the most recent and accurate state-level APS data on elder abuse. The project was a follow-up to the 2000 report, *A Response to the Abuse of Vulnerable Adults: The 2000 Survey of State Adult Protective Services* and provides data, where comparable, to identify trends. The first part of this report compares the 2004 data concerning abuse of adults of all ages with the 2000 data to provide a context for the age 60 and older specific information.

National Trends: Abuse of Vulnerable Adults of All Ages

- APS received a total of 565,747 reports of elder and vulnerable adult abuse for persons of all ages (50 states, plus Guam and the District of Columbia). This represents a 19.7% increase from the 2000 Survey (472,813 reports).

Excerpted from "The 2004 Survey of State Adult Protective Services: Abuse of Adults 60 Years of Age and Older," National Center on Elder Abuse, Administration on Aging, February 2006.

- APS investigated 461,135 total reports of elder and vulnerable adult abuse for persons of all ages (49 states). This represents a 16.3% increase from the 2000 Survey (396,398 investigations).

- APS substantiated 191,908 reports of elder and vulnerable adult abuse for victims of all ages (42 states). This represents a 15.6% increase from the 2000 Survey (166,019 substantiated reports).

- The average APS budget per state was $8,550,369, compared to an average of $7,084,358 reported in the 2000 Survey (42 states).

Statewide Reporting Numbers

- APS received a total of 253,426 reports on persons aged 60 and older (32 states).

- APS investigated a total of 192,243 reports on persons aged 60 and older (29 states).

- APS substantiated 88,455 reports on persons aged 60 and older (24 states).

- APS received a total of 84,767 reports of self-neglect on persons aged 60 and older (21 states).

- APS investigated a total of 82,007 reports of self-neglect on persons aged 60 and older (20 states).

- APS substantiated 46,794 reports of self-neglect on persons aged 60 and older (20 states).

- The most common sources of reports of abuse of adults 60 and older were family members (17.0%), social services workers (10.6%), and friends and neighbors (8.0%).

Categories of Elder Abuse, Victims Aged 60 and Older

- Self-neglect was the most common category of investigated reports (49,809 reports or 26.7%), followed by caregiver neglect (23.7%), and financial exploitation (20.8%) (19 states).

- Self-neglect was the most common category of substantiated reports (26,752 reports or 37.2%), followed by caregiver neglect (20.4%), and financial exploitation (14.7%) (19 states).

Substantiated Reports, Victims Aged 60 and Older

- States reported that 65.7% of elder abuse victims were female (15 states).

- Of the victims aged 60 and older, 42.8% were 80 years of age and older (20 states).

- The majority of victims were Caucasian (77.1%) (13 states).

- The vast majority (89.3%) of elder abuse reports occurred in domestic settings (13 states).

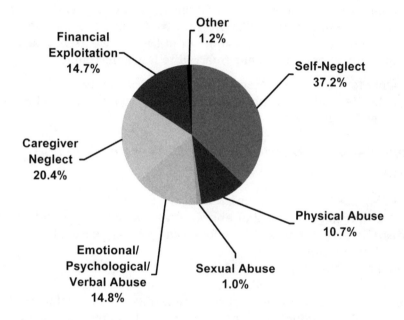

Figure 40.1. *Substantiated Reports by Category for Adults 60 and Older (n=19 states)*

Substantiated Reports, Alleged Perpetrators of Victims Aged 60 and Older

- States reported that 52.7% of alleged perpetrators of abuse were female (11 states).

- Over three-fourths (75.1%) of alleged perpetrators were under the age of 60 (seven states).

- The most common relationships of victims to alleged perpetrators were adult child (32.6%) and other family member (21.5%) (11 states).

- Twenty-one states (40.4%) maintain an abuse registry or database of alleged perpetrators, while 31 (59.6%) do not.

Interventions and Outcomes, Victims Aged 60 and Older

- Over half (53.2%) of cases were closed because the client was no longer in need of services or the risk of harm was reduced (eight states). Other reasons for closure were the death of the client, client entering a long-term care facility, client refusing further services, client moving out of the service area, unable to locate client, and client referred to law enforcement.

- Only four states, Colorado, Connecticut, Louisiana, and Massachusetts, and Guam provided information on outcomes of APS involvement.

Conclusions: Abuse of Adults 60 Years of Age and Older

Self-neglect made up approximately one-third of both investigated and substantiated reports of abuse of adults aged 60 and older (20 states). Self-neglect was closely followed by caregiver neglect and financial exploitation.

As borne out by previous surveys and extant research literature (Bonnie and Wallace, 2003; Teaster and Colleagues, 2003), the most common reporters of elder abuse were family members, followed by social services agency staff and friends and neighbors (11 states). Medical staff, including nurses and nurses' aides, home health staff, and physicians constituted less than 5% of total report sources. New categories of reporters arose in the other category, notably the abusers themselves, municipal agents, postal service workers, utility workers, and hospital discharge planners. Also, as borne out by the research literature (Bonnie and Wallace, 2003), the reporters can also arise from family members who are reporting on the abuse of other family members.

Over 65% of victims aged 60 and older were women (15 states). Over 40 percent of victims in the 60 and older age category were 80 years of age and older (20 states). Domestic settings were the most common location of the occurrence of abuse in substantiated reports (13 states), likely because all state APS programs investigate in domestic settings. The majority of victims aged 60 and older were Caucasian (71.1%); however, only 13 states were able to provide data on racial composition. Only three states could compare Hispanic and non-Hispanic victims.

Slightly more than half of alleged perpetrators of abuse of victims aged 60 and older were women (11 states). The largest age category of alleged perpetrators was between thirty and fifty years of age (seven states). Most alleged perpetrators were adult children or other family members (11 states).

Chapter 41

Caregiver Stress
and Elder Abuse

Although the overwhelming majority of informal caregivers provide adequate to excellent care, reports of abuse are not uncommon and appear to be on the rise. Abuse by caregivers may be physical, emotional, or financial. It may involve intentional or unintentional neglect. These various forms of abuse may be motivated by many factors. The motive behind financial abuse and intentional neglect, for example, is often greed. Domestic violence by a caregiving spouse or intimate partner is motivated by the abuser's need to exercise power and control. Abuse by caregivers may be triggered or exacerbated by alcohol or substance abuse, or psychiatric illness. Although all of these forms of abuse by caregivers are of critical concern, this chapter focuses on caregiver abuse that is related to the stresses associated with caregiving and the relationship between caregiver stress and physical elder abuse.

Caregiver Stress and Physical Abuse

Studies of physical abuse by caregivers have yielded divergent results reflecting variations in methodology and how caregiving was defined. An early study of abuse by non-spousal caregivers, for example, revealed that 23 percent engaged in some form of physical abuse. A survey administered to a sample of 342 callers to a help line

Excerpted from "Preventing Elder Abuse by Family Caregivers," National Center on Elder Abuse, March 2002. Reviewed in November 2008 by Dr. David A. Cooke, M.D., Diplomate, American Board of Internal Medicine.

371

for caregivers found that 12 percent of the callers had physically abused the person in their care at least once. Other studies have revealed rates of physical abuse by caregivers at six percent. Other inconsistencies have also been observed. For example, one research team identified adult offspring caregivers as the most likely to commit acts of violence; others suggest that spousal caregivers are proportionately more likely to abuse.

Assuming that caregiver abuse is related to caregiver stress, several researchers have attempted to discern whether or not the predictors of stress also predict abuse. This line of reasoning has yielded some promising results. Depression, which is highly predictive of caregiver stress, has also been found to be a strong predictor of elder abuse, particularly when caregivers' level of depression reaches near-clinical levels. Similarly, cohabitation has been found to be highly predictive for both caregiver stress and caregiver abuse, although some suggest that this is only true in cases of non-spousal caregiver abuse.

Several researchers who have taken a closer look at the process by which caregiver stress turns to violence have observed intervening factors or links between stress and violence. Bendek and his colleagues, for example, postulated that stress, in and of its self, did not cause caregivers to become abusive; rather, it leads to mood disturbances, which may lead to abuse. When caregivers lack adequate income, problem-solving skills, or social support, or when they believe that the situation is beyond their control, it triggers a sequence of events that lead to mood disturbances and a loss of rational behavior. It is these mood disturbances that culminate in mistreatment. Garcia and Kosberg identified anger as the intermediary step or link between stress and abuse.

Just as the early literature on caregiving assumed that stress was directly related to burden (defined in terms of care receivers' disabilities and the amount of care they require), early researchers in elder abuse also assumed that the risk of abuse increased in direct relation to the amount of care required. There is some evidence to support this assumption. Coyne and his colleagues observed, for example, that the risk of abuse is elevated when caregivers provide high levels of care (defined in terms of hours of care per day and the number of years that care is provided), and that victims function at lower levels than their non-abused counterparts. However, other studies of caregiver abuse have mirrored the literature on caregiver stress in suggesting that these objective measures of burden are less important than subjective factors. Some, in fact, believe that victims of caregiver abuse are no more impaired and require no more care than non-abused care receivers. Many now believe that it is the quality of past relationships between caregivers and care receivers, caregivers' perceptions of burden, and caregivers' patterns of coping that explain why stress leads some caregivers, but not others, to abuse.

Just as caregivers who have had close and positive relationships with patients in the past are less likely to experience stress, so too are they less likely to become violent. It has also been observed that care receivers who were violent toward their caregivers prior to the onset of their illnesses, are more likely to suffer abuse at the hands of their caregivers.

The likelihood that caregivers will abuse also appears to be strongly linked to how they perceive their situations. Abusive caregivers are more likely than non-abusive caregivers to feel that they aren't receiving adequate help from their families, social networks, or public entities. Anetzberger found that these perceptions may be ungrounded. Abusive caregivers who perceived themselves to be socially isolated, for example, were not, in fact, found to be more isolated than their non-abusive counterparts when objective measures of isolation were employed. Abusive caregivers report that certain behaviors are particularly stressful to them. These include verbal aggression, refusal to eat or take medications, calling the police, invading the caregiver's privacy, noisiness, vulgar habits, disruptive behavior, embarrassing public displays, and physical aggression.

Caregivers' low self-esteem has also emerged as a significant risk factor in predicting abuse, although, as some researchers point out, the causal relationship between abuse and self-esteem is not clear. It has not been determined whether low self-esteem is the cause or the result of abuse.

Families at Risk and Interactive Violence

Whereas, patient aggression and caregiver abuse have, in the past, been viewed as separate and unrelated phenomena, the two are increasingly being seen as interrelated. Several researchers have proposed that caregiving creates stresses that affect both caregivers and patients, and that these stresses may trigger aggression in one or the other partner, or both. Some even suggest that a more useful approach to understanding the risk of abuse in caregiving relationships is to look at families at risk, as opposed to individuals at risk.

Studies of families at risk have looked at pairs, or dyads, of caregivers and care receivers in which one or both members are abusive.

These studies have revealed that caregivers in abusive dyads report higher levels of emotional and mental burnout, poorer physical health, and stronger reactions to care receivers, regardless of whether it is the caregiver or the care receiver who is violent. Depression and living together have been found to be predictive of abuse in either direction. Paveza and his colleagues further suggest that when abuse is mutual, which they found to be the case in 3.8 percent of the families, it reflects a reactive pattern or feedback loop between caregivers and patients; patients' verbal and physical abuse prompts caregivers to abuse.

Fear of Becoming Violent

The research on caregiver stress and abuse has revealed that a surprisingly high proportion of caregivers (20 percent) live in fear that they will become violent. This rate increases to 57 percent among caregivers who have experienced violence from those they care for. The fear of becoming abusive also appears to be affected by living arrangement. Caregivers who live with care receivers are more likely to experience fear, particularly when the caregiver is a spouse and the marital relationship has been stressful. Fearful caregivers have also been found to have lower self-esteem and to be older than non-fearful caregivers. Pillemer and Suiter went further in exploring whether the fear of becoming abusive actually leads to or predicts violence. In looking at 236 caregivers, they found that 14 percent feared they would become violent. Of these, six percent actually engaged in violent behavior. When fearful, non-abusive caregivers were compared with fearful abusive caregivers, several differences were observed. The violent caregivers were more likely to have experienced violence from care receivers, leading the researchers to conclude that "violence by care receivers is not only a risk factor for fear of violence but also appears to move persons who are fearful of becoming violent to actually commit violent acts."

Non-Physical Abuse Associated with Caregiver Stress

Although it has been assumed by many that caregivers who experience high levels of stress may engage in other forms of mistreatment (besides physical abuse), only a few studies have looked at the relationship between stress and non-physical abuse. An early study on elder abuse by Steinmetz in 1988, suggests that one in six caregivers resort to emotional or psychological abuse and about one-third use verbally abusive methods to gain control. Compton in 1997 estimated that as many as 26.3 percent of caregivers were verbally abusive. Neither study, however, established a direct link between stress and abuse. An Australian study by Rahman in 1996, on stress, coping, and abuse in which 30 female caregivers were interviewed, revealed that some caregivers "felt so helpless that it made them lose their power of concentration, leading to accidents" (for example, falls). According to Rahman, however, these caregivers did not feel responsible for the accidents or blame themselves.

Services and Techniques for Reducing Caregiver Stress

As the population ages and caregiving becomes a fact of life for many families, a myriad of new services have been developed to meet caregivers' need for support and assistance. These programs and services have been designed to help caregivers and their families reduce their stress and isolation, handle difficult behaviors, improve their coping skills, and delay or prevent nursing home placement. Services for caregivers are typically funded by states through general revenue funds or as part of multipurpose, publicly funded home and community-based care programs that serve both care recipients and their family caregivers. Fifteen states now have comprehensive state-funded caregiver support programs, which typically offer respite care and four or more other services, including specialized information and referral, family consultation or care planning, support groups, care management, and education and training. The states vary considerably in how they deliver and fund these services, and how they define eligibility. Other states have developed smaller, innovative programs. Policy makers at the national level are increasingly recognizing the needs of caregivers.

Chapter 42

Coordinating Care for Victims of Late-Life Domestic Violence

State and area agencies' aging and direct service providers—especially long term care ombudsmen, adult protective services workers, legal assistance providers, and information and referral specialists—are likely to be in contact with older domestic violence victims, if not now, then, in the future as the baby-boom generation ages. For the victims, coordinated response by the aging network with domestic violence service providers will very likely prove vital. Similar to how the aging network is structured, the types and availability of domestic violence intervention services vary among states and often within states. To be of greatest help to victims, members of the aging network need to know more about the support and programs for victims of late-life violence in their respective states, common indicators of abuse in late life, potential victim reactions, and areas where there is potential for interagency collaboration.

What Is the Relationship Between Elder Abuse and Domestic Violence?

Some experts view late life domestic violence as a subset of the larger elder abuse problem. Elder abuse, broadly defined, includes physical, sexual and emotional abuse, financial exploitation, neglect and self-neglect, and abandonment. The distinctive context of domestic

Excerpted from "Late Life Domestic Violence: What the Aging Network Needs to Know," Nation Center on Elder Abuse, February 2006.

abuse in later life is the abusive use of power and control by a spouse, partner, or other person known to the victim.

Domestic violence programs are likely to have skills and procedures in place to help many older victims of abuse. On the other hand, the elder abuse network or adult protective services systems have legal responsibility and authorities to protect vulnerable elders and adults. They have special skills for assisting victims with diminished decisional capacity or those who are unable to protect themselves from further abuse. They also have access to a number of supportive services for older victims.

The aging network is encouraged not to try to draw fine lines between the two service systems, for example, not to try to answer: Is this domestic violence? Or, is it elder abuse? Rather, efforts should be made to maximize the capacity of both systems by partnering to meet older victims' unique needs.

Domestic Violence Prevention Programming

While service availability can vary from one community to another, most domestic violence programs offer some or all of the following services:

- **24-hour help/crisis lines** are available in communities and states across the country. They have specially trained counselors who are available by phone to help victims.

- **Peer and individual counseling** services are available for victims of domestic violence to assist the decision-making process.

- **Support groups** allow individuals an opportunity to express their feelings and experiences with domestic abuse, and to support others in similar situations. A few domestic violence programs in the country have formed groups specifically for older women.

- **Legal advocacy** services assist victims in understanding and navigating the legal system. Some domestic violence centers hire their own lawyers to assist. Some have trained non-lawyers to support women at criminal and civil hearings and helping with pro se proceedings, such as getting a court order of protection. ("Pro se" means you act as your own lawyer.) The availability of legal advocacy varies greatly depending on the size of the program.

- **Emergency housing** for victims leaving domestic abuse situations includes battered women's shelters, safe homes, or other temporary emergency shelter where a victim can stay while she decides what to do next.

- **Information and referral** is routinely provided by domestic violence service providers to victims about their rights, available sources of support, and additional resources and services that can help (for example: economic support, housing, health care, mental health, and aging network services).

- **An emergency safety plan** can help a person who is being abused or threatened to protect herself in the event of further violence. Domestic violence safety plans generally consider such issues as which rooms are safest in case of an assault, how to reach out for help if the abuser shows up, and what a victim should pack if she needs to leave in an emergency.

Keep in Mind

Most domestic violence programs were designed for younger women; however, around the country some agencies offer specialized services for older women. Most also offer some services and referrals for male and child victims and may offer batterer intervention programming.

Sexual Assault

Sexual assault service availability also varies from area to area. In larger communities, the sexual assault crisis center may be a separate agency from the domestic violence program. Most of them offer some services and referrals for male victims. Sexual assault services include 24-hour crisis lines; peer counseling; support groups; legal advocacy; information; referrals; safety planning; and medical advocacy.

Sexual assault nurse examiners (SANE) are key providers of medical advocacy services. These nurses are specially trained to provide survivors first response care, both emotional and medical. The SANE nurses collaborate with the local rape crisis or sexual assault center advocates to provide counseling support; with the local hospital or sexual assault clinic to provide follow-up care; and with law enforcement to assist in cases of legal prosecution.

When a patient arrives, the SANE nurse will ask her questions about the assault, listen to her, and explain the available options. Generally the SANE nurse will also examine and care for minor injuries; consult with the emergency doctor about any injury or illness concerns; collect forensic evidence that may be used in court to prosecute the perpetrator; and provide information and treatment to help prevent sexually transmitted diseases.

Working with Domestic Violence Organizations

Aging network professionals are encouraged to reach out and learn more about state and local domestic violence intervention services, develop referral procedures, and promote joint efforts with domestic violence networks.

Cross-referral is crucial to victim safety. There will be instances when aging network staff will identify a victim or potential victim and want to make a referral to a domestic violence program. Ideally aging network professionals and domestic violence program advocates know each other and will have been trained on elder abuse together. If this has not occurred, opportunities for networking and joint training should be arranged.

Domestic violence programs may be particularly appropriate for older persons who do not fit the intake criteria for adult protective services, but who need help in addressing violence and abuse in their lives. In addition, domestic violence staff can be partners in outreach, linking older victims to adult protective, advocacy, community and supportive services such as, transportation, legal assistance, senior activities, and health promotion.

Additional considerations in assisting victims of late life violence:

- **When to call a domestic violence program:** Many states mandate reporting cases of suspected elder abuse, which often involves domestic violence, to adult protective services. A victim of late life violence may be referred to a local domestic violence program, whether or not a report has been made to adult protective services. Many victims will benefit from the support they can offer.

- **Accepting referrals:** Unlike adult protective services or law enforcement, domestic violence programs do not investigate allegations of abuse. Most domestic violence programs use a self-help model, meaning the victim needs to call the program and ask for help. Outside referrals from concerned friends, family, or professionals may not be accepted. It is permissible to suggest that a victim call the domestic violence program herself.

Another option is to make the call while the individual is in the room so the victim can talk to the advocate. If the victim is unwilling to talk to an advocate, aging network staff can ask the domestic violence program to send materials to share with the victim.

- **Eligibility:** Most domestic violence programs offer services to victims free of charge. In general, victims of domestic violence who seek help are not required to prove they have experienced abuse. Most domestic abuse and sexual assault services were developed to provide services to women although most can provide information, referrals, or services for men. Some work exclusively with victims of intimate partner violence. If a victim has been abused by an adult child or other family member or caregiver, they may not be eligible for services at those agencies. Check with your local program for eligibility criteria.

- **Advocacy approach:** Domestic violence advocacy is based on a self-empowerment philosophy. Victims are given support, information, and options so they are able to make choices that will work for them. Advocates do not tell victims what they should do, and they do not judge or question a victim's decisions.

- **Confidentiality:** Domestic violence programs have strict confidentiality policies to protect victims. Too often abusers will lie or attempt to manipulate staff to get information about victims. Therefore, domestic violence staff members do not provide any information about their clients. One possible scenario: In the event an aging network staff calls a domestic abuse program to reach an older victim, she or he may be told that the domestic violence staff cannot confirm whether the program is working with the woman or if they know her. It is best to leave a message for the victim to return the call. Also, keep in mind that some domestic violence shelters keep the location of their building confidential so abusers do not show up to harass victims. Aging network staff will need to work with the local program to understand how to best work collaboratively with elder victims and how to meet with staff and/or victims.

- **Training and community education:** Beyond direct services to victims domestic violence programs offer professional training and community education on a variety of topics pertaining to domestic violence and abuse. These programs may be involved in task forces and multidisciplinary teams. Staff members are also available to consult about domestic violence situations, even if a victim does not choose to accept services.

Building Awareness: Common Indicators of Domestic Violence in Later Life

Aging network professionals may encounter older victims of domestic violence in their work. Most often victims will not readily disclose their situation to friends, family, or professionals. Abusers use violence to get their way, or to control or punish their victims. Many victims will do what abusers want to avoid being hurt. Professionals in the aging network need to be aware of possible behavioral indicators of abuse and common reactions of victims.

Part Six

Domestic Violence Prevention

Chapter 43

Choose Respect: Develop Healthy Relationships

Overview

Choose Respect is an initiative to help youth form healthy relationships to prevent dating abuse before it starts. This national effort is designed to motivate youth to challenge harmful beliefs about dating abuse and take steps to form respectful relationships.

The Need

Unhealthy relationship behaviors can start early and last a lifetime. According to research from the Centers for Disease Control and Prevention (CDC), one in eleven youth reports being a victim of physical dating abuse. Even more startling, youth who report experiencing dating abuse are also more likely to report binge drinking, suicide attempts, physical fighting, and current sexual activity.

The Goal

Choose Respect is designed to encourage positive action on the part of youth to form healthy, respectful relationships. Research for the initiative showed that most youth have positive, healthy attitudes about their relationships with others. Choose Respect seeks to reinforce and sustain these positive attitudes among youth as they get

This chapter includes text from the "Choose Respect Press Kit," Centers for Disease Control and Prevention (CDC), 2006.

older and begin to enter dating relationships by providing effective messages for youth, parents, caregivers, and teachers that encourage them to establish healthy and respectful relationships; and by creating opportunities for youth and communities to support healthy and respectful relationships.

The Audience

Choose Respect reaches out to youth ages 11–14 because they're still forming attitudes and beliefs that will affect how they are treated and how they treat others. The initiative also connects with parents, teachers, youth leaders, and other supportive adults who influence the lives of youth.

Materials

Choose Respect messages are supported by online games and interactive learning tools, television and radio spots, streaming video clips, and interactive quizzes that inspire youth to think about choosing respect.

Roles for Youth and Adults

Healthy relationships are built on a foundation of respect. This means that both people can talk openly, honestly, and freely to each other—without feeling pressure to act or think in a certain way. People in healthy relationships practice give and take. They support each other, take turns making decisions, and talk things through to make sure both people are heard.

Being a youth can be tough. Adolescence is a time when youth learn how to make decisions about relationships with their friends, family, and girlfriends or boyfriends. What they learn now about how to treat others will affect relationships throughout their lives. But youth cannot do this by themselves. They need adults—parents, teachers, coaches, and others—to help them choose respect.

Did you know that one in eleven youth reports experiencing physical dating abuse? Even something as subtle as putting someone down or trying to change how someone dresses can be a sign of an unhealthy relationship. That's why adults need to talk to youth now about the importance of developing healthy, respectful relationships. Adults can start by helping youth learn some key skills that will help them give and get respect in any relationship they have.

Choosing Respect

Healthy relationships are a choice. But to get respect you have to give it. Youth can start by learning key skills that will help them give and get respect in all their relationships.

Anger control: Think before speaking, especially when angry. Take a deep breath or walk away until calmer. Never express anger through physical abuse. Be aware that anger can be a cover-up for other emotions and look for the underlying reason.

Problem solving: Break the problem down into manageable pieces. Identify possible solutions. Consider the likely outcome(s) for each possible solution.

Negotiation and compromise: Look at problems objectively, acknowledging differing points of view. Strive to find win-win solutions. Realize that healthy relationships involve give and take on both sides.

Assertiveness: Be clear and open about feelings and expectations. Respect one's own needs as well as those of others. Don't confuse assertiveness with aggression. Aggression is an abusive way to express feelings and expectations. In contrast, assertiveness is an honest and courageous way to express oneself.

Fighting fair: Recognize that all relationships have disagreements, but how a couple deals with conflict is important to the health of the relationship. Stick to the subject, avoid insults, and do not bring up past hurts. Understand that it's okay to excuse oneself and return to the discussion when calmer.

Understanding: Take a minute to understand what others might be feeling—put yourself in their shoes. It can improve your communications skills and help form healthy relationships.

Listening: Do not just talk, listen. Keep the lines of communication open. Allow others to express their opinions without forcing yours on others to win an argument.

Being a role model: Take every opportunity to show respect for others. Help others to see where they agree and disagree. This will help everyone know how to choose respect.

By using these skills, youth choose respect—and choose to treat others the way they want to be treated.

Chapter 44

Self-Defense and Safety Awareness

Self-Defense

You've seen it in movies: A girl walks through an isolated parking garage. Suddenly, an evil-looking guy jumps out from behind an SUV. Girl jabs bad guy in the eyes with her keys—or maybe she kicks him in a certain sensitive place. Either way, while he's squirming, she leaps into her car and speeds to safety.

That's the movies. Here's the real-life action replay: When the girl goes to jab or kick the guy, he knows what's coming and grabs her arm (or leg), pulling her off balance. Enraged by her attempt to fight back, he flips her onto the ground. Now she's in a bad place to defend herself—and she can't run away.

Many people think of self-defense as a karate kick to the groin or jab in the eyes of an attacker. But self-defense actually means doing everything possible to avoid fighting someone who threatens or attacks you. Self-defense is all about using your smarts—not your fists.

This chapter includes: "Self-Defense," February 2006, reprinted with permission from www.kidshealth.org. Copyright © 2006 The Nemours Foundation. This information was provided by KidsHealth, one of the largest resources online for medically reviewed health information written for parents, kids, and teens. For more articles like this one, visit www.KidsHealth.org, or www.TeensHealth.org. Also, under the heading "Safety Awareness," text is excerpted from "Self-Defense and Safety Awareness," available at http://hr.od.nih.gov/worklife/documents/SelfDefenseHandout.pdf, from the National Institutes of Health (NIH), May 10, 2006.

Use Your Head

People (guys as well as girls) who are threatened and fight back "in self-defense" actually risk making a situation worse. The attacker, who is already edgy and pumped up on adrenaline—and who knows what else—may become even more angry and violent. The best way to handle any attack or threat of attack is to try to get away. This way, you're least likely to be injured.

One way to avoid a potential attack before it happens is to trust your instincts. Your intuition, combined with your common sense, can help get you out of trouble. For example, if you're running alone on the school track and you suddenly feel like you're being watched, that could be your intuition telling you something. Your common sense would then tell you that it's a good idea to get back to where there are more people around.

Attackers aren't always strangers who jump out of dark alleys. Sadly, teens can be attacked by people they know. That's where another important self-defense skill comes into play. This skill is something self-defense experts and negotiators call de-escalation.

De-escalating a situation means speaking or acting in a way that can prevent things from getting worse. The classic example of de-escalation is giving a robber your money rather than trying to fight or run. But de-escalation can work in other ways, too. For example, if someone harasses you when there's no one else around, you can de-escalate things by agreeing with him or her. You don't have to actually believe the taunts, of course, you're just using words to get you out of a tight spot. Then you can redirect the bully's focus ("Oops, I just heard the bell for third period"), and calmly walk away from the situation.

Something as simple as not losing your temper can de-escalate a situation. Learn how to manage your own anger effectively so that you can talk or walk away without using your fists or weapons.

Although de-escalation won't always work, it can only help matters if you remain calm and don't give the would-be attacker any extra ammunition. Whether it's a stranger or someone you thought you could trust, saying and doing things that don't threaten your attacker can give you some control.

Reduce Your Risks

Another part of self-defense is doing things that can help you stay safe. Here are some tips from the National Crime Prevention Council and other experts:

- Understand your surroundings. Walk or hang out in areas that are open, well lit, and well traveled. Become familiar with the buildings, parking lots, parks, and other places you walk. Pay particular attention to places where someone could hide—such as stairways and bushes.

- Avoid shortcuts that take you through isolated areas.

- If you're going out at night, travel in a group.

- Make sure your friends and parents know your daily schedule (classes, sports practice, club meetings, and so forth). If you go on a date or with friends for an after-game snack, let someone know where you're going and when you expect to return.

- Check out hangouts. Do they look safe? Are you comfortable being there? Ask yourself if the people around you seem to share your views on fun activities—if you think they're being reckless, move on.

- Be sure your body language shows a sense of confidence. Look like you know where you're going and act alert.

- When riding on public transportation, sit near the driver and stay awake. Attackers are looking for vulnerable targets.

- Carry a cell phone if possible. Make sure it's programmed with your parents' phone number.

- Be willing to report crimes in your neighborhood and school to the police.

Take a Self-Defense Class

The best way—in fact the only way—to prepare yourself to fight off an attacker is to take a self-defense class. We'd love to give you all the right moves in an article, but some things you just have to learn in person.

A good self-defense class can teach you how to size up a situation and decide what you should do. Self-defense classes can also teach special techniques for breaking an attacker's grasp and other things you can do to get away. For example, attackers usually anticipate how their victim might react—that kick to the groin or jab to the eyes, for instance. A good self-defense class can teach you ways to surprise your attacker and catch him or her off guard.

One of the best things people take away from self-defense classes is self-confidence. The last thing you want to be thinking about during

ck is, "Can I really pull this self-defense tactic off?" It's much
o take action in an emergency if you've already had a few dry
runs.

A self-defense class should give you a chance to practice your
moves. If you take a class with a friend, you can continue practicing
on each other to keep the moves fresh in your mind long after the class
is over.

Check out your local YMCA, community hospital, or community
center for classes. If they don't have them, they may be able to tell
you who does. Your physical education (PE) teacher or school counselor may also be a great resource.

Safety Awareness

Protection from Stalking

- Have a home security survey.

- Make sure your address marker is clearly visible from the
  street. This can help save valuable time in the event that an
  emergency response is necessary.

- Use exterior lighting.

- Do not allow strangers into your home.

- Get an unlisted phone number. Keep a notebook by your phone
  and note times of prank or hang-up calls. Have emergency numbers posted near each phone. Consider acquiring the caller ID
  option available from the phone company.

- If you have an answering machine, your greeting should indicate that you are unavailable. Never say, "I'm not home right
  now." Remember answering machines can be used to screen
  calls before answering.

- Be careful not to develop patterns—vary walking and travel
  routes. Be aware of your surroundings at all times.

- Children should be accompanied to bus stops or school.

- Always secure your car. Do not park in garages that require you
  to leave the car unlocked and surrender the keys. If this cannot
  be avoided, provide only the ignition key.

- Equip gas tank with a locking gas cap. To prevent tampering,
  the hood release should be controlled from inside the vehicle.

- Lock the doors when traveling in your car. Be aware of traffic around you. If you are being followed, go to a busy place where people can be found. Sound your horn to attract attention. Get help and phone the police immediately. A car phone can be useful to call for help in an emergency.

- Take precautions to safeguard personal information such as your address.

Protection from Rape

Common Sense Indoors

- Make sure all doors (include sliding glass doors) and windows have dead bolt locks, and use them. Install a peephole in the door. Keep entrances well-lighted.

- Never open your door to strangers. Offer to make an emergency call while someone waits outside. Check the identification of any sales or service people before letting them in. Don't be embarrassed to phone for verification.

- Be wary of isolated spots—apartment laundry rooms, underground garages, parking lots, offices after business hours. Walk with a friend, co-worker, or security guard, particularly at night.

- Know your neighbors so you have someone to call or go to if you're scared.

- If you come home and see a door or window open, or broken, don't go in. Call the police from a cell or public phone.

Common Sense Outdoors

- Avoid walking or jogging alone, especially at night. Stay in well-traveled, well-lighted areas.

- Wear clothes and shoes that give you freedom of movement.

- Be careful if anyone in a car asks you for directions—if you answer, keep your distance from the car.

- Have your key ready before you reach the door—home, car, or office.

- If you think you're being followed, change direction and head for open stores, restaurants, theaters, or a lighted house.

Car Sense

- Park in area that will be well-lighted and well-traveled when you return.

- Always lock your car—when you get in and when you get out.

- Look around your car and in the back seat before you get in.

- If your car breaks down, lift the hood, lock the doors, and turn on flashers. If someone stops, roll the window down slightly and ask the person to call the police or a tow service.

- Don't hitchhike, ever. Don't pick up a hitchhiker.

When the Unthinkable Happens

How should you handle a rape attempt? It depends on your physical and emotional state, the situation, the rapist's personality. There are no hard and fast, right or wrong answers. Surviving is the goal.

- Try to escape. Scream. Be rude. Make noise to discourage your attacker from following.

- Talk, stall for time, and assess your options.

- If the rapist has a weapon, you may have no choice but to submit. Do whatever it takes to survive.

- If you decide to fight back, you must be quick and effective. Target the eyes or groin.

Chapter 45

Intervention Programs for Abusers

Perpetrator Intervention Programs for Abusers

Abusers can enter voluntarily or be court ordered to perpetrator intervention programs. It is important to note that there are no guarantees that he will change his violent behavior. He is the only one that can make the decision—and commitment—to change.

For example, in Alabama, there are certification guidelines for perpetrator intervention programs. Certified programs have completed a standards review process to ensure they meet guidelines. You can contact the Alabama Coalition Against Domestic Violence for information on these standards, 334-832-4842, or your local domestic violence shelter for information about your state.

An intervention program should include these factors:

- Victim's safety is the priority
- Meets minimum standards for weekly sessions (16 weeks)
- Holds him accountable
- Curriculum addresses the root of his problem
- Makes no demand on the victim to participate
- Is open to input from the victim

This chapter includes text from "Why do abusers batter?" © Alabama Coalition Against Domestic Violence (www.acadv.org). Reprinted with permission.

What programs teach:

- Education about domestic violence
- Changing attitudes and beliefs about using violence in a relationship
- Achieving equality in relationships
- Community participation

In the program, an abuser should become aware of his pattern of violence and learn techniques for maintaining nonviolent behavior, such as "time outs," buddy phone calls, support groups, relaxation techniques, and exercise.

How do you know if he is really changing?

Positive signs include the following:

- He has stopped being violent or threatening to you or others.
- He acknowledges that his abusive behavior is wrong.
- He understands that he does not have the right to control and dominate you.
- You don't feel afraid when you are with him.
- He does not coerce or force you to have sex.
- You can express anger toward him without feeling intimidated.
- He does not make you feel responsible for his anger or frustration.
- He respects your opinion even if he doesn't agree with it.
- He respects your right to say "no."

Am I safe while he is in the program?

For your own safety and your children's safety, watch for these signs that indicate problems while he is in the program:

- Tries to find you if you've left.
- Tries to get you to come back to him.
- Tries to take away the children.
- Stalks you.

If you feel you are in danger, contact a crisis line for assistance.

Lies

Six Big Lies

If you hear your partner making these statements while he is in a treatment program for abusers, you should understand that he is lying to himself, and to you.

- "I'm not the only one who needs counseling."
- "I'm not as bad as a lot of other guys in there."
- "As soon as I'm done with this program, I'll be cured."
- "We need to stay together to work this out."
- "If I weren't under so much stress, I wouldn't have such a short fuse."
- "Now that I'm in this program, you have to be more understanding."

Counseling

Couples' Counseling Does Not Work in Violent Relationships

If you are struggling with a relationship, some people may advise you to get marriage counseling, or couples' counseling. While this can be good advice in some relationships, it is not good for couples where there is violence. In fact, in many cases, couples' counseling has increased the violence in the home.

Couples' counseling does not work because:

- Couples' counseling places the responsibility for change on both partners.
  - Domestic violence is the sole responsibility of the abuser.
- Couples' counseling works best when both people are truthful.
  - Individuals who are abusive to their partners minimize, deny, and blame, and therefore are not truthful in counseling.
- Couples resolve problems in counseling by talking about problems.
  - His abuse is not a couple problem, it is his problem. He needs to work on it in a specialized program for abusers. A victim

who is being abused in a relationship is in a dangerous position in couple's counseling. If she tells the counselor about the abuse, she is likely to suffer more abuse when she gets home. If she does not tell, nothing can be accomplished.

If you think you will benefit from joint counseling, go after he successfully completes a batterer's intervention program and is no longer violent.

Red Flags of Abuse

You may be involved with a perpetrator if any of the following "red flags" exist in the relationship:

- Quick involvement—the perpetrator pushes for a commitment or major event to occur very early in the relationship.

- Isolation—the perpetrator begins asking you to spend less time with your friends and family and more time with him. You end up no longer maintaining close relationships with friends or family members.

- Suggestions for change—the perpetrator has lots of suggestions on how you can improve your appearance, behavior, and so forth. You begin to make changes solely based on these suggestions.

- Controlling behaviors—the perpetrator influences your decisions on hobbies, activities, dress, friends, daily routines, and so forth. You begin to make fewer and fewer decisions without the perpetrator's opinion or influence.

- Information gathering and pop-ins—the perpetrator wants to know the specific details of your day and rarely leaves you alone when you are not with him, such as when you are at work or out with friends.

- Any forms of abuse—the perpetrator may use name calling, intimidation, humiliation, shoving, pushing, or other forms of abuse to get you to do whatever they want you to do.

These red flags may indicate that you are involved with a perpetrator of domestic violence. These red flags may occur early in the relationship and be explained by the perpetrator as caring or loving behaviors such as "I just check on you because I miss you" or "I just want what is best for you" or "I just want us to work on our relationship and spend more time together."

If You Have Concerns about Your Relationship or Your Safety

National Domestic Violence Hotline
P.O. Box 161810
Austin, TX 78716
Toll-Free Hotline: 800-799-SAFE (7233)
Toll-Free TTY: 800-787-3224
Website: http://www.ndvh.org

National Sexual Assault Hotline
Rape, Abuse & Incest National Network (RAINN)
2000 L Street, NW, Suite 406
Washington, DC 20036
Toll-Free: 800-656-HOPE (4673)
Phone: 202-544-3064
Fax: 202-544-3556
Website: http://www.rainn.org
E-mail: info@rainn.org

Chapter 46

Working with Men to Prevent Violence against Women

Chapter Contents

Section 46.1

What Works in Men's Violence Prevention?

Excerpted from: Berkowitz, A. (2004, October). Working With Men to Prevent Violence: An Overview (Part One). Harrisburg, PA: VAWnet (www .vawnet.org), a project of the National Resource Center on Domestic Violence/Pennsylvania Coalition Against Domestic Violence. © 2004. Reprinted with permission. The complete document is available online at http://new.vawnet.org/category/Main_Doc.php?docid=413.

There is a growing awareness that men, in partnership with women, can play a significant role in ending violence against women. This has led to an increase in programs and activities that focus on men's roles in violence prevention. Men should take responsibility for preventing violence against women because of the untold harm it causes to women in men's lives and the ways in which it directly hurts men. Violence against women hurts men when it results in women being afraid of or suspicious of men due to fear of potential victimization and when it perpetuates negative stereotypes of men based on the actions of a few. The behaviors and attitudes that cause violence against women may also be a cause of men being violent towards other men. These same behaviors and attitudes may also keep men from having close and meaningful relationships with each other. Finally, while only a minority of men is violent, all men can have an influence on the culture and environment that allows other men to be perpetrators. For example, men can refuse to be bystanders to other men's violent behavior.

For all of these reasons, men have a stake in ending violence against women. To do this, men must accept and examine their own potential for violence and take a stand against the violence of other men. In recent years, a number of authors have argued persuasively that men need to take responsibility for preventing men's violence against women, both in the United States, and internationally.

Defining Men's Roles in Prevention

Men can prevent violence against women by not personally engaging in violence, by intervening against the violence of other men, and by addressing the root causes of violence. This broad definition provides roles for all men in preventing violence against women. Men's involvement can take the form of primary or universal prevention (directed at all men, including those who do not appear to be at risk of committing violence and those who may be at risk for continuing a pattern of violence), through secondary or selective prevention (directed at men who are at-risk for committing violence), and/or through more intensive tertiary or indicated prevention (with men who have already been violent).

For violence prevention these distinctions may be somewhat artificial because it can be argued that all men are at risk for perpetration by virtue of their socialization as men, because men can commit violence without defining it as such, and because men who have been violent can successfully participate in programs to prevent other men's violence. Prevention is defined here as any program or activity that reduces or prevents future violence against women by men. Programs for men who already have a documented history of violence against women, such as batterer's or perpetrator treatment programs, will not be discussed here.

Prevention programs can take the form of one session, a series of sessions, or ongoing interactive educational workshops, leadership training, social marketing and social norms media campaigns, or through participation in one-time or ongoing public events. These may focus directly on the issue of violence or on its specific forms (for example, sexual assault, domestic violence, dating violence and/or harassment, and stalking), or indirectly through men's involvement in consciousness raising, fatherhood and/or skill-building programs that foster attitudes and behaviors that may protect against violence, or by providing healthy resocialization experiences about what it means to be a healthy, nonviolent man. In its broadest definition, violence prevention for men includes any activity that addresses the root causes of men's violence including social and structural causes as well as men's gender role socialization and men's sexism.

Among men's violence prevention programs, those for school-aged boys have tended to focus on issues of sexual harassment and dating violence, those for college age men have tended to focus on sexual assault, and those for men not in college or older have tended to focus on domestic violence in longer-term partnerships. In actuality, it is important for all men to be involved in the prevention of all forms of violence against women, even when it may be developmentally or strategically appropriate to foster this involvement by focusing initially on one form of men's violence.

What Works in Men's Violence Prevention?

Due to evaluation literature that is limited in scope, it is difficult to assess the effectiveness of violence prevention programs for men. For example, most prevention program assessments measure changes in attitudes that are associated with a proclivity to be violent rather than actual violent behavior. Reviews of the literature suggest that sexual assault prevention programs for college men can be effective in improving attitudes that may put men at risk for committing violence against women, although these attitudinal changes are often limited to periods of a few months. In contrast, programs that focus only on providing information have not been found to be effective. Among pre-college aged males, dating violence and harassment prevention programs offered to mixed gender groups in school settings can result in both attitude and behavior change for a few months or longer.

Despite the limited research, there is an emerging consensus regarding what constitutes effective violence prevention for men. Violence prevention programs that have been found effective in evaluation studies tend to share one or more of the following assumptions. Practitioners who work with men to prevent violence have also concluded that effective violence prevention programs for men share some or all of these assumptions:

- Men must assume responsibility for preventing men's violence against women.

- Men need to be approached as partners in solving the problem rather than as perpetrators.

- Workshops and other activities are more effective when conducted by peers in small, all-male groups because of the immense influence that men have on each other and because of the safety all-male groups can provide.

- Discussions should be interactive and encourage honest sharing of feelings, ideas, and beliefs.

- Opportunities should be created to discuss and critique prevailing understandings of masculinity and men's discomfort with them, as well as men's misperceptions of other men's attitudes and behavior.

- Positive anti-violence values and healthy aspects of men's experience should be strengthened, including teaching men to intervene in other men's behavior.

- Work with men must be in collaboration with and accountable to women working as advocates, educators, and prevention specialists.

What is the logic of these assumptions?

First, research and experience have shown that putting men on the defensive or using blame is not effective and can even result in negative outcomes. Thus, in Lonsway's review of the literature she stated: "although educational programs challenging rape culture do require confrontation of established ideologies, such interventions *do not necessitate a style of personal confrontation*" (Italics added, 1996, p. 250). Thus, men should take responsibility for acting as perpetrators and bystanders of violence, and the best way to accomplish this is to encourage men to be partners in solving the problem rather than by criticizing or blaming men. Most men are not coercive or opportunistic, do not want to victimize others, and are willing to be part of the solution to ending sexual assault. (In contrast, while men who are predatory or who have a history of perpetration may benefit from exposure to some education and prevention programs, more intensive treatment is likely required for these men to change previous patterns of perpetration).

The majority of men may already hold attitudes that can be strengthened to prevent and reduce violence and encourage men to intervene with other men. For example, research has demonstrated that most men are uncomfortable with how they have been taught to be men, including how to be in relationship with women, homophobia, heterosexuality, and emotional expression, and that they are uncomfortable with the sexism and inappropriate behavior of other men. Because many men already feel blamed and are on the defensive about the issue of men's violence (even when this defensiveness is misplaced), effective approaches create a learning environment that can surface the positive attitudes and behaviors that allow men to be part of the solution. This can be accomplished in the context of a safe, nonjudgmental atmosphere for open discussion and dialogue in which men can discuss feelings about relationships, sexuality, aggression, and so forth, and share discomfort about the behavior of other men.

What types of discussions are effective?

Literature reviews have suggested that the quality and interactive nature of the discussion may be more important than the format in which it is presented, a dimension that Davis (2000) has called program process. Because men are influenced by other men and by what men think is true about other men, this influence can be positively channeled in all-male groups. Thus, effective violence prevention for men acknowledges the important influence that male peer groups have on men's actions, corrects misperceptions that men have about each other's attitudes and behavior, and channels this influence towards positive change.

The common element in successful prevention programs for men is the opportunity to participate in an experience where men are encouraged to honestly share real feelings and concerns about issues of masculinity and men's violence. The opportunity for men to hear the attitudes and views of other men is powerful, especially because it empowers men who want to help and provides them with visible allies. This strategy encourages the majority of men to take the necessary steps to avoid perpetrating and to confront the inappropriate behavior of male peers.

Are all male or mixed gender programs more effective?

Research suggests that these goals can be accomplished most effectively with male facilitators in all-male groups. For example, Brecklin and Forde (2001) conducted a comprehensive meta-analysis of forty-three college rape prevention program evaluations and concluded that both men and women experienced more beneficial change in single-gender groups than in mixed-gender groups. This was also the conclusion reached in five other literature reviews of rape prevention programs that all recommended that rape prevention programs be conducted in separate-gender groups when possible.

While there are advantages to programs facilitated by men, skilled female facilitators can also work very effectively with men. Women working with men need to be aware that men may view their leadership as reinforcing the assumption that violence prevention is a women's issue not relevant to men, and must also find ways to prevent participants from attributing honest dialogue simply to the presence of a female. It is also beneficial for men to see women and men co-facilitating in a respectful partnership. Examples of programs for men that have been developed and led by women include those by Hong (2000) and Mahlstedt (1999).

One of the main arguments for separate gender workshops is that the goals for violence prevention are different for men and women. Despite this being true in some settings, it may be necessary or more appropriate to offer violence prevention in mixed groups. Trainers must still take into account the gender differences that make such separation desirable, avoid the polarization that can occur in mixed-gender groups, avoid potential victim-blaming, not give information about victim-risk that could be useful to perpetrators, and avoid approaches that are blaming of men (Schewe, 2002). While mixed gender workshops have been evaluated as successful with boys in school settings, these programs have not been compared with similar programs offered in all-male settings.

Partnerships with Women and Accountability to Women

Attention to men's roles in preventing violence against women is only possible because of the decades of tireless work and sacrifice by female victim advocates, social activists, researchers, academicians, survivors, and leaders. These courageous women have successfully challenged society to take notice of this problem and to begin to fund efforts to solve it. Men's work to end violence against women must include recognition of this leadership and must never be in competition with or at the expense of women's efforts. Thus, prevention programs for men should be developed to exist alongside of victim advocacy, legal and policy initiatives, academic research, rape crisis and domestic violence services, and educational programs for women. Male anti-violence educators must recognize that we are accountable to the women who are the victims of the violence we hope to end, and must work to create effective collaborative partnerships and alliances that provide a role for women in men's programs (Flood, 2003). To do this requires an understanding and exploration of men's privilege, sexism, and other biases, and an openness to learning from women and to working with them as allies.

Challenges to Men's Involvement

Finally, it is important to acknowledge that there are many challenges and barriers for men who do this work. Men who work to end violence against women are challenging the dominant culture and the understandings of masculinity that maintain it. Thus, male activists are often met with suspicion, homophobia, and other questions about their masculinity. Men and women who feel threatened by this work often discredit male activists' efforts and persons. At the same time many men are grateful for the example set by male activists and for modeling a different way of being male. Men who do this work are also frequently and unfairly given more credit for their efforts than women who do similar work. Men engaged in violence prevention need to personally recognize these challenges and take responsibility to change these dynamics both personally and professionally.

Cultural Issues and Masculinities

While men in North America may share some common socialization experiences and definitions of what it means to be male, there are also important differences in terms of race, ethnicity, social class, sexual orientation, religion, and other identities that must be addressed in violence prevention efforts. In addition, there are cultural differences regarding the appropriate context for prevention including how violence should be addressed. Currently there is extensive literature documenting the need for culturally relevant and tailored programs in medical, psychological, and public health literatures, along with evidence for the ineffectiveness of approaches derived from dominant groups or paradigms. Providing culturally competent programming should not be considered optional, but is a necessity for effectiveness.

Relevance is a critical component of program success. It has been determined to be an important component of effective prevention programs. Because men from different identities have different experiences, relevant programming must address these differences, including experiences of racism among men of color; of homophobia for gay, bisexual, and transgender men; the effects of economic inequalities for working class and poor men; and, the cultural context for violence prevention within different communities. As with every other issue, there is a danger of imposing definitions and understandings from more established violence prevention efforts (which, like the larger culture, is predominantly white and middle class) upon other cultures and communities.

An example of the importance of culturally relevant programs comes from research on the differential impact of programs on men from different racial backgrounds. In one study, a generic race-neutral program was effective for European heritage men but not men of color, while a modified program with a co-presenter of color and relevant information (including statistics on violence in ethnic communities and dispelling of ethnically based rape myths) were effective for both groups. In other research conducted on perpetrators from different ethnic backgrounds, differences were found in personality characteristics and motivations for perpetration that may have important implications for designing culturally sensitive prevention programs for men.

Violence prevention efforts need to acknowledge these kinds of differences and also correct stereotypes and myths about the prevalence of violence among different groups of men. Finally, men from different cultural groups have different experiences with the educational and criminal justice systems that may influence receptivity to violence prevention. Violence prevention efforts that are community based, sensitive to ethnic and class issues, and accountable to the larger community, have been developed in many communities and show promise. All of these strongly suggest the critical importance of developing programs that are either tailored to the needs of a particular group, or conducted in a way that is inclusive and welcoming of all backgrounds. A critical oversight is the lack of research examining the needs of gay, bisexual, and transgendered men with respect to violence prevention programming.

Summary

In recent years, there has been expanded interest in developing programs and strategies that focus on men's responsibility for ending violence against women. These programs create a safe environment for men to discuss and challenge each other with respect to information and attitudes about men's violence. The literature suggests that these programs can produce short-term change in men's attitudes that are associated with a proclivity for violence, encourage men to intervene against the behavior of other men, and in some cases reduce men's future violence. As these programs become more popular and as more men take leadership on this issue, we are hopeful that the epidemic of men's violence against women will be significantly reduced and that all of our relationships will come closer to embodying ideals of respect, mutual empowerment, growth, and co-creation.

Section 46.2

Coaching Boys into Men

Your Role in Ending Violence against Women

Now more than ever, the boys in your life need your time and energy. Your son, grandson, nephew, younger brother—the boys you teach and coach—rely on you to grow into healthy young men.

Boys need advice, especially on how to behave toward girls. They are watching how you treat women. Help them learn that men don't hurt women, that violence does not equal strength, and that there is honor in taking a stand for respect and against violence.

If you want to stop violence against women, reach out to a boy in your life.

What You Can Do

Be there: If it comes down to one thing you can do, this is it. Just being with boys is crucial. They might not say this directly, but boys want a positive male presence around them, even if few words are exchanged.

Know he's watching you: He's watching everything you say and do—your way of talking, your sense of humor, how you deal with stress, conflict, and anger, and how you treat women. He takes cues from you, both good and bad.

Show respect: Make respect your way of dealing with people. Boys will learn what respect means by watching how you treat others. That means in traffic, in stores, in restaurants, on the basketball court, and around the dinner table.

Teach him about honor: Let him know from an early age that honor and integrity are marks of a great man. Tell him what they are and that there is no honor or integrity in abusing women and girls.

Give him options: Share strategies for handling violent situations and staying safe. Tell him what he can do if he sees any signs of violence against girls or women.

Ask about his world: Find out who his role models are—sports figures, celebrities, or people in your neighborhood and community. Ask him who he respects and why. Let him know that people who disrespect women are not admirable and point him to men who are.

Listen: When he gets frustrated and mad, tell him he can walk it off or talk it out. Let him know he can come to you anytime he feels like things are getting out of hand.

Discuss the rules: Young people need to understand limits. Family rules and school rules about treating others with respect need to be talked about and reinforced. And when it comes time for dating, be sure he knows that treating girls with respect is important.

Remember, we all make mistakes. Boys (and parents) aren't always perfect. The goal is to learn from the past to make a better future.

Your Message Matters

Boys are swamped with messages from television, friends, school, the neighborhood, online, music, and movies. Everything they see and hear tells them what it means to "be a man"—that they have to be tough, be in control, or that they need to boss others around, including their girlfriends.

You can give positive messages—ones about respect, honor, and responsibility.

The benefits of investing time in boys' lives and talking with them about violence are clear: they will know what is and is not okay in relationships with girls and women, and they will know they can come to you with problems and questions.

You can make a real difference in boys' lives.

Chapter 47

Prevent Domestic Violence: Tips for Parents

Tips for Being a Nurturing Parent

A healthy, nurturing relationship with your child is built through countless interactions over the course of time. It requires a lot of energy and work, but the rewards are well worth it. When it comes to parenting, there are few absolutes (one, of course, being that every child needs to be loved) and there is no one right way. Different parenting techniques work for different children under different circumstances. These tips provide suggestions as you discover what works best in your family. Do not expect to be perfect; parenting is a difficult job.

Help Your Children Feel Loved and Secure

We can all take steps to strengthen our relationships with our children:

- Make sure your children know you love them, even when they do something wrong.

- Encourage your children. Praise their achievements and talents. Recognize the skills they are developing.

This chapter includes text from "Safe Children and Healthy Families Are a Shared Responsibility," 2006 Community Resource Packet, Children's Bureau, U.S. Department of Health and Human Services (HHS), 2006. Also, the sections titled "Time Out," "The Power of Choice," and "Setting Rules and Consequences with Teens," are reprinted with permission of Elizabeth Pantley. © 2006 Elizabeth Pantley. All rights reserved.

- Spend time with your children. Do things together that you both enjoy. Listen to your children.

- Learn how to use nonphysical options for discipline. Many alternatives exist. Depending on your child's age and level of development, these may include simply redirecting your child's attention, offering choices, or using time out.

Realize That Community Resources Add Value

Children need direct and continuing access to people with whom they can develop healthy, supportive relationships. To assist this, parents may try the following:

- Take children to libraries, museums, movies, and sporting events.

- Enroll children in youth enrichment programs, such as sports or music.

- Use community services for family needs, such as parent education classes or respite care.

- Communicate regularly with childcare or school staff.

- Participate in religious or youth groups.

Seek Help If You Need It

Being a parent is difficult. No one expects you to know how to do it all. Challenges such as unemployment or a child with special needs can add to family tension. If you think stress may be affecting the way you treat your child, or if you just want the extra support that most parents need at some point, try the following:

- Talk to someone. Tell a friend, healthcare provider, or a leader in your faith community about what you are experiencing. Or, join a support group for parents.

- Seek respite care when you need a break. Everyone needs time for themselves. Respite care or crisis care provides a safe place for your children so you can take care of yourself.

- Call a helpline. Most states have helplines for parents. Childhelp USA® offers a national 24-hour hotline at 800-4-A-CHILD (800-422-4453) for parents who need help or parenting advice.

- Seek counseling. Individual, couple, or family counseling can identify and reinforce healthy ways to communicate and parent.

- Take a parenting class. No one is born knowing how to be a good parent. It is an acquired skill. Parenting classes can give you the skills you need to raise a happy, healthy child.

- Accept help. You do not have to do it all. Accept offers of help from trusted family.

Soothing a Crying Infant

One of the most stressful experiences for new parents is dealing with a crying baby. Babies cry for all sorts of reasons, and it's sometimes difficult to figure out why your baby is crying and how to soothe your baby. It's important to remember that crying is one of the main ways that babies communicate, and their crying can mean lots of different things. With a new baby, it may be difficult to distinguish different types of crying; as babies get older, parents may be able to tell wet-diaper crying from I'm hungry crying.

Here are some things to check for when a baby cries:

- Is the baby sick? Take the baby's temperature, and call a health care provider if there is a fever or if you're not sure about any other symptoms. If your baby cries for hours at a time, be sure to have him or her checked out by a pediatrician.

- Is the baby hungry? Try feeding the baby. Newborns like to eat frequently. Even if the baby isn't hungry, he or she may respond to sucking on a pacifier.

- Is the diaper wet or dirty? This is a common cause for crying.

- Is the room too hot or cold, or is the baby overdressed or underdressed?

- Is the baby lonely or afraid? Try holding the baby and comforting him or her.

- Is the baby overstimulated? Try turning down the lights and the noise level.

Calming the Baby

Often, a parent has made sure that the problem is not hunger or sickness or a wet diaper—but the baby is still crying. What are some other ways to calm a crying baby?

- Swaddle the baby in a soft blanket and hold the baby next to you. Sing or hum to the baby.

- Rock the baby in a chair or swing, or gently sway your body while holding the baby close.

- Take the baby for a ride in the stroller or car. Motion often puts a baby to sleep.

- Distract the baby by making faces or quiet noises.

- Give the baby a warm bath to relax him or her.

- Use some white noise such as running a vacuum cleaner or hair dryer to help lull the baby to sleep.

Calming Yourself

There are few things more stressful than a crying baby. It is normal for babies to cry—sometimes as much as 2–4 hours a day—and sometimes nothing parents try to soothe the baby will work. Coupled with a parent's own lack of sleep and the general adjustment to having a new baby in the house, a crying baby can seem overwhelming. There are some things parents can do to maintain control over the situation, even when the baby continues to cry.

- Take a break. Put the baby safely in a crib, and take a few minutes for yourself in another room.

- Call a friend or relative who will listen to your problem and be sympathetic.

- Ask a trusted friend or neighbor to watch your child while you take a short break or a brief nap.

- If you feel as though you are losing control and might hurt your child, call a hotline, such as the 24-hour National Child Abuse Hotline 800-4-A-CHILD (800-422-4453).

- It's normal for babies to cry sometimes, and it's certainly normal for parents to feel frustrated by the crying. Different babies respond to different soothing techniques, and parents will eventually learn what works best with their baby. In the meantime, it's helpful for new parents to have some support in the form of friends, relatives, and neighbors who can lend a sympathetic ear or even baby sit.

Dealing with Temper Tantrums

Almost every parent of a toddler has experienced the frustration of dealing with a child throwing a floor-thumping, hair-pulling temper tantrum. Even though this can be embarrassing and challenging for parents, this is normal behavior for most young children.

Why do they do it?

Toddlers are not yet able to use words to express their feelings and emotions. When they are tired, frustrated, or angry, and unable to express themselves with words, they may throw a temper tantrum. Some children throw tantrums because their emotions run out of control, and they aren't yet old enough to know how to contain them. Finally, some children continue to throw tantrums if they are rewarded for doing so (that is, if they learn that parents will give them what they want to stop the tantrum).

How can parents prevent tantrums?

It is often easier to prevent tantrums than to deal with them once they have begun. Parents may notice some signals that children give as a warning that a tantrum may be brewing. If a parent suspects that a tantrum is coming, or if a child gets in the habit of having a tantrum after a particular experience or at a particular time of day, here are some prevention tips to keep in mind:

- Distract or redirect your child's attention to something else.
- Use a sense of humor to distract your child. This may help you cope, too.
- Give your child control over small things by giving him or her a choice.
- Take your child to a quiet place and speak softly to him or her.
- Encourage your child to express emotions and feelings with words.
- Stick to a daily routine that gives your child enough rest and enough activity.
- Reward your child when he or she requests something without having a tantrum.

How can parents deal with tantrums, especially public temper tantrums?

Parents can be caught off guard when a child throws a tantrum in public. It can be embarrassing, and parents may be tempted to give in to the child just to stop the tantrum. But giving in just teaches the child that tantrums work. Instead, try some of the following tips to deal with tantrums that happen in the home or in public:

- Remain calm. Don't lose control because your child has lost control. Instead, try to model behavior that is calm and controlled.

- Hugging or holding your child until the tantrum subsides may help a younger child through a tantrum.

- Put the child in time out or in a quiet place (even strapped in to a stroller) where he or she can calm down. Time out should be one minute for each year of the child's age.

- Older children who throw tantrums may be seeking attention. Try ignoring them until the tantrum is over.

What can parents do after the tantrum?

As children get older, they will grow out of temper tantrums. In the meantime, try to take some time and talk over the experience with your child after it happens. Helping your child identify and talk about feelings will help your child to express feelings with words rather than with tantrums. Finally, congratulate yourself for getting through your child's tantrum while remaining calm. A calm parent provides a child with a great behavior model for the child to follow.

Time Out

Time out can be a valuable tool in disciplining a child. As we go about the business of teaching our children proper behavior, there are times when emotions threaten to get out of control. When this happens, it's wise to separate yourself from your child so that you can both cool off. Time out can be used as an effective, positive tool. There are three different ways to use time out, each having a different purpose.

1. **To give the child time and space to cool off and calm down.** The key here is in the attitude of the parent. In advance, let your child know that when her behavior is out of control she'll be asked to go to her room. Tell her that when she is calm and under control she may join the family. How she chooses to use the time is her business, as long as it's respectful of people and property. Screaming or pounding on the door is not acceptable, but reading a book or other activities are fine. This is a valuable life skill that will prevent your child from flying off the handle and saying and doing things she might regret later.

Never drag a child to his time out. This robs you of the upper hand and makes you look foolish. Let him know in advance that when asked to remove himself he needs to do so immediately. If he does not, he'll be choosing to give up a privilege (one you have specified in advance), in addition to time out.

2. **To give the parent time and space to cool off and calm down.** There are times when we get so angry at our children that we want to scream, hit, or ground them for life! This is the time to use a four-letter-word: E X I T. Make a brief statement, "I'm so angry, I need a minute to think." Then go to your room or send the child to his room so that you can calm down and regroup. This will help you get yourself under control, and it provides good modeling for your children.

3. **As a method for stopping a specific misbehavior.** This can be an excellent way to put an immediate stop to a child's action. It brings a strong message, "This behavior is unacceptable and it will stop now." There are several keys:

   - **Be quick:** Catch your child in the act. Delayed reactions dilute the effect.

   - **Use selectively:** Use for hitting, talking back, and whining, or other specific problems. Don't overuse.

   - **Keep calm:** Your anger only adds fuel to the fire and changes the focus from the behavior of the child to your anger. This prevents you from being in control.

   - **Stick with it:** Once you say, "time out," don't back down or be talked out of it. If you decide to use time out to control hitting, for example, use it every time your child hits, even if he spends most of the day in time out. Eventually, he'll decide that it's more fun to play without hitting than to sit alone in his room.

Time out is one more effective discipline tool for parents. When used with other positive parenting methods it helps you feel good about the job you are doing with your kids.

The Power of Choice

Would you like to get your kids to cooperate willingly? Stop the daily battles? Teach your kids valuable life skills? If your answer is "Yes, yes, yes" then read on...

419

There are so many things we must get our children to do and so many things we must stop them from doing: Get up. Get dressed. Don't dawdle. Do your homework. Eat. It goes on and on. We can get our kids to cooperate and at the same time allow them to learn self-discipline and develop good decision-making skills. How? By offering choices.

Giving a choice is a very powerful tool that can be used with children who are toddlers and children who are teenagers. This is one skill that every parent should have tattooed on the back of his or her hand as a constant reminder. Parents should use this skill every day, many times a day. Giving children choices is a very effective way to enlist their cooperation because children love having the privilege of choice. It takes the pressure out of your request and allows a child to feel in control. This makes a child more willing to comply.

Using choice is an effective way to achieve results, and when you get in the habit of offering choices you are doing your children a big favor. As children learn to make simple choices (milk or juice?), they get the practice required to make bigger choices (buy two class T-shirts or one sweatshirt?) which gives them the ability as they grow to make more important decisions (save or spend? drink beer or soda? study or fail?). Giving children choices allows them to learn to listen to their inner voice. It is a valuable skill that they will carry with them to adulthood.

You should offer choices based on your child's age and your intent: A toddler can handle two choices, a grade-school child three or four. A teenager can be given general guidelines. Only offer choices that will be acceptable to you. Otherwise, you are not being fair. For example, a parent might say, "Either eat your peas or go to your room," but when the child gets up off his chair, the parent yells, "Sit down and eat your dinner, young man!" (So that wasn't really a choice, was it?) Here are some ways in which you can use choice:

- Do you want to wear your Big Bird pajamas or your Mickey Mouse pajamas?

- Do you want to do your homework at the kitchen table or the desk?

- Do you want to wear your coat, carry it, or put on a sweatshirt?

- Would you prefer to let the dog out in the yard or take him for a walk?

- Do you want to run up to bed or hop to bed like a bunny?

- What do you want to do first, take out the trash or dry the dishes?

A typical problem with choices is the child who makes up his own choice. For example, "Taylor, do you want to put on your pajamas first, or brush your teeth?" To which little Taylor answers, "I want to watch TV." What to do? Just smile sweetly and say, "That wasn't one of the choices. What do you want to do first, put on your pajamas or brush your teeth?"

If your child is still reluctant to choose from the options that you offer, then simply ask, "Would you like to choose or shall I choose for you?" If an appropriate answer is not forthcoming, then you can say, "I see that you want me to choose for you." Then follow through. Make your choice and help your child—by leading or carrying him—so that he can cooperate.

Setting Rules and Consequences with Teens

Rules and consequences are critical to negotiating your way through the teen years. Both the rules and the consequences may change as your teen's needs (and desires) develop. It helps to ask yourself some questions about your rules periodically.

General Questions to Ask about Rules

- Are they reasonable?
- Have the reasons for the rules been explained thoroughly?
- Are there too many?
- Are they enforceable?
- Has my teen been involved in making any of the rules?
- Are they consistent with other parents' (you respect) rules?
- Whose needs are the rules designed to meet?

Depending on the answers to these questions and what you've decided is your bottom line, you may be able to negotiate a relaxation of these rules, as your teen is more able to make mature decisions. Or you may find that the rules are entirely unenforceable, meaning either that you need to make changes in your life in order to enforce them or you need to give them up. For example, you may decide that you should arrange your schedule to allow being home more of the time, or simply that you need to be more aware when you are at home. Remember, no matter how reasonable the rules are, it is normal for teens to challenge them. This means that you need to be prepared to impose consequences.

Consequences Need to Meet Certain Conditions in Order to Be Effective

Consequences should:

- Be related to the behavior so they make sense. (Being grounded for every infraction doesn't allow connection to a specific behavior, but if your teen damages someone else's property, part of the consequence might be to help pay for the damage.)

- Teach your teen how to express feelings and desires in acceptable ways. (You don't damage other people's property just because you're angry; anger can be expressed with words.)

- Not be so severe or unenforceable that there is no hope of compliance. (Being grounded for six months will contribute to non-compliance.)

- Be useful in changing behavior. They need to be unpleasant enough that your teen doesn't want to repeat the consequence. They should not include things that you want your child to learn to enjoy, like going to Grandma's for a weekend.

- Teach self-control. (Help your teen see the benefits of more freedom, less control, or something tangible like driving.)

What kinds of consequences might be useful with your teen?

The answer to this varies, depending on your values and the personality, intensity, and interests of your teen. Sometimes he or she can help you find workable consequences. However, be careful because children will sometimes be harsher on themselves than you might think necessary. The goal is to prevent unacceptable behavior and teach your teen to make mature decisions. Think through consequences in advance and take time to manage your own anger or frustration before talking to your teen.

Chapter 48

What Schools Can Do to Help Prevent Domestic Violence

Chapter Contents

Section 48.1

Effectiveness of Programs for the Prevention of Violent and Aggressive Behavior

This section includes text from "Curbing Teen Dating: Evidence from a School Prevention Program," © 2006 RAND Corporation (www.rand.org). Reprinted with permission. And, excerpts from "The Effectiveness of Universal School-Based Programs for the Prevention of Violent and Aggressive Behavior," *MMWR*, August 10, 2007, Centers for Disease Control and Prevention (CDC).

Curbing Teen Dating Violence: Evidence from a School Prevention Program

Violence between dating partners represents a significant public health problem. Approximately 20 percent of U.S. teens report dating someone who became violent with them. Victims face the threat of injury and also an elevated risk of substance abuse, poor health, sexually risky behavior, pregnancy, and suicide. Several school-based programs designed to prevent dating violence have been developed, but few have been assessed to determine what works. In particular, no study has examined the effectiveness of prevention programs for Latino teens, a large and growing group in public schools. Latinos may suffer disproportionate harms from dating violence because they may be less likely to report the problem or to seek help. A study led by RAND Corporation psychologist Lisa Jaycox assessed the effectiveness of a school-based program tailored to Latino students in inner city public high schools. The study found that the intervention created a long-term improvement in students' knowledge of dating violence, reduced tolerance for aggressive or violent behavior, and improved teens' perceptions about getting help if they experienced dating violence. The study also found that Latino teens are most likely to turn to peers for help, and consequently, peer counselors are a promising source for assistance.

"Ending Violence:" A Law-Centered Intervention

The study evaluated "Ending Violence," a three class session prevention program. Developed by a Los Angeles-based nonprofit group called Break the Cycle, the program focuses on the law, highlighting legal rights of victims of domestic violence, and legal responsibilities of perpetrators. The teachers are bilingual, bicultural attorneys. This program has three distinctive features: it is brief (three class sessions), it is compatible with existing health curricula, and it focuses on the legal dimension of dating violence. This perspective is usually new to teens—especially Latino teens in families that have recently immigrated—who may be unfamiliar with their rights under U.S. law or how to exercise them. The program also informs students about its legal services program, in which attorneys are available to teens at no cost to help them with dating violence issues.

The evaluation was conducted in ninth-grade health classes in 11 Los Angeles Unified School District high schools. All of the school populations had more than 80 percent Latino students. Classes were assigned randomly to receive the Ending Violence curriculum or the standard health curriculum. A total of 2,540 students from ten schools and 110 classes participated. Researchers assessed the program's immediate impact and longer-term impact (six months later) on student knowledge and judgments about dating violence, student propensity to seek help, and the level of victimization and dating violence experienced by students after the intervention.

The Intervention Improved Student Knowledge and Changed Views about Seeking Help

The evaluation found that the intervention had modest but significant effects in three areas: student knowledge, attitudes about female-on-male violence, and attitudes about seeking help.

- Teens who participated in the program had greater knowledge of laws related to dating violence and retained this knowledge six months later.

- Participating teens were less accepting of female-on-male violence.

- The intervention did not change attitudes toward male-on-female violence, which were already strongly negative.

- The intervention also did not change the frequency of teens' violent or fearful dating experiences in the six months after the program.

- Students in the intervention group reported increased likelihood of seeking help from certain sources if they experienced dating violence.

Getting and Giving Help

A striking finding emerged from baseline surveys: Although students viewed various institutional sources of support as helpful, they would be far more likely to turn to informal sources, such as friends, parents, or family members, for help should they ever experience dating violence. Each student was asked to rate how helpful a particular source would be in addressing dating violence, and then was asked how likely he or she would be to talk to such a source for help. Students responded using a 5-point scale—rating a particular source's helpfulness from zero (not at all helpful) to four (extremely helpful), and rating the likelihood of talking to that source from not at all likely to talk to the source (zero) to extremely likely to talk to the source (four).

Notably, teens expressed positive views about the helpfulness of police, teachers, priests, and lawyers, but those views did not translate into a corresponding likelihood that they would turn to these sources for help if needed. The intervention improved teens' perceptions of police, lawyers, teachers, and school nurses as helpful, but the intervention improved their likelihood of seeking help only with respect to lawyers.

To explore student views of help-seeking behavior in greater depth, the research team conducted focus groups following the intervention. The sessions also explored attitudes about giving help to peers involved in dating violence. The focus groups underscored teens' propensity to turn to peers for help rather than to formal, institutional sources. Furthermore, most teens reported that they do not confide in or trust the adults in their social network. Teens also expressed reluctance to intervene in dating violence situations and did not perceive that their help would be effective.

Implications for Strengthening Interventions

Survey results also showed that teens who experience or witness aggression in their family life and among peers hold less negative attitudes about dating violence, so finding opportunities for reducing aggression in teens' daily lives may be helpful. In schools, a focus on reducing school and peer aggression and violence might bolster prevention efforts aimed at dating violence. Improving legal knowledge about dating violence may be a promising prevention element and could encourage victims of dating violence to seek help.

The results also suggest that another way to strengthen interventions is to target teen attitudes about seeking and giving help. Given

Latino teens' inclination to seek help from peers, a promising avenue for intervention is the use of teens as peer educators to teach other teens about identifying and preventing dating violence. In addition, these teens can act as counselors who can link students with more formal sources of support, such as attorneys, police, and school personnel.

When giving help, teens would also benefit from a better understanding of how to aid others in an abusive relationship. The surveys and focus groups showed that teens are less likely to intervene in dating violence situations if they know the perpetrator. Intervention programs can educate teens about the importance of intervening when they witness an incident of violence or abuse among their friends and the best methods of doing so.

Table 48.1. Intervention Effects: Increased Knowledge and Value of Getting Help from Attorneys Persisted Six Months after Intervention

	Effects	
Outcomes Measured	Was There a Positive Change Immediately after the Program?	Did the Change Persist Six Months after the Program?
Knowledge about violence and about dating violence	Yes	Yes
Acceptance of dating violence:		
Female-on-male violence	Yes	No
Male-on-female violence	No	No
Abusive or fearful dating experiences	No	No
Usefulness of seeking help from:		
Attorney	Yes	Yes
Police	Yes	No
Teacher	Yes	No
School counselor	Yes	No
School nurse	No	No
Parents/family	No	No
Friends	No	No
Doctors	No	No

Effectiveness of Universal School-Based Programs for the Prevention of Violent and Aggressive Behavior

During 2004–2006, the Task Force on Community Preventive Services review assessed the effectiveness of universal school-based programs in reducing or preventing violent and aggressive behavior among children and adolescents. These programs teach all students in a school or school grade about the problem of violence, and its prevention or about one or more of the following topics or skills intended to reduce aggressive or violent behavior: emotional self-awareness, emotional control, and self-esteem; positive social skills; social problem solving; conflict resolution; and teamwork.

As used in this report, universal means that programs are administered to all children in classrooms regardless of individual risk, not only to those who already have manifested violent or aggressive behavior or risk factors for these behaviors. Although meriting separate review because youths who manifest violence or aggressive behavior at young ages are at greater risk for later violence, programs that target youths who already have manifested problems of violence or are considered at high risk for violence were not evaluated in this review.

Universal programs might be targeted by grade or school in high-risk areas (defined by residents' low socioeconomic scale, commonly indicated by the proportion of school children receiving subsidized lunches, or high crime rates). Programs are delivered to all children in those settings. Programs also might be implemented in special schools (for example, schools for children with specific disabilities). Prekindergarten, kindergarten, elementary, middle, and junior and senior high school settings were included in this review.

Universal school-based programs are founded on multiple theoretical approaches. Theories of behavior change vary in their focus on individuals; interpersonal relations; the physical and social environment, including social norms; and combinations of these. Certain programs focus on providing information about the problem of violence and approaches to avoiding violence, on the assumptions that providing this information to students will lead to its application and subsequently to reduced violence and that information is necessary, if not sufficient, to change behavior. For example, the Violence Prevention Curriculum for Adolescents is designed to teach students about the causes of violence; knowledge of violence resistance skills is taught through discussion. Other programs assume that self-concept and self-esteem derive from positive action and its rewards, so if children's behavior can be made more positive and sociable, they will develop better attitudes toward themselves and then continue to make positive choices. In the Second Step program, teaching and discussion are accompanied by role playing, modeling, skill practice, feedback, and reinforcement.

The present review was produced by the systematic review development team (the team) and a multidisciplinary team of specialists and consultants representing various perspectives on violence. This review included studies that assessed directly measured violent outcomes, specifically self- or other-reported or observed aggression or violence, including violent crime. The review also included studies that examined any of five proxies for violent outcomes that include not only clearly violent behavior but also behavior that is not clearly violent. These include:

- measures of conduct disorder (the psychiatric condition, in which the rights of others or major societal norms or rules are violated);

- measures of externalizing behavior (for example: rule-breaking behaviors and conduct problems, including physical and verbal aggression, defiance, lying, stealing, truancy, delinquency, physical cruelty, and criminal acts);

- measures of acting out (aggressive, impulsive, or disruptive class behaviors) or conduct problems (includes talking in class, stealing, fighting, lying, not following directions, teasing, and breaking things);

- measures of delinquency (which might include violent behavior and behavior not regarded as violent); and,

- school records of suspensions or disciplinary referrals.

The purpose of this review was to assess the effectiveness of school-based programs in reducing or preventing violent behavior.

The findings of this review were compared with a recently updated meta-analysis with a similar approach to intervention definition and outcomes assessed, although certain differences existed in the literature and methods used. Expanded versions of both reviews, including a detailed exploration of similarities and differences, have been published. The meta-analysis indicated that the associations reported in the present review were not greatly confounded. School-based programs for the prevention of violence are effective for all school levels, and different intervention strategies are all effective. Programs have other effects beyond those on violent or aggressive behavior, including: reduced truancy and improvements in school achievement, problem behavior, activity levels, attention problems, social skills, and internalizing problems (anxiety and depression).

Use of the Recommendation in States and Communities

U.S. schools provide a critical opportunity for changing societal behavior because almost the entire population is engaged in this institution for many years, starting at an early and formative period. With approximately 71 million children in primary and secondary schools in 2003 and an overall high school graduation rate of 85%, this opportunity is difficult to overestimate. The potential benefits of improved school function alone are notable. The broader and longer-term benefits in terms of reduced delinquency and antisocial behavior are yet more substantial. Universal school-based violence prevention programs represent an important means of reducing violent and aggressive behavior in the United States. The findings of this review suggest that universal school-based violence prevention programs can be effective in communities with diverse ethnic compositions and in communities whose residents are predominantly of lower socioeconomic scale or that have relatively high rates of crime.

Section 48.2

Classroom Abuse Prevention Program for Youth with Disabilities

This material was reprinted from the National Resource Center on Domestic Violence publication entitled: *Kid&TeenSAFE: An Abuse Prevention Program for Youth with Disabilities* by Wendie H. Abramson and Iracema Mastroleo, © 2002. The National Resource Center on Domestic Violence deems that this information is current as of November 2008.

Goals

Kid&TeenSAFE works to:

- reduce the risk of sexual, physical and/or emotional abuse or exploitation faced by many children and youth with disabilities;

- increase the ability of children and youth with disabilities to identify, prevent, and report abuse;

- enhance awareness and strengthen skills of family members, teachers, and other professionals to prevent, detect, and report abuse of children with disabilities; and,

- promote ongoing abuse prevention education for children and youth with disabilities.

Staffing

Staffing for this project originally included one part-time education coordinator, one part-time public relations coordinator, the program director, administrative support, a social work intern, and volunteers. After a year, the program reorganized the two part-time positions into one full-time position (Kid&TeenSafe educator) that combined the responsibilities of marketing, coordinating, and delivering abuse prevention sessions to students with disabilities. The social work intern would be responsible for developing educational materials for families and teachers, as well as providing case management and resource referral for families as needed. Volunteers would assist with role plays and evaluation activities during educational sessions.

Components

I. Classroom presentations: Staff and volunteers provide a series of three to four educational presentations for children with disabilities in kindergarten through 12th grade on topics such as personal safety, abuse prevention, healthy sexuality, bullying, and harassment.

II. Professional and family training: Staff provides training and workshops for special education teachers and other professionals who work in the disability field, as well as family members. The sessions focus on providing information on risk factors related to abuse, incidence and indicators of abuse, detecting and reporting abuse, and strategies to reduce the risk of abuse of children with disabilities.

III. National Resource Library: Access to over 350 items related to violence against people with disabilities, abuse prevention, sexuality, personal safety, healthy relationships, and other pertinent topics is offered through the project's library. Educational materials include curricula, books, videos, journals, anatomically correct models and dolls, and other resources.

Classroom Presentations

The Kid&TeenSAFE project provides school-based abuse prevention education to empower children and youth with disabilities about their rights to personal safety and to teach them skills to protect themselves from abuse. Sessions are offered to elementary, middle/junior, and high school students with disabilities and usually last three to four sessions.

Presentations are customized to the learning needs of each group, for example, visual materials are described for those who are blind, information is presented in concrete terminology for persons with cognitive disabilities, and so forth. Classes are held primarily in special education classrooms and residential schools for students who are blind or deaf, but are also offered at the local children's shelter, the state hospital, summer camps, group homes for children with disabilities, and non-profit agencies that serve children with disabilities and their families.

The main teaching concepts include:

- building awareness of emotions and personal boundaries;
- identifying various types of touches;
- asserting an individual's right to say "no" to unwanted touches;
- escaping abusive or potentially abusive people and situations;
- identifying and telling trusted adults if abuse occurs; and,
- other relevant topics that may be identified by youth, families, or service providers.

Participants include children with physical, cognitive, learning, sensory, psychiatric, behavioral, and/or multiple disabilities. The program has served children who have the following diagnoses: mental retardation, cerebral palsy, muscular dystrophy, autism, Down syndrome, pervasive developmental disorder, attention deficit hyperactive disorder, traumatic brain injury, deaf, blind, visually impaired, behavioral or emotional disorder, and speech impairment.

Prior to the first session, the educator obtains the following information from the teacher: size of the class, age of students (for determining age appropriate topics and role plays), types and severity of students' disabilities; best learning strategies for specific students; language to utilize in the classroom (medical terminology versus other phrases when teaching about the private parts of the body); examples of actual situations to address during role play activities; as well as concerns about past, present, or suspected abuse. The educator requests information on the disciplinary, sexual harassment and bullying policies of the host school (or school district) prior to teaching so that the information can be incorporated into the training. The educator also requests that a special education teacher and/or aide be present during the sessions to assist with children who have behavioral challenges, or to talk privately with any child who may become upset. Some children with disabilities need information repeated many times, so it is also helpful for the teacher to be present so that he or she can reinforce the teaching concepts throughout the school year.

Teaching abuse prevention in a group setting will also demonstrate that abuse or assault is not a shameful secret, but can and should be discussed frankly and honestly. As a result of these sessions, children with disabilities build awareness, knowledge, or skills in the following areas:

- Emotions and personal boundaries
- Types of touches

- Rights to personal safety
- Strategies for safety in potentially dangerous situations
- What to do if abuse occurs

A typical abuse prevention series will frequently model the following schedule:

Day 1

- Define personal safety
- Identify and discuss feelings
- Identify and discuss types of touches and words
  - "okay" touches and "okay" words
  - "not okay" touches and "not okay" words
  - confusing touches (optional)
- Overview of safety rules
  - say "no"
  - go away and/or yell
  - other ways of communicating
  - tell trusted adults

Day 2

- Review previous lesson
- Identify body parts, including private parts
- Discuss secrets: fun secrets and hurtful, "special" secrets
- Address bullying and sexual harassment in a safe manner

Day 3

- Role-plays using safety rules

Day 4 (For Teens)

- Healthy sexuality education or other suggested topics (for example: puberty, dating, violence at home)
- Additional topics may be added, based on student interests, age, and needs

Daily sessions usually last 30–60 minutes, depending upon the attention span of the students. The educator utilizes an interactive format that focuses on non-violent ways to respond to abuse, bullying, or harassment. Teaching strategies for children and youth with disabilities include discussions, drawings, the use of anatomically correct dolls/models, and role-playing activities. The educator encourages participation, but also respects and honors a student's choice not to actively participate. The educator primarily uses the following curricula and teaching aids (as determined by chronological age):

- No-Go-TELL!
- Safe and Okay
- Teach a Body Doll
- LifeFacts: Sexual Abuse Prevention
- LifeFacts: Sexuality
- LifeFacts: Managing Emotions
- Changes in You

Strategies for Educators

The following are strategies that the educator utilizes in teaching students with disabilities:

Teaching about Feelings, Touches, and Words

- Define feelings. With student input, develop a list of basic emotions, such as happy, sad, scared, angry, and safe. Provide examples of situations when people may have these feelings.

- With student participation, create a list of touches that are okay and can make us feel good. Make linkages to the relationship that is appropriate for each touch, for example, a hug from Mom is okay, but not from a stranger.

- Explain that there are touches that are not okay and can make us feel bad or confused. Provide concrete examples.

- Tell the group that it is not okay for anyone to touch them without their permission unless it is to protect their health or safety; talk about sexual touches as part of this discussion.

- Explain the exceptions to touches on the private parts of the body (such as health care reasons).

- Acknowledge the fact that both males and females can receive abusive touches and that both males and females can be persons who give abusive touches.

- Use similar strategies for discussing words that are okay versus not okay.

Teaching No-Go-TELL!

The ability to assertively say "no" to inappropriate requests, advances, and perceived harm, even to an authority figure, is an important skill. In some potentially abusive situations, if a child can say no effectively, the offender may leave that child alone.

- Teach the child that saying no can mean using other forms of communication, such as sign language, facial expressions, head shaking, a direct look in the offender's eyes, or leaving the environment.

- Practice these assertiveness skills with the child. The strategy of just saying no is not always effective for stopping abuse; however, all children should have the opportunity to practice the skills, including saying no.

- Having the verbal ability or the assistive devices to make loud noises is an important safety measure for students who cannot leave or remove themselves independently from a potentially dangerous environment. For students who are non-verbal and have no other forms of communication, adaptive devices to call attention to potentially dangerous situations are recommended. Some suggestions are a horn, whistle, or a communication device (may require an assessment by a speech therapist).

- Assist those students who use communication boards or other augmentative communication devices in updating the board or device with words or symbols to communicate about issues relating to personal safety.

- Teach children to tell a trusted adult(s) about abuse, bullying, or harassment. This may help prevent future victimization and increase the child's safety, if the adult takes action. Unfortunately, adults do not always believe children who disclose abuse or may not take action to prevent a situation from escalating. If the child tells more than one person about an abusive incident, there is a higher likelihood that someone will believe the child and intervene. It is important that a child is able to identify several trusted adults to tell if someone hurts or tries to hurt him or her.

- Ask students whom they would tell if someone tried to hurt them. If a child says that she or he would tell a brother or sister, ask how old the sibling is. Explain that they also need to tell an adult (someone 18 years or older) who is able to help them in a non-violent way.

- If the child says that he or she would call 9-1-1, practice role-playing as the 9-1-1 operator and allow the child to practice calling 9-1-1. If the student is deaf or has a speech impairment and would need to use a TTY or other communication device to disclose abuse, make sure he or she has access to a device at school and home and knows how to operate it.

Teaching about Body Parts

- Check with the school about district policies for educating students about the private parts of the body. Obtain parental permission, if required.

- Ask students what their preference is for separating males and females in the class. Some teenagers feel more comfortable and are more open to looking at pictures, asking questions, and participating, if they are among same-gender peers.

- Use curricula designed for teaching children with disabilities about anatomy or abuse prevention.

- Encourage the students to participate by asking them to name the various parts of the body.

- Include the names of body parts that are the same for males and females such as eyes, nose, arms, hands, back, legs, feet, and navel.

- When teaching students who are blind about the body parts, bring anatomically correct dolls or models of males and females for students who need a tactile learning experience.

- Teach students the names of the private parts for both genders.

- If the group is separated, bring the group back together after the information has been presented to briefly recap the information and to ensure an atmosphere of respect and trust for both genders.

437

- As children develop vocabulary for the body parts, they may be able to discuss related health concerns with physicians or nurses and be better able to disclose if abuse occurs.

Teaching about Sexual Harassment and Bullying

The goal of teaching about harassment and bullying is for students to understand what sexual harassment is, the difference between teasing and bullying, the difference between telling and being a tattletale, as well as what to do if one is being harassed, teased, or bullied.

- Check with the school district or school administration about policies and procedures for responding to sexual harassment or bullying incidents. The procedures (or lack thereof) vary from campus to campus. Some schools need help in developing procedures, others with enforcing existing rules or policies.

- Hold a discussion about the topics and ask students to define the concepts of sexual harassment and bullying and provide examples.

- Discuss the consequences of sexual harassment and bullying.

- Expand upon student examples by explaining that bullies and harassers are people who pick on other people and use aggressive behavior to intentionally harm or hurt someone.

- Encourage students to have confidence, to speak up, and protect themselves and others if, or when, bullying or harassment occurs. Participating in role-plays in the safety of the classroom can help students develop responses in the event they are teased, bullied, sexually harassed, or if they observe someone else being bullied or harassed.

Role-Play Examples

- A student calls another student ugly, fat, stupid, retarded, sissy, or another offensive name.

- A boy uses force to back a girl up against her locker.

- A male student teases another to wrestle with him.

- An adult exposes himself to a girl outside the school.

- A man asks a girl to take a surprise from his pocket.

- A stranger in a store offers to buy a game or compact disc (CD) for the student.

- The student is on the internet in a chat room and someone asks to meet her or him in person.

Teaching Healthy Sexuality Education

It is recommended that sexuality be included as a component of abuse prevention so the child learns that it is not shameful to discuss sexuality and personal safety issues. Sexuality education also helps children with disabilities learn about socially appropriate behaviors, and provides them with a sense of ownership of their bodies.

- Check with the school about district policies for providing information related to healthy sexuality education to students. Sometimes written parental permission is necessary prior to providing sexuality education.

- Strive to create an educational atmosphere in which students can feel comfortable and safe talking about and asking questions related to sexuality.

- Direct student questions about sexuality to family members or other trusted adults, should your community prohibit teaching about sexuality. Also suggest, when appropriate, researching in encyclopedias or science books at the school or public library. If students have questions about their ability to have erections, orgasms, menstruation, or to get pregnant or impregnate, encourage them to ask a family member, doctor, or nurse.

- Take advantage of natural teaching moments that come about based on where the students are developmentally. For example, younger children may ask where babies come from or older children may ask about something they have seen or heard from other kids. These are opportunities to answer honestly, with a developmentally appropriate response, and engage the child(ren) in discussions on topics they are interested in, or curious about.

Evaluation Methods and Results

Evaluation Checklist

Staff developed an evaluation checklist to collect data on each student's knowledge and skills in the following areas:

- Identification of touches that are okay

- Identification of touches that are not okay
- Identification of own gender
- Identification of anatomically correct private parts for males and females
- Ability to recall and demonstrate the No-Go-TELL! prevention strategy sequence
- Identification of a trusted adult(s)
- Communicative ability (spoken or sign language) to refuse an unwanted touch
- Behavioral ability to refuse an unwanted touch
- Ability to verbally or behaviorally report an unwanted touch

Child Evaluations

During calendar year 1999–2000, 849 children participated in abuse prevention education sessions and information was collected on 94 percent of the children. Not all participants were included because some were absent on the last session, some were non-responsive throughout the sessions or to particular questions by choice, and some students had disabilities that were too severe.

Prior to the training, the educator asks each student what she or he would do if someone tries to hurt them. A correct response is coded if the student indicates (without prompting) that she or he would tell the person "no," leave the situation, tell an adult, or a similar reply. The same question is asked after the abuse prevention information is taught. Responses indicated that 21 percent of students showed increased knowledge of personal safety strategies after the training when asked what they would do if someone tried to hurt them.

At the end of the sessions, the following were able to respond correctly without prompting:

- 68 percent could identify "okay or all right" touches;
- 77 percent could identify "not-okay or not-all right" touches;
- 88 percent could identify their own gender (male or female);
- 64 percent could identify anatomically correct private areas;
- 73 percent could recall/demonstrate the No-Go-TELL! prevention strategy sequence; and,
- 86 percent could identify one known, trusted adult.

Teen Evaluations

Also, during the same time period, 93 teens took part in abuse prevention education sessions. A separate evaluation tool was administered to those able to complete a written survey (primarily students who do not have a cognitive disability label). Students were asked to complete the survey that was distributed at the end of the final class to gauge whether participants had learned new information about abusive behaviors and respectful relationships as a result of the training. A majority—74 percent—of students indicated that they learned new information about abuse, and 73 percent reported that they gained knowledge about respectful relationships as a result of participating in the training. Some teens also offered written suggestions of other related topics to include in future sessions. Others provided written comments indicating the most important information they learned from classes. Examples included:

• There is such a thing as marital abuse or marital rape.

• Abuse is not okay.

• A definition of sexual harassment.

• There are different types of abuse that exist.

• Respect others' space and body.

• Ask before touching someone else.

• No, means no.

• Have respect for others.

Challenges in Working with Children and Youth with Disabilities

Kid&TeenSAFE works with children and youth with any type or severity of disability. Thus, the educator must be able to work with children with diverse learning needs. Language may need to be adapted and used in basic, concrete terms for students with mental retardation or other cognitive disabilities. This can become complex in a classroom that includes several students with different types of disabilities and distinct learning needs. Some students have learning needs that require an individualized presentation and further adaptation of materials.

It is common to encounter children and youth with disabilities who have speech impairments or are non-verbal and yet do not have communication devices. It then becomes very difficult to have an interactive session with these children. Some children with disabilities take medications to prevent seizures, manage spasticity, and so forth. This can present a problem if children are heavily medicated and fall asleep during the presentation.

Some children disclose abuse during the presentation. This can be a complex situation because the educator wants to acknowledge the child for disclosing abuse, but does not want to engage other students in a discussion about the child's experience. When this situation arises, the educator acknowledges the situation and offers to discuss the matter privately after the class session ends. Kid&TeenSAFE does not offer a counseling component, but does make referrals to the parent organization's (SafePlace) Children's Counseling Program, as appropriate.

The project also relies on volunteers to participate in role-plays and assist in evaluation activities with students. Classes are scheduled according to the availability of teachers, so there is no consistency in the day of the week or time that abuse prevention sessions are held. Some weeks the educator has full days of presentations scheduled throughout the week; at other times, classes may be scheduled only on a particular morning or afternoon. As with any project that utilizes volunteers, it can be challenging to recruit and maintain participation in activities due to such irregular scheduling.

Chapter 49

Workplace Violence: How You Can Help Prevent It

Violence rarely occurs without some signs that things are not going well for an individual. Often these signs are apparent to co-workers and supervisors who notice that a person's behavior is changing. Change itself is often an important factor. If we are aware of potential signs of problems, we may be able to help our colleagues and keep our workplaces violence-free.

What to Notice

Job Performance Changes

- Excessive tardiness or absences, especially if this was not the case in the past

- Reduced productivity, especially of a previously efficient and productive colleague

- Significant changes in work habits, including alternating high and low productivity or quality

- Violation of safety or security procedures, including a sudden increase in accidents

This chapter includes text from "Civil Conversations #1 and #3," National Institutes of Health (NIH), reviewed in 2008.

Personal Characteristics

- Changes in health or hygiene such as a colleague suddenly disregards personal health or grooming
- Strained relationships at work including disruptive or isolating behavior different from the past
- Apparent signs of drug or alcohol abuse
- Stress which may be indicated by excessive phone calls, yelling, crying, or personal difficulties
- Inability to concentrate when that was not a problem before
- Unshakable depression, often having low energy, little enthusiasm, or making despairing remarks
- Unusual behavior for that individual, different from the past
- Unusual fascination with weapons or stories of violence in the media
- Threatening, intimidating, or harassing behavior

What to Do

If you feel comfortable talking with your colleague, you may indicate your concerns to him or her, based on what you have observed. Let your colleague know what resources the workplace has that might help. If you are not comfortable speaking directly with your colleague, you should notify your supervisor or seek information through the employee assistance program.

If you notice several of the potential signs, you should pay attention. You may observe these changes in yourself or in your colleagues, and you should take action. These indicators do not mean that someone will behave violently; however, when violent incidents have occurred throughout our country, some of these signs were usually present ahead of time. If each of us helps ourselves and others, we can help make our places of work a safer place for all.

Supervisors: Your Role in Preventing Workplace Violence

Your Behavior and Management Style Can Affect the Office

By exhibiting certain behaviors, or allowing certain behaviors to be exhibited by your employees, you may contribute to a hostile or unhealthy work environment.

Remember:

1. Allowing aggressive or inappropriate conduct without taking action can foster a hostile or threatening work environment in which employees feel harassed or intimidated.

2. Decision-making without employee input or participation can lead to frustrated employees who don't feel valued as anything but "worker bees."

3. Your staff looks to you to assist in resolving conflicts. You are better equipped to resolve workplace conflicts if both you and your staff have had conflict resolution training.

4. If you are inconsistent or unpredictable, your employees will be unsure of your expectations and become frustrated.

5. Engaging in relationships with your employees that are personal or too informal may lead to misunderstandings, as well as other employees feeling alienated.

Be a Good Leader

You can set the direction for establishing a harmonious, productive workplace, which can prevent the potential for workplace violence. Good leadership includes the following:

- Setting a good example for your employees

- Communicating clear standards

- Providing clear rationale underlying your decisions

- Ensuring your employees have the resources and training to do their job

- Getting to know your employees

- Conducting performance counseling

- Assisting employees who are having performance problems

- Addressing misconduct promptly

- Availing yourself of advice from human resources when you have any questions or concerns, even prior to the need to pursue disciplinary and performance-based actions

- Treating employees fairly and equitably, and applying rules consistently

Be on the Lookout for Signs That Can Lead to Workplace Violence

- A usually outgoing, communicative employee becomes withdrawn and quiet
- An employee frequently comes in late for work, then is argumentative with co-workers and behaves erratically
- An employee voices a keen interest in weapons or explosives
- An employee persists in expressing romantic interest towards a co-worker who is obviously not interested
- An employee suddenly takes no interest in maintaining his or her personal appearance or hygiene
- An employee makes comments about violent means of dealing with, or coping with, a particular situation
- An employee talks about having nothing to lose or not caring about anything anymore

In addition to recognizing and responding to potential signs of workplace violence from your employees, remember that customers, patients, relatives or acquaintances of employees or patients, and outsiders can be perpetrators of violent acts or threats.

Be Ready to Act

In emergency situations, dial 911.

When inappropriate behavior occurs, you need to deal with the situation. You need to:

- gather all of the facts,
- analyze the immediate situation,
- involve whatever parties are appropriate to assist you,
- formulate a plan,
- and intervene.

If you know that someone is in danger, you need to act quickly, but remember that acting too quickly without having the necessary facts can fuel the situation.

Chapter 50

What Faith Communities Can Do to Help Prevent Domestic Violence

This information applies to people of all faiths, regardless on how or where they practice.

What is domestic violence?

Domestic violence is a pattern of coercive behavior used by one person in order to maintain power and control in an intimate relationship. Domestic violence includes actual or threatened physical, sexual, psychological, or economic abuse. It occurs between persons who are current or former sexual or intimate partners or who live in the same household, regardless of sexual orientation. Victims and abusers come from all age groups and social classes. Ninety-five percent of victims of domestic violence are women.

I find it difficult to believe that this is happening in my faith community. Is that possible?

Unfortunately, domestic violence is so prevalent that it is almost certain that there are both victims and abusers in every faith community, including yours. According to a very recent study, nearly one in three women reported being physically abused by a spouse or boyfriend at some point in her life. Hard as it is to believe or understand,

---

Text in this chapter is from "Resources–Faith Communities," © West Virginia Coalition Against Domestic Violence. Reprinted with permission.

the fact is that victims and abusers can be found within all institutions within the community, including faith communities.

How can my faith community help those who are affected by domestic violence?

Faith communities have great potential to help both victims and abusers. However, it is important to intervene in a way that does not make a difficult situation worse. The most important thing your community can do is develop a relationship with the domestic violence program that serves your area, and work collaboratively with that program to ensure that both the spiritual and secular needs of victims and abusers in your faith community are met.

I am the leader of my faith community. If I refer one of my members to a domestic violence program, how can I be sure that person's spiritual needs will be met?

Domestic violence programs are experts in meeting the secular needs of victims, their children, and abusers. They are not experts in spiritual matters, however, and this is an area in which faith communities can be of great help. If you refer a member of your faith community to a domestic violence program, you should be willing to work with staff there to help address the member's spiritual needs. Do not expect the domestic violence program to be able to do that without your help. Offer yourself as a resource.

What if both the victim and the abuser are members of my faith community?

You must attend to the needs of both, but the victims' safety must always be your first priority. Avoid the temptation to offer marital counseling. Until the violence has stopped, marital counseling will only give the abuser another forum in which to use abusive tactics to control the victim.

How can I learn more about this important topic to share with my faith community?

The domestic violence program that serves your area is an invaluable resource for training and consultation on this complex issue. The toll-free 24-hour National Domestic Violence Crisis Hotline number is 800-799-SAFE (7233).

More Suggestions for Communities of Faith

Adapted in part from the Nebraska Domestic Violence and Sexual Assault Coalition and the Center for the Prevention of Sexual and Domestic Violence, Seattle, Washington.

The religious community provides a safe haven for women and families in need. In addition, it exhorts society to share compassion and comfort with those afflicted by the tragedy of domestic violence. Leaders of the religious community have identified actions to share with the nation to create a unified response to violence against women.

- **Become a safe place:** Make your church, temple, mosque, or synagogue a safe place where victims of domestic violence can come for help. Display brochures and posters which include the telephone number of the domestic violence and sexual assault programs in your area. Publicize the National Domestic Violence Hotline number, 800-799-SAFE (7233) or 800-787-3224 (TDD).

- **Educate the congregation:** Provide ways for members of the congregation to learn as much as they can about domestic and sexual violence. Routinely include information in monthly newsletters, on bulletin boards, and in marriage preparation classes. Sponsor educational seminars on violence against women in your congregation.

- **Speak out:** Speak out about domestic violence and sexual assault from the pulpit. As a faith leader, you can have a powerful impact on peoples' attitudes and beliefs.

- **Lead by example:** Volunteer to serve on the board of directors at the local domestic violence or sexual assault program or attend a training to become a crisis volunteer.

- **Offer space:** Offer meeting space for educational seminars or weekly support groups, or serve as a supervised visitation site when parents need to visit their children safely.

- **Partner with existing resources:** Include your local domestic violence or sexual assault program in donations and community service projects. Adopt a shelter for which your church, temple, mosque, or synagogue provides material support, or provide similar support to families as they rebuild their lives following a shelter stay.

- **Prepare to be a resource:** Do the theological and scriptural homework necessary to better understand and respond to family violence and receive training from professionals in the fields of sexual and domestic violence.

- **Intervene:** If you suspect violence is occurring in a relationship, speak to each member of the couple separately. Help the victim plan for safety. Let both individuals know of the community resources available to assist them. Do not attempt couples counseling.

- **Support professional training:** Encourage and support training and education for clergy and lay leaders, hospital chaplains, and seminary students to increase awareness about sexual and domestic violence.

- **Address internal issues.** Encourage continued efforts by religious institutions to address allegations of abuse by religious leaders to insure that religious leaders are a safe resource for victims and their children.

Chapter 51

Recovering from Childhood Abuse Helps Prevent Domestic Violence

Chapter Contents

Section 51.1

Recovering Man's Guide to Coping with the Effects of Childhood Abuse Issues

"Helping Yourself Heal: A Recovering Man's Guide to Coping with the Effects of Childhood Abuse," Substance Abuse and Mental Health Services Administration (SAMHSA), DHHS Publication No. (SMA) 06–4134, updated 2006.

Men who are in treatment for substance abuse experience many different feelings. Because of the way most men were brought up, it may be difficult for them to experience, express, understand, and cope with their feelings—or even admit to having them. Now that you are in treatment, you may feel relieved, optimistic, and proud of yourself for taking the first step toward recovery. Yet, at times, you also may feel:

- ashamed,
- anxious,
- embarrassed,
- depressed,
- angry,
- guilty,
- bad about yourself,
- that you can't connect with family or friends,
- that you're crazy,
- numbness or nothing at all,
- fearful, or
- helpless.

Believe it or not, some of these feelings are common for any man who starts treatment for a substance use disorder, but for a man who also was abused in childhood these feelings can be even stronger. The feelings can be so painful or overwhelming that he may do many things to avoid them, including using drugs or alcohol or both.

Some men in treatment for substance abuse don't clearly remember being abused (or don't realize that the way they were treated as children was abusive), but they have some of the feelings mentioned here. Some men push their memories of abuse so far away that they can't explain why they have intense anger or fear, feel embarrassed around a particular person, have nightmares, or always feel as if something bad is about to happen. Sometimes, after people stop drinking or using drugs and are in treatment, memories may surface that had been too painful to think about before or that were blocked from memory by drugs or alcohol.

Working through the bad memories and experiences from childhood you've tried to forget can help you when you're in substance abuse treatment because facing old feelings can help you focus on your present life.

What Is Childhood Abuse?

Child abuse can occur in any family, regardless of its race, religion, or income level.

Abuse has many definitions, and sometimes it can be hard to know whether what you went through as a child was abuse. At the time, the way you were punished or treated may have seemed normal because you were too young to know differently. Here are some questions to think about. These questions ask about only a few experiences that are generally considered abuse. You may have had other experiences that are not on this list but are still considered abuse. Do you remember anyone in a position of authority:

- Using extreme discipline or punishment on you?

- Spanking or hitting you so hard that you had bruises, cuts, or broken bones?

- Beating or punching you?

- Acting in a way that made you feel uncomfortable or powerless?

- Calling you names or abusing you verbally?

- Criticizing or making fun of your physical characteristics, such as your hair, your skin color, your body type, or a disability?

- Talking to you in a sexual way, watching you undress or bathe, making you watch pornographic pictures or movies, or photographing you in inappropriate ways?

- Touching you sexually or making you touch yourself or someone else sexually?
- Forcing you to watch or talking you into watching others acting in a sexual way?
- Forcing you to have or talking you into having sex?

What Symptoms Could You Have If You Were Abused?

The effects of childhood abuse may still be with you as an adult. These effects might be part of the reason you feel angry, anxious, ashamed, or depressed and may be part of the reason you abuse substances. You may:

- have flashbacks of the abuse;
- have frequent nightmares;
- be sensitive to noise, being touched, or being close to people;
- always expect something bad to happen;
- become angry easily;
- not remember periods of your life;
- abuse others;
- feel numb;
- feel depressed, even suicidal; or,
- let people abuse or take advantage of you.

These problems may get worse or become more intense when you're stressed or in situations that trigger memories of the abuse, such as when you fight with someone close to you or see a movie or television program that reminds you of a past experience. Know that you are okay—the feelings may seem overpowering, but you can get through them.

But, if you ever feel like hurting yourself or others or are thinking about suicide, tell your substance abuse counselor immediately, call 911, or call the National Suicide Prevention Lifeline at 800-273-8255 (TTY: 800-799-4889). These thoughts and feelings need immediate attention from your counselor or a mental health professional.

How Can You Address Childhood Abuse Issues While You're in Treatment?

During the early stages of substance abuse treatment, you'll be focusing on getting the drugs or alcohol out of your system, clearing your head, and learning how to establish healthy patterns of thinking and behaving. You may want to put off addressing painful past abuse until you're comfortable being drug and alcohol free and have built relationships with your counselor, other clients, and others who are in recovery.

However, if the feelings are too overwhelming and painful or make you feel overly aggressive, you must address them right away. You can raise the issue with your counselor or other clients whenever you want or need to. No matter what stage of recovery you're in, help is available for you. And remember: Many other men have worked through these feelings and now lead happy, productive, substance-free lives.

It's up to you to decide when to discuss abuse with your counselor, but it is important for you to raise the subject when you're ready. This may be the first time you've ever told anyone about what happened to you as a child. You may feel embarrassed talking about what happened to you; you also may feel guilty or disloyal talking about a family member or another person close to you. You may fear how your family will react to you after you've talked about what happened. These feelings and fears are very normal; talk about them with your counselor. Sometimes, it's hard to remember the difference between what you felt as a child who was abused and the choices you have as an adult in counseling. You couldn't protect yourself then, but you can now. As an adult, you can talk about what happened to you and you can begin to heal.

How Can Your Counselor Help?

In general, everything that you tell your counselor is confidential. Your counselor will inform you of the few situations in which he or she would have to break confidentiality. For example, if you were to tell your counselor that you intended to harm yourself or someone else, he or she would be required to take action. It's also important that you know that mental health and substance abuse counselors generally are required to report the abuse of children. If this concerns you and you are younger than 18, talk to your counselor about the guidelines he or she must follow. If you're an adult, your counselor generally is not required to report childhood abuse. The exception is when the abuser still has access to children and may harm them.

As you talk to your counselor or therapist about your experiences, you may find that your talks become more difficult when painful and embarrassing memories and feelings arise and you look more closely at the past. Sometimes, these overwhelming feelings contribute to a drug or alcohol relapse. Your counselor can help you understand the relationship between the abuse in your past and your substance use. He or she can help you understand and cope with your feelings and will help you find self-help groups, such as Survivors of Incest Anonymous. If you grew up in a family in which one or more people had substance use problems, groups like Adult Children of Alcoholics (ACA) or Co-Dependents Anonymous (CoDA) also might be very helpful to you.

Your substance abuse counselor also may help you find a counselor or therapist who specializes in working with people who have been abused as children. Addressing childhood abuse issues takes time; you'll need to develop a relationship with a therapist who can work with you now and who will continue to work with you after you've finished treatment for your substance use disorder.

A Final Note

As a man in recovery from substance use disorder, you've faced great challenges. It is a tribute to your strength that you have survived and have now made the courageous choice to enter a substance abuse treatment program. You deserve the chance to heal and to live a happy, healthy life.

You will face more challenges, but you will have the ability to cope with them, too. Remember: You are not alone. Use the many resources and support networks that are available to help you and to keep you moving toward your goal. As you stay sober, your options grow. As you create a trusting relationship with your counselor or therapist, you begin to heal. And the courage you find to help yourself heal might one day help another person who is lost in addiction and pain. Be patient with yourself. Healing takes time, but it's worth it.

Section 51.2

Recovering Woman's Guide to Coping with Childhood Abuse Issues

"Helping Yourself Heal: A Recovering Woman's Guide to Coping with Childhood Abuse Issues," Substance Abuse and Mental Health Services Administration (SAMHSA), DHHS Publication No. (SMA) 03–3789, 2003.

Now that you're in treatment for substance abuse, you may begin to have many different feelings. At times, these feelings may be painful, and you may have a hard time understanding or coping with them. You may feel:

- fearful,
- helpless,
- guilty,
- ashamed,
- anxious,
- depressed,
- angry,
- bad about yourself,
- as if you can't connect with family or friends,
- as if you're crazy,
- numbness or nothing at all, or
- as if you want to die.

Some of these feelings are common for any woman who starts treatment for substance abuse, but the same feelings may be stronger for many women who were abused in childhood. The pain may be so great that a woman may do anything to cope with her feelings, including using drugs or alcohol.

Some women in treatment for substance abuse don't clearly remember being abused, but they have some of the feelings mentioned here. Some women may have pushed the memories of the abuse so far away that they may not be able to explain why they feel intense anger, fear a particular person, have nightmares, or always believe something bad is about to happen. Sometimes, after people stop drinking or using drugs and are in treatment, memories may surface that were too painful to remember before or that were blocked from memory by drugs and alcohol.

Working through childhood memories or memory lapses can help you when you're in substance abuse treatment because facing past pain can help you focus on your present life.

What Is Childhood Abuse?

Abuse has many definitions, and sometimes it can be hard to know whether what you went through as a child was abuse. At the time, the way you were punished or treated may have seemed normal. Here are some questions to think about. These questions ask about just a few experiences that are generally considered abuse. You may have had other experiences that are not on this list but are still considered abuse.

Do you remember anyone when you were a child:

- Using extreme discipline or punishment on you?
- Spanking or hitting you so hard that it left bruises, cuts, or broken bones?
- Beating or punching you?
- Acting in a way that made you feel uncomfortable or powerless?
- Calling you names or abusing you verbally?
- Among family members or others close to you, criticizing or making fun of your physical characteristics, such as your hair, your skin color, your body type, or a disability?
- Talking to you in a sexual way, watching you undress or bathe, showing you pornographic pictures or movies, or photographing you in inappropriate ways?
- Touching you sexually or making you touch yourself or someone else sexually?
- Forcing you to watch others acting in a sexual way?
- Forcing you to have sex?

What Symptoms Could You Have If You Were Abused?

The effects of childhood abuse may be with you as an adult. As well as feeling angry, anxious, ashamed, or depressed, you may:

- have flashbacks of the abuse,
- have frequent nightmares,
- be very sensitive to noise or to being touched,
- always expect something bad to happen,
- let people abuse or take advantage of you,
- not remember periods of your life, or
- feel numb.

These feelings may get worse or become more intense when you're stressed or in situations that trigger memories of the abuse, such as when you fight with someone close to you. If you feel like hurting yourself, or are thinking about suicide, tell your counselor immediately, or call an emergency hotline or 911.

How Can You Address Childhood Abuse Issues While You Are in Treatment?

For the first month or so of substance abuse treatment, you'll be focusing on getting the drugs or alcohol out of your system, clearing your head, and establishing healthy patterns of thinking and behaving. You may want to put off addressing painful past abuse until you are comfortable being drug and alcohol free, establish a strong relationship with your counselor, make new friends, and build relationships with people who do not abuse drugs or alcohol. Then you may begin to feel safe enough to think about this issue.

However, if the feelings are too overwhelming and painful, or if you feel that you must address them right away, know that you can raise the issue whenever you want or need to. No matter what stage of recovery you're in, help is available for you. And remember: Many other women have worked through their pain and now lead happy, fulfilling, drug-free lives.

It's up to you to decide when to discuss abuse with your counselor, but it is important for you to raise the subject when you are ready. This may be the first time you've ever told anyone about what happened to you as a child. You may feel guilty or disloyal talking about a family member or another person close to you. You may fear how your family will react to you after you've talked about what happened. All of these feelings and fears are very normal; talk about them with your counselor.

Sometimes, it's hard to remember the difference between what you felt as a child victim and the choices you have as an adult in counseling. You could not protect yourself then, but you can now. As an adult, you can talk about what happened to you and you can begin to heal.

How Can Your Counselor Help?

It's important that you know that all states require mental health and substance abuse counselors to report abuse. If you're younger than 18, talk to your counselor about your state's requirements. If you're an adult, your counselor generally is not required to report the childhood abuse. The exception is when the abuser still has access to children and may harm them.

As you and your counselor or therapist talk about your experiences, your talks may become more difficult when painful memories and feelings arise and you look more closely at the past. Sometimes, these overwhelming feelings contribute to a drug or alcohol relapse. A counselor or therapist can help you understand the relationship between the abuse in your past and your substance abuse. He or she can help you cope with your feelings better so that you won't become overwhelmed.

Your substance abuse counselor also can help you find a counselor or therapist who specializes in working with people who have been abused as children. Addressing child abuse issues takes time; you'll need to develop a relationship with a therapist who can work with you now and who will continue to work with you after you've finished your treatment for substance abuse.

In addition to helping you find a skilled therapist, your substance abuse counselor can help you find self-help groups, such as Survivors of Incest Anonymous. If you grew up in a family in which one or more members had addiction issues, groups like Adult Children of Alcoholics (ACA) or Co-Dependents Anonymous (CoDA) might also be very helpful for you.

A Final Note

As a woman in recovery from substance abuse, you've faced great challenges and survived. It is a tribute to your strength that you've made the courageous choice to enter a substance abuse treatment program. You deserve the chance to heal and to live a happy, healthy life.

You will face challenges, but you have the ability to make things better. You can do this, as many have before you. Remember: You are not alone. Use the many resources and support networks available to help you feel safe and to keep you moving toward your goal. As you stay sober, your options grow. As you create a trusting relationship with your counselor or therapist, you begin to heal. And the courage you find to help yourself heal may one day help another person who is lost in addiction and pain.

Be patient with yourself. Healing takes time, but it's worth it— because you are.

Part Seven

Domestic Violence Survivor Assistance

Chapter 52

What to Do the First 24 Hours after Domestic Violence

In the immediate aftermath of a violent crime, it can be difficult to know what to do, where to go or even how to begin coping with something so overwhelming. This chapter provides a step-by-step guide of what to do in those critical first 24 hours following violent trauma.

If you have any questions or concerns, please feel free to contact Witness Justice for more information or for assistance. If you need immediate assistance, following are some resources that can help.

National Center for Victims of Crime
Toll-Free 24-Hour Hotline: 800-FYI-CALL (800-394-2255)

National Domestic Violence Hotline
Toll-Free: 800-799-SAFE (800-799-7233)
Toll-Free TDD: 800-787-3224

National Hopeline Network
Toll-Free: 800-SUI-CIDE (800-784-2433)

Step-by-Step Guide

If you or someone you know has just been victimized, there are some important steps you should consider to help protect yourself, treat any injuries, and set the stage for more effective prosecution of

---

"First 24 Hours," © 2008 Witness Justice (www.witnessjustice.org). Reprinted with permission.

your offender(s), in the event that you decide to pursue justice through the justice system. Following are some key considerations, compiled from victims' first-hand experiences and input from law enforcement and mental health experts.

Establish Safety for Yourself

Most importantly, get to a safe place, away from danger. If you need help determining a safe place or in getting there, ask someone to help you.

Care for Your Injuries

Go to a hospital or physician to have physical injuries treated and documented. It is important to tell medical personnel that your injuries are the result of a crime before you are treated so that forensic evidence can be collected and photographs taken. Do not shower, change clothes, or do anything else that might compromise physical evidence which could be crucial in apprehending and convicting the perpetrator(s), unless such action is necessary to preserve your immediate safety or well-being.

Get Help

Call the police (or ask medical personnel to phone the police) as soon as possible, so that they can provide assistance. Try to preserve a crime scene to the extent possible. Avoid cleaning or moving anything so that detectives can collect evidence. Then, call a trusted friend or family member to be with you as you interact with the police, physicians, and investigators. In the days following, consider consulting a counselor to help you cope with the mental health concerns that so often accompany trauma, such as acute stress disorder, posttraumatic stress disorder, and substance abuse.

Document the Crime

Though it may be the last thing you feel like doing, it is very important to write down exactly what happened as soon as possible following the crime while the details are still fresh in your mind. Writing down what took place is perhaps the best way to preserve your memory and to avoid potential inconsistencies that a criminal defense attorney might exploit to diminish your credibility in a court of law.

Do not be discouraged if you omit something or cannot remember all of the details in your initial written account. Even under the best of circumstances, it is difficult to remember all of the details of any given event. However, writing down what has taken place can help serve as a catalyst for remembering additional details later. In the event that you need to testify in court against the perpetrator(s), having a full, accurate, and consistent account of the crime will be very important. A written account also can help to validate your feelings as you work through the healing process, and perhaps even assist a counselor in working with you, should you seek one and choose to share the information with him or her. Following are some examples of details to include in your written account.

- **The nature of the incident:** Step by step, record what happened, whether you were assaulted, how you were assaulted, and what was said by whom and when, as well as how it was said. Include how you arrived at a place of safety and which direction the perpetrator(s) may have escaped.

- **Stolen or missing items:** A detailed list of any items that were stolen from you or are missing will help the police in their investigation and may be needed for insurance purposes.

- **The location and context of the crime:** Document where the crime occurred, as well as important landmarks or other notable information, such as the presence of any potential witnesses.

- **The time of the crime:** As accurately as possible, record exactly when the crime took place, as well as any warning signs you may recall. If you have difficulty remembering the time, try to think of clues that might shed light on the time of the incident. For example, was a particular television show on at the time? Did you notice stores or night clubs opening or closing at or around the time of the incident? Do you recall a city transit bus making a stop at a certain location at or around the time of the crime?

- **A description of your assailant(s):** Describe hair color and style, eye color, shape of face, height, weight, voice, clothing, tattoos or other identifying marks, or anything else that may help identity of the perpetrator(s).

- **Description of other items:** Try to recall the details of any items that were used or present during the crime, such as a handgun or car.

467

Protect Yourself against Further Harm

If your home was robbed or if you had your wallet or purse stolen, it is common to feel the need to have your home checked before returning to it. Consider asking the police to check your home for you and to make sure that you arrive there safely. Many survivors also feel a need to have someone with them for a while after returning home, especially if the perpetrator(s) have not been apprehended.

It is important for survivors to reestablish a sense of safety in their lives again and to understand that doing so likely will not come quickly or easily. Establishing a renewed sense of safety is unique to each person. Some survivors feel the need to acquire security devices or weapons. Others need to relocate to another city or state for a period of time or permanently. Generally, experts agree that the being aware of your surroundings at all times is the single best action you can take to protect yourself.

Short-Term Planning

You may feel bombarded with countless details, decisions, and tasks following a violent encounter. It is important to recognize that in all likelihood you simply will not be able to continue with your normal activities without skipping a beat. In addition to what was probably a very busy schedule for you prior to your violent encounter, you are now faced with the added tasks of working through the healing process and, if you so choose, the criminal justice process, both of which require time and effort. Following are some practical suggestions to consider for the short term to begin the processes on solid footing.

- **Contact your employer** or have a friend call if you are unable to return to work right away. Remember that you just survived a serious trauma, and even if you weren't physically injured, you may need some time away from work to cope.

- **Notify your health insurance company** or primary care provider so that you will be covered for your medical care and counseling needs. If you have lost a loved one, you or a friend or family member should notify the life insurance company.

- **Cancel your credit and debit cards if they were stolen or are missing.** This will help prevent added headaches with regard to your finances and might also help lead to the apprehension of someone trying to use them.

- **Learn about the investigation of your case** from law enforcement officials. Ask them what they will be doing, what the process is, how you will be notified of developments, and what your expected role will be.

- **Inform family and friends that you have experienced a violent encounter** so that they can offer their support. It is often difficult for family and friends to know how to assist victimized loved ones, but providing them with an idea of what you have experienced is essential to allowing them to help you.

For More Information

Witness Justice
P.O. Box 475
Frederick, MD 21705-0475
Toll-Free: 800-4WJ-HELP (95-4357)
Phone: 301-846-9110
Fax: 301-846-9113
Website: http://www.wintessjustice.org

Chapter 53

When You Call the Police

Chapter Contents

Section 53.1

Police Reports and Actions

This section includes text from "Response and Follow-Up by Responding Police Officers," "Response and Follow-Up by Domestic Violence Detectives," and "Resources and Services Available by Domestic Violence Counselors," © 2008 Metropolitan Nashville Police Department, Domestic Violence Division. Reprinted with permission.

Response and Follow-Up by Responding Police Officers

If you believe you are the victim of an abusive relationship or domestic violence, then call the police and allow them to assist you, the victim. As the responding officers are in route to your address remember that they are there to help you and your children. Following are but a few of the issues that the officers will address and what you can expect.

When the police arrive:

- tell what has happened and who is involved;
- tell the location of the suspect (if known);
- tell if weapons were involved and their location(s) (don't approach the officer with a weapon); and,
- indicate injuries you sustained (photos may have to be taken).

The officer's responsibilities include the following:

- The officer will write a report of the incident that occurred.
- The officer will ask and/or determine if medical attention is needed.
- The officer will help you if you wish to prosecute or wish to obtain an order of protection.

The officer can assist you with the following:

- In obtaining a warrant or order of protection. (The suspect's address, work location, or other possible locations is needed.)
- They can provide transportation to obtain a warrant, order of protection, or shelter.
- The officer can assist in locating a victim's shelter.
- They can refer other social services as needed.

Response and Follow-up by Domestic Violence Detectives on Assigned Cases

The detective will:

- photograph any injuries, property damage, or other evidence;
- ask for any written or taped statements of the incident; and,
- collect evidence and reports concerning the incident.

The detective can assist in the following:

- Obtaining warrants or filing an order of protection
- Calling or locating a shelter for you and your children's safety
- Referral to counseling or other social services
- Go over a safety plan, which helps you make yourself safer
- Answering any other questions you have about the process by explaining the prosecution and how it proceeds

Resources and Services Available by Domestic Violence Counselors

Some police departments provide domestic violence counseling; but, most do not. However, counseling and advocacy services to the victims of domestic violence are available and the police can direct you to local agencies for assistance. When a domestic crime occurs, the family is also affected by the crime. Therefore, non-perpetrating family members may also be entitled to services. Every victim of domestic violence has:

- the right to these services regardless of whether or not they may prosecute the offender;
- the right to be respected and to be treated fairly, regardless of race, religion, creed or sexual orientation;

- the right to confidentiality (exceptions will be discussed by the counselor); and,
- the right to victim's compensation information, when applicable.

Domestic violence counselors are committed to providing all services in a culturally sensitive environment.

Domestic violence can affect you emotionally. The following are a few examples of how you may feel:

- Like you are "walking on eggshells"
- Difficulty concentrating at school or work
- Fearful
- Sadness, feeling trapped, or angry
- Guilt feelings

Domestic violence can affect your children. A few examples include the following:

- Eating and sleeping disorders (nightmares)
- Separation anxieties
- Regressive or aggressive behaviors (angry)
- Difficulty in concentration
- Anxiety, fear, shame, guilt
- Taking responsibility for the abuse
- Constant anxiety (that another beating will occur)
- Guilt for not being able to stop the abuse or for loving the abuser
- Fear of abandonment

Domestic violence services are personalized, compassionate, and confidential. They may include the following:

- Short-term individual counseling and support for victims, their children, and non-perpetrating family members
- Limited court support
- Resource and referral services
- Safety planning

- Group counseling for victims and children
- Education seminars to community groups on domestic violence
- Grief counseling

Section 53.2

Reporting Rape

"Reporting Rape," © 2008 Rape, Abuse & Incest National Network (www .rainn.org). Reprinted with permission. For immediate crisis intervention, and information about recovery, prosecution, and local resources, call the National Sexual Assault Hotline at 1-800-656-HOPE, or visit the National Sexual Assault Online Hotline at https://online.rainn.org to receive live help over the RAINN website. The National Sexual Assault Hotlines are free, confidential, and secure services of RAINN and affiliated crisis centers across the country.

Should I report my attack to the police?

We hope you will decide to report your attack to the police. While there's no way to change what happened to you, you can seek justice while helping to stop it from happening to someone else.

Reporting to the police is the key to preventing sexual assault: every time we lock up a rapist, we're preventing him or her from committing another attack. It's the most effective tool that exists to prevent future rapes. In the end, though, whether or not to report is your decision to make.

Am I required to report to police?

No, you are not legally obligated to report. The decision is entirely yours, and everyone will understand if you decide not to pursue prosecution. You should be aware that the district attorney's office retains the right to pursue prosecution whether or not you participate, though it is uncommon for them to proceed without the cooperation of the victim. There are also times when a third party, such as a doctor or teacher, is a mandatory reporter of suspicion of sexual abuse.

Many victims say that reporting is the last thing they want to do right after being attacked. That's perfectly understandable—reporting can seem invasive, time consuming, and difficult.

Still, there are many good reasons to report, and some victims say that reporting helped their recovery and helped them regain a feeling of control.

How do I report the rape to police?

Call 911 (or ask a friend to call) to report your rape to police. Or, visit a hospital emergency room or your own doctor and ask them to call the police for you. If you visit the emergency room and tell the nurse you have been raped, the hospital will generally perform a sexual assault forensic examination. This involves collecting evidence of the attack, such as hairs, fluids, and fibers, and preserving the evidence for forensic analysis. In most areas, the local rape crisis center can provide someone to accompany you, if you wish. Call 800-656-HOPE (4673) to contact the center in your area.

Is there a time limit on reporting to the police?

There's generally no legal barrier to reporting your attack even months afterwards. However, to maximize the chances of an arrest and successful prosecution, it's important that you report as soon as possible after the rape. If you aren't sure what to do, it's better to report now and decide later. That way, the evidence is preserved should you decide to pursue prosecution. Some states have statutes of limitations that bar prosecutions after a certain number of years.

What if I need time to think about whether I want to pursue prosecution?

Understandably, many people aren't ready to make the decision about prosecution immediately after an attack. It's normal to want time to think about the decision and talk it over with friends and family.

If you think you might want to pursue prosecution, but haven't decided for sure, we recommend that you make the police report right away, while the evidence is still present and your memory is still detailed. The district attorney will decide whether or not to pursue prosecution; however, it is unusual for cases to proceed without the cooperation of the victim. And, if prosecution is pursued, the chance of success will be much higher if you reported and had evidence collected immediately after the attack.

There's one additional consideration: If you are planning to apply for compensation through your state's victim compensation fund, you will generally first have to report your attack to police to be eligible. Contact your local rape crisis center at 800-656-HOPE (4673) to learn about the rules in your state.

Can I report to police even if I have no physical injuries?

Yes. In fact, most rapes do not result in physical injuries. So, the lack of such injuries should not deter you from reporting.

It's also important to get medical care and to be tested for sexually transmitted infections and pregnancy, even if you think you aren't injured. And keep in mind that rape can cause injuries, often internal, that aren't visible. Many hospitals have special equipment that can detect such hidden injuries.

The rapist got scared away before finishing the attack. Can I still report it?

Yes. Attempted rape is still a serious crime and should be reported.

I knew the person who raped me and invited him (or her) in. Can I still report it?

Yes. About two-thirds of victims know their attacker. And the fact that you were voluntarily together, or even invited him or her home with you, does not change anything. Rape is a serious crime, no matter what the circumstances.

Do I have to go through the police interview alone?

In most areas, a trained volunteer from your local rape crisis center can accompany you to the police interview. The volunteer can also answer your questions about the process and explain how it will work.

What's the reporting process?

In most cases, the police will come to you and take a statement about what occurred. It helps to write down every detail you can remember, as soon as possible, so you can communicate the details to the police.

In addition to taking a statement, police will collect physical evidence. Also, your nurse or doctor may conduct an exam to collect hair, fluids, fibers, and other evidence.

The police interview may take as long as several hours, depending on the circumstances of your case. Some questions will probably feel intrusive, and the officer will probably go over the details of your attack several times. The extensive questioning isn't because the police don't believe you; it is the officer's job to get every detail down precisely, to make the strongest possible case against your rapist.

Most local crisis centers have staff trained to help you through the reporting process. They can answer your questions and, if necessary, advocate on your behalf.

Do most rape victims report their attack to police?

Just over half of rape victims don't report the crime. However, reporting is up substantially in the last decade. Our goal is have every rape reported to police, just as every murder is reported and investigated. It's the best way to get rapists off the streets and make sure they can't find new victims.

Why don't more people report their rape?

The most common reason given by victims (23%) is that the rape is a "personal matter." Another 16% of victims say that they fear reprisal, while about 6% don't report because they believe that the police are biased.

I'm Not Sure My Rape Is Serious Enough to Report to Police

The Federal Bureau of Investigation (FBI) ranks rape as the second most violent crime, behind only murder. Every rape is a very serious crime that should be prosecuted, even if no physical injuries occur during the assault.

I'm Afraid That If I Report, I Will Regret It

That's certainly possible. It's true that some people have a bad experience and wish they had never reported. But, it is also the case that many people who don't report later regret that decision. In the end, this is a personal decision that only you can make.

I'm Afraid That My Actions Will Be Scrutinized, and I'll Have to Testify about Intimate Details of My Personal Life

Many successful prosecutions end in a plea agreement, without trial, which means that the victim will not have to testify. However, if your case does go to trial, you will generally have to testify. Although there are no guarantees, prosecutors have legal tools they can use to protect you in court. One tool is called a rape shield law, which limits what the defense can ask you about your prior sexual history. The prosecutor can also file legal motions to try to protect you from having to disclose personal information

If you are worried about having to testify about intimate matters such as your own sexual history, let the police or prosecutor know about your concerns. They can explain the laws in your state and help you understand what might happen if you do go to trial.

I'm Afraid the Police Won't Take It Seriously

There has been great investment in police training in recent years. While there are occasional exceptions, most law enforcement officers are understanding and on your side. Many police departments participate in what are known as SART (Sexual Assault Response Teams), which provide a victim-sensitive, coordinated response to sexual assault that incorporates medical personnel, law enforcement, and a crisis center representative to organize questioning, reduce repetition, and facilitate communication among all the agencies involved.

If you do encounter someone who isn't taking your case seriously, it's important to complain to his or her supervisor. You should also tell your local rape crisis center which has people trained to advocate on your behalf.

I'm Afraid of Getting in Trouble

Sometimes victims, particularly youth, are afraid of getting in trouble for doing something they weren't supposed to be doing when the assault took place, such as drinking or sneaking out. While there's a possibility that you can get in trouble, most authorities (and parents) will be understanding, particularly about minor infractions.

What if I decide not to report?

Reporting is a very personal decision, and you should make the decision that's right for you. While we encourage you to report, if you decide not to, for whatever reason, that's perfectly understandable, and there's no reason to feel bad about your decision.

Chapter 54

Documenting Domestic Violence: How Health Care Providers Can Help Victims

Physicians and other health care providers know that often the first thing victims of domestic violence need is medical attention. They also know they may have a legal obligation to inform the police when they suspect the patient they are treating has been abused. What they may not know is that they can help the patient win her case in court against the abuser by carefully documenting her injuries.[1]

In the past decade, a great deal has been done to improve the way the health care community responds to domestic violence. One way that effort has paid off is in medical documentation of abuse. Many health care protocols and training programs now note the importance of such documentation. Only if medical documentation is accurate and comprehensive can it serve as objective, third party evidence useful in legal proceedings.

For a number of reasons, documentation is not as strong as it could be in providing evidence, so medical records are not used in legal proceedings to the extent they could be. In addition to being difficult to obtain, the records are often incomplete or inaccurate and the handwriting may be illegible. These flaws can make medical records more harmful than helpful.

Excerpts from "Documenting Domestic Violence: How Health Care Providers Can Help Victims," by Nancy E. Isaac and V. Pualani Enos, U.S. Department of Justice, September 2001. The full report of the study summarized here is on the website of the Domestic Violence Institute, Northeastern University School of Law, http://www.dvi.neu.edu/ers/med_doc. Reviewed in November 2008 by Dr. David A. Cooke, M.D., Diplomate, American Board of Internal Medicine.

Health care providers have received little information about how medical records can help domestic violence victims take legal action against their abusers. They often are not aware that admissibility is affected by subtle differences in the way they record the injuries. By making some fairly simple changes in documentation, physicians and other health care professionals can dramatically increase the usefulness of the information they record and thereby help their patients obtain the legal remedies they seek.

Why Thorough Documentation Is Essential

The victim's attorney, or the victim acting on her own behalf as a pro se litigant, can submit medical documentation as evidence for obtaining a range of protective relief (such as a restraining order). Victims can also use medical documentation in less formal legal contexts to support their assertions of abuse. Persuasive, factual information may qualify them for special status or exemptions in obtaining public housing, welfare, health and life insurance, victim compensation, immigration relief related to domestic violence, and in resolving landlord-tenant disputes.

For formal legal proceedings, the documentation needs to be strong enough to be admissible in a court of law.[2] Typically, the only third-party evidence available to victims of domestic violence is the police report, but this can vary in quality and completeness. Medical documentation can corroborate police data. It constitutes unbiased, factual information recorded shortly after the abuse occurs, when recall is easier.

Medical records can contain a variety of information useful in legal proceedings. Photographs taken in the course of the examination record images of injuries that might fade by the time legal proceedings begin, and they capture the moment in a way that no verbal description can convey. Body maps[3] can document the extent and location of injuries. The records may also hold information about the emotional impact of the abuse. However, the way the information is recorded can affect its admissibility. For instance, a statement about the injury in which the patient is clearly identified as the source of information is more likely to be accepted as evidence in legal proceedings. Even poor handwriting on written records can affect their admissibility.

Overcoming Barriers to Good Documentation

There are several reasons medical record-keeping is not generally adequate. Health care providers are concerned about confidentiality and liability. They are concerned about recording information that might inadvertently harm the victim. Many are confused about whether, how, and why to record information about domestic violence, so in an effort to be neutral, some use language that may subvert the patient's legal case and even support the abuser's case.

Some health care providers are afraid to testify in court. They may see the risks to the patient and themselves as possibly outweighing the benefits of documenting abuse. Even health care providers who are reluctant to testify can still submit medical evidence. Although the hearsay rule prohibits out-of-court statements, an exception permits testimony about diagnosis and treatment. In addition, some states also allow the diagnosis and treatment elements of a certified medical record to be entered into the evidentiary record without the testimony of a health care provider. Thus, in some instances, physicians and other health care providers can be spared the burden of appearing in court.

The patient's excited utterances or spontaneous exclamations about the incident are another exception to the prohibition of hearsay. These are statements made by someone during or soon after an event, while in an agitated state of mind. They have exceptional credibility because of their proximity in time to the event and because they are not likely to be premeditated.

Excited utterances are valuable because they allow the prosecution to proceed even if the victim is unwilling to testify. These statements need to be carefully documented. A patient's report may be admissible if the record demonstrates that the patient made the statement while responding to the event stimulating the utterance (the act or acts of abuse). Noting the time between the event and the time the statements were made or describing the patient's demeanor as she made the statement can help show she was responding to the stimulating event. Such a showing is necessary to establish that a statement is an excited utterance or spontaneous exclamation, and thus an exception to the hearsay rule.[4]

What the Records Lack

It appears that at present, many medical records are not sufficiently documented to provide adequate legal evidence of domestic violence. A study of 184 visits for medical care in which an injury or other evidence of abuse was noted revealed major shortcomings in the records:

- For the 93 instances of an injury, the records contained only one photograph. There was no mention in any records of photographs filed elsewhere (for example, with the police).

- A body map documenting the injury was included in only three of the 93 instances. Drawings of the injuries appeared in eight of the 93 instances.

- Doctors' and nurses' handwriting was illegible in key portions of the records in one-third of the patients' visits in which abuse or injury was noted.

All three criteria for considering a patient's words an excited utterance were met in only 28 of the more than 800 statements evaluated (3.4%). Most frequently missing was a description of the patient's demeanor, and often the patient was not clearly identified as the source of the information.

On the plus side, although photographs and body maps documenting injuries were rare, injuries were otherwise described in detail. And, in less than one percent of the visits were negative comments made about the patient's appearance, manner, or motive for stating that abuse had occurred.

What Health Care Providers Can Do

Medical records could be much more useful to domestic violence victims in legal proceedings if some minor changes were made in documentation. Clinicians can do the following:

- Take photographs of injuries known or suspected to have resulted from domestic violence.

- Write legibly. Computers can also help overcome the common problem of illegible handwriting.

- Set off the patient's own words in quotation marks or use such phrases as patient states or patient reports to indicate that the information recorded reflects the patient's words. To write, "patient was kicked in abdomen," obscures the identity of the speaker.

- Avoid such phrases as "patient claims" or "patient alleges," which imply doubt about the patient's reliability. If the clinician's observations conflict with the patient's statements, the clinician should record the reason for the difference.

- Use medical terms and avoid legal terms such as alleged perpetrator, assailant, and assault.

- Describe the person who hurt the patient by using quotation marks to set off the statement. The clinician would write, for example: The patient stated, "My boyfriend kicked and punched me."

- Avoid summarizing a patient's report of abuse in conclusive terms. If such language as "patient is a battered woman," "assault and battery," or "rape" lacks sufficient accompanying factual information, it is inadmissible.

- Do not place the term domestic violence or abbreviations such as DV in the diagnosis section of the medical record. Such terms do not convey factual information and are not medical terminology. Whether domestic violence has occurred is determined by the court.

- Describe the patient's demeanor, indicating, for example, whether she is crying or shaking or seems angry, agitated, upset, calm, or happy. Even if the patient's demeanor belies the evidence of abuse, the clinician's observations of that demeanor should be recorded.

- Record the time of day the patient is examined and, if possible, indicate how much time has elapsed since the abuse occurred. For example, the clinician might write: Patient states that early this morning her boyfriend hit her.

Notes

1. Although men as well as women are victims of domestic violence, terms referencing women are most often used in this report because women are more frequently injured, in heterosexual relationships.

2. The evidentiary laws of each state define the scope and degree of use of medical records in legal proceedings.

3. A body map is a drawing of the human figure used by physicians. In domestic violence protocols, body maps are used to mark the locations, size, and age of injuries observed during a medical examination.

4. The rules of evidence adopted in most states include this exception to the general rule that statements made outside the courtroom are inadmissible. The exception is premised on the notion that if a speaker makes a statement while responding to an exciting or emotionally charged experience, that

substantially reduces the likelihood that the speaker had time to fabricate the statement. This makes the statement more reliable.

Additional Information and Resources

National Criminal Justice Reference Service
P.O. Box 6000
Rockville, MD 20849-6000
Toll-Free: 800-851-3420
Phone: 301-519-5500
Website: http://www.ojp.usdoj.gov/nij
E-mail: askncjrs@ncjrs.org

Chapter 55

Programs and Tools That Improve Health Care for Domestic Violence Victims

Up to 25 percent of U.S. women have been the victims of domestic violence, which can result in immediate injury and/or chronic health problems. When victims seek medical care, clinicians often do not screen for and identify domestic violence. In fact, the U.S. Preventive Services Task Force indicates that very few research studies exist that can help guide clinicians on how to screen for domestic violence and manage care for identified victims. Further, health care providers need to be able to refer victims to programs and counseling that will be effective in helping them end the violence in their lives. Assessing the quality and effectiveness of these programs, however, has been difficult.

Research funded by the Agency for Healthcare Research and Quality (AHRQ) has:

- identified gaps in research on domestic violence indicating a need to build a stronger evidence base for screening, detecting, and treating victims;

- helped health care providers screen for and identify victims of domestic abuse;

- created tools that help providers counsel and treat victims; and,

---

This chapter includes text from "Women and Domestic Violence: Programs and Tools That Improve Care for Victims," *Research in Action Issue 15*, by Barbara L. Kass-Bartelmes, M.P.H., C.H.E.S., Agency for Healthcare Research and Quality (AHRQ), 2004.

- developed a tool that evaluates the quality of domestic violence programs.

Background

Each year in the United States, about two million women are physically assaulted by their intimate partners. These assaults result in injuries that lead to over 73,000 hospitalizations and 1,500 deaths. In addition to the physical injuries domestic violence causes, it is also a major risk factor for depression. For example, one study found that 61 percent of women diagnosed with depression had also experienced domestic violence—a rate two times that of the general population. Victims of domestic violence have more physical problems, including headaches, chronic pain, sleep problems, vaginal infections, digestive problems, sexually transmitted diseases, and urinary tract infections, and they are more likely to rate their health as only fair or poor.

Even though injuries and health problems are apparent and well documented, health care providers often do not ask about domestic violence or intervene on behalf of their patients who experience it. One study found that only six percent of physicians ask their patients about possible domestic violence, yet 88 percent admitted that they knew they had female patients who had been abused. Another study indicated that 48 percent of women supported routine screening of all women, with 86 percent stating it would make it easier to get help.

Health care providers have said that they do not screen for domestic violence because they lack the necessary training, time, tools, and resources, and they do not feel they can make a difference. An AHRQ-funded survey found that many primary care clinicians, nurses, physician assistants, and medical assistants lack confidence in their ability to manage and care for victims of domestic abuse.

- Only 22 percent had attended any educational program on domestic violence within the previous year.

- Over 25 percent of physicians and nearly 50 percent of nurses, physician assistants, and medical assistants stated that they were not at all confident in asking their patients about physical abuse.

- Less than 20 percent of clinicians asked about domestic violence when treating their patients for high-risk conditions such as injuries, depression or anxiety, chronic pelvic pain, headache, and irritable bowel syndrome.

- Only 23 percent of physicians, nurses, physician assistants, and medical assistants believed they had strategies that could assist victims of domestic abuse.

Impact of AHRQ Research: More Research Is Needed on Screening and Treating Domestic Violence Victims

In an extensive review of research literature, the U.S. Preventive Services Task Force (USPSTF) did not find enough evidence to recommend for or against routine screening for domestic violence among the general population. However, the USPSTF reinforced the necessity for health care providers to be able to identify the signs and symptoms of domestic violence, document the evidence, provide treatment for victims, and refer victims to counseling and social agencies that can provide assistance. Essentially, the USPSTF found the following:

- When domestic violence is suspected, health care providers need to conduct the appropriate history and examinations, offer treatment, document their findings, and refer the victim for counseling and support.

- None of the research has indicated that screening patients who have no symptoms of domestic violence has reduced harm.

- More research is needed to develop screening tools that are effective in the general population, along with programs that can improve health outcomes and reduce violence.

- Several screening instruments have demonstrated good "internal consistency," indicating that all the items on the instrument are consistent with one another. However, the best methods to administer screening instruments in various settings have not been determined.

- Definitions of abuse varied among the studies, which limited the ability to combine and compare studies in different settings. Refining these definitions, along with measurements of severity and the chronic occurrence of abuse, would allow development of standardized instruments and evaluation tools.

- No research has been done to determine if there were any adverse effects of screening or interventions.

Training Helps Providers Identify and Manage Victims of Domestic Violence

Training sessions funded by AHRQ improved primary care providers' confidence in asking and treating victims of domestic violence. Providers who participated in the training increased their screening for domestic violence from 3.5 percent prior to the training program to 20.5 percent after training. Upon completion of the training sessions, participants stated they:

- felt less fear of offending patients by asking about domestic violence;

- had less fear for their own safety;

- asked patients more often about possible domestic violence;

- offered strategies to abusers to seek help;

- provided strategies so victims could change their situation;

- had better access to information on managing domestic violence;

- had methods to ask abusers about domestic violence while minimizing the risk to the victims.

This domestic violence training program uses a systems approach, helping health care providers working in primary care settings identify and manage domestic violence. In addition, its randomized design allows assessment of outcomes and effectiveness. Specifically, one can measure:

- changes in providers' knowledge, attitudes, and beliefs;

- how often they ask about domestic violence (documented);

- case findings; and,

- completeness of case management.

An interdisciplinary team provided training for receptionists, medical assistants, nurses, physician assistants, and physicians. The team included a nurse, an epidemiologist, primary care physicians, and personnel from treatment programs, social work, and a women's shelter, as well as a former domestic violence victim and a prosecuting attorney.

There were two 4-hour training sessions. At the first training session, participants received basic information about domestic violence, including prevalence, indications, how to get information from their patients, how patients change behaviors, documentation, and patient safety.

Specifically, participants were taught how to do the following:

- Ask direct questions

- Acknowledge what the patient said

- Assess the patient's safety needs

- Refer the patient to social and mental health workers as well as community and state domestic violence agencies and hotlines

- Document their findings in the patient's chart

- Arrange to have the patient follow up with them

The first training session also included a discussion about abusers—those who commit domestic violence. Participants learned the following:

- How to identify abusers by noticing injuries to the abuser's hands, problems with alcohol, depression, employment problems, stress disorders, and problems with anger and hostility

- How to interview abusers by asking questions about what happens during disagreements with their partners and if anyone gets hurt

- The indications of increasing risk of domestic violence, including a history of escalating violence, multiple forms of violence, threats of serious harm, increased drug and alcohol use, depression, mental illness, suicide threats or attempts, jealousy, and obsession with the victim on the part of the abuser; expressions of fear for safety from victims; separation; and divorce

- Methods to help ensure their safety when meeting with abusers

- What to say to the abuser: for example, this behavior is not acceptable, violence will not go away by itself, violence has harmful effects on the family, and the abuser has a responsibility to get help

- Where to refer the abuser to get help

During the second training session, participants learned how to manage the care for victims of domestic violence. They participated

491

in role playing, talked with a former victim of domestic violence, and received presentations from a prosecuting attorney and a community domestic violence agency.

After the two half-day workshops, during the following year, newsletters were sent four times to all participants to reinforce what they had learned and were applying in practice. Additional educational sessions were held on skill improvement and community resources, and participants were told about early results of the study to encourage their efforts. Posters were placed in clinic waiting areas to allow patients to feel more comfortable about talking with providers about domestic violence. Providers also carried cue cards in their pockets to help reinforce the processes they had learned.

An Assessment Tool Helps Providers Counsel Victims

The Domestic Violence Survivor Assessment (DVSA) tool helps health care providers and abused women identify issues and feelings created by domestic violence and helps guide counseling. Social workers have said that the DVSA is "easy to understand, quick to complete, and provided a valuable holistic viewpoint." It enabled them to see visually the various states a woman was experiencing about different issues and could help them identify areas where she was "stuck" and required counseling to be able to move forward.

The DVSA instrument has been adopted as an outcome measure for counseling in two community-based and one hospital-based domestic violence counseling program. It is also being piloted for possible adoption by a state for measuring outcomes of domestic violence counseling programs.

Researchers funded by AHRQ collaborated with the United Family Services of Central Maryland and the House of Ruth of Baltimore, Maryland, to develop and implement the DVSA in order to guide interventions and measure outcomes. The instrument is based on the Trans Theoretical Model of Change and Landenburger's Theory of Domestic Violence Recovery. It measures where a woman perceives herself regarding eleven issues commonly experienced by survivors of domestic violence. Five of these issues concern her relationship with the abuser:

- Triggers of abusive incidents
- Managing partner abuse
- Attachment to the abuser

- Views of the relationship and options
- Managing loyalty to norms and her own beliefs

Six of the issues concern her as an individual:

- Accessing help
- Feelings
- Self-identity
- Self-efficacy (ability to be on her own)
- Mental health
- Medical care for domestic violence injuries and stress

Based on interviews with the client, the clinician identifies the state the woman is in with regard to resolving each of the eleven issues. For example, when a woman denies and excuses the abuse or ignores her injuries, she is still in a state of being committed to continuing the relationship. Once she is able to reject self-blame and realizes she cannot prevent her partner's abuse, she is considering change and begins looking at the abuse and her options, although she may delay getting medical care for her injuries. Finally, she makes the decision not to tolerate the abuse and either leaves the relationship or, if she stays, becomes mindful of the need for her partner to change and seeks medical treatment as needed.

The complete, updated DVSA can be obtained from:

University of North Carolina at Charlotte
Department of Adult Health Nursing
9201 University City Boulevard
Charlotte, NC 28223
E-mail: jadienem@uncc.edu

A Critical Pathway for Intimate Partner Violence Provides Guidance for Patient Care

Researchers who developed the DVSA instrument also created a critical pathway for intimate partner violence (IPV). The critical pathway encompasses physical health, mental health, and social assessment and treatment for victims of domestic violence. The IPV critical pathway has been validated using the Delphi technique of gathering feedback from experts.

A Tool for Hospital-Based Domestic Violence Programs Helps Assess Quality

The Delphi Instrument for Hospital-Based Domestic Violence Programs, funded by AHRQ, can be used to assess the quality of a hospital's performance in implementing a domestic violence program and can be used to create program goals, assess performance over time, and compare one program to another. Eventually, it can be linked to outcomes to determine what parts of the program create the best outcomes for victims of domestic violence. The instrument examines the physical structure of the programs, such as facilities, equipment, personnel, and organizational structure. It also examines the provider's process of care, such as chart documentation and treatment.

The Delphi Instrument has had both local and international impact. It was used at the University of North Carolina (UNC) Chapel Hill Medical School to evaluate the domestic violence program at UNC hospitals. Foyle Women's Aid and the Consultancy Mentoring Works research team, based in Northern Ireland, used the Delphi Instrument in a study to investigate care for victims of domestic violence at Altnagelvin Hospital. The findings from that study led researchers to recommend the Delphi Instrument as an "excellent template... for any organization, agency or public body to monitor their services in respect to domestic violence."

The tool measures nine different categories of performance. A panel of 18 experts on domestic violence (researchers, program planners, and advocates) evaluated and agreed on 37 performance measures in these nine categories that can be used to evaluate hospital-based domestic violence programs. Each performance measure within a category is assigned a score and the scores are added to obtain a total for the category. The raw scores for each category are then weighted and the weighted scores added to obtain a total score, with 100 being the best possible score. Guidelines, instructions, and the tool itself can be found on AHRQ's website at http://www.ahrq.gov/research/domesticviol.

Chapter 56

Creating a Safety Plan

Personalized Safety Plan

Your safety is the most important thing. Listed are tips to help keep you safe. The resources in this chapter can help you to make a safety plan that works best for you. It is important to get help with your safety plan.

If You Are in an Abusive Relationship, Think About

1. Having important phone numbers nearby for you and your children. Numbers to have are the police, hotlines, friends, and the local shelter.

2. Friends or neighbors you could tell about the abuse. Ask them to call the police if they hear angry or violent noises. If you have children, teach them how to dial 911. Make up a code word that you can use when you need help.

3. How to get out of your home safely. Practice ways to get out.

4. Safer places in your home where there are exits and no weapons. If you feel abuse is going to happen, try to get your abuser to one of these safer places.

"Personalized Safety Plan," © 2008 North Carolina Coalition Against Domestic Violence (www.nccadv.org). Reprinted with permission.

5. Any weapons in the house. Think about ways that you could get them out of the house.

6. Even if you do not plan to leave, think of where you could go. Think of how you might leave. Try doing things that get you out of the house—taking out the trash, walking the pet, or going to the store. Put together a bag of things you use everyday (see the following checklist). Hide it where it is easy for you to get.

7. Going over your safety plan often.

If You Consider Leaving Your Abuser, Think About

1. Four places you could go if you leave your home.

2. People who might help you if you left. Think about people who will keep a bag for you. Think about people who might lend you money. Make plans for your pets.

3. Keeping change for phone calls or getting a cell phone.

4. Opening a bank account or getting a credit card in your name.

5. How you might leave. Try doing things that get you out of the house—taking out the trash, walking the family pet, or going to the store. Practice how you would leave.

6. How you could take your children with you safely. There are times when taking your children with you may put all of your lives in danger. You need to protect yourself to be able to protect your children.

7. Putting together a bag of things you use everyday. Hide it where it is easy for you to get. Items to take, if possible, include the following:

   - Children (if it is safe)
   - Money
   - Keys to car, house, work
   - Extra clothes
   - Medicine
   - Important papers for you and your children
   - Birth certificates
   - Social security cards

- School and medical records
- Bankbooks, credit cards
- Driver's license
- Car registration
- Welfare identification
- Passports, green cards, work permits
- Lease/rental agreement
- Mortgage payment book, unpaid bills
- Insurance papers
- Protective order, divorce papers, custody orders
- Address book
- Pictures, jewelry, things that mean a lot to you
- Items for your children (toys, blankets, and so forth)

8. Think about reviewing your safety plan often.

If You Have Left Your Abuser, Think About

1. Your safety—you still need to.

2. Getting a cell phone.

3. Getting a protective order from the court. Keep a copy with you all the time. Give a copy to the police, people who take care of your children, their schools and your boss.

4. Changing the locks. Consider putting in stronger doors, smoke and carbon monoxide detectors, a security system and outside lights.

5. Telling friends and neighbors that your abuser no longer lives with you. Ask them to call the police if they see your abuser near your home or children.

6. Telling people who take care of your children the names of people who are allowed to pick them up. If you have a protective order protecting your children, give their teachers and babysitters a copy of it.

7. Telling someone at work about what has happened. Ask that person to screen your calls. If you have a protective order that

includes where you work, consider giving your boss a copy of it and a picture of the abuser. Think about and practice a safety plan for your workplace. This should include going to and from work.

8. Not using the same stores or businesses that you did when you were with your abuser.

9. Someone that you can call if you feel down. Call that person if you are thinking about going to a support group or workshop.

10. Safe way to speak with your abuser if you must.

11. Going over your safety plan often.

Warning: Abusers try to control their victim's lives. When abusers feel a loss of control—like when victims try to leave them—the abuse often gets worse. Take special care when you leave. Keep being careful even after you have left.

Chapter 57

Protecting Your Identity after Domestic Violence

Chapter Contents

Section 57.1

Steps to Protect Your Identity

Protecting Your Identity

Identity theft is rampant in the United States. Survivors of domestic violence must take extra precautions to protect themselves from abusers who use identity as a means of power and control. Abusers may use survivors' credit cards without their permission, open fraudulent new credit cards in survivors' names (ultimately ruining their credit), or open credit cards in children's names. Misuse of survivors' social security numbers is also common in the context of domestic violence. Abusers may fraudulently use survivors' social security numbers to stalk, harass, or threaten survivors. Read more to learn how to protect yourself if you are experiencing this type of abuse.

Survivors experiencing abuse should contact their local domestic violence program for immediate support. Check your local yellow pages or call the National Domestic Violence Hotline (operated by the Texas Council on Family Violence) at 800-799-SAFE (7233) to be connected to the program in your area.

Steps to Take to Protect Your Identity

- **Relocate:** Moving across town, across the state, or across the country puts physical distance between you and the abuser. Be sure to obtain an unlisted phone number and be aware of the Full Faith and Credit provisions in your restraining order, which make the order valid when you travel to another state or tribal jurisdiction.

- **Apply to the address confidentiality program in your state:** These types of programs allow individuals who have experienced domestic violence, sexual assault, stalking, or other types of crime to receive mail at a confidential address, while

500

keeping their actual address undisclosed. Rules and eligibility vary from state to state.

- **Open a post office box to receive mail:** Abusers may be able to open fraudulent credit cards by responding to credit card offers received in the mail. A post office box may prevent this if only you have access to it. Be wary of the confidentiality policies of non-government post office box centers such as Mail Boxes, Etc., and the fact that it may not be possible to remain anonymous in rural towns while accessing the post office.

- **Protect your incoming and outgoing mail:** Shred all credit card offers that come in the mail along with other documents that have your name, address, and/or social security number on them. Mail your bills and other sensitive documents directly from the post office instead of from the mailbox on your porch or at the end of your driveway. Call 800-5OPT-OUT (678-688) to stop receiving credit card offers in the mail.

- **Guard your social security number:** Do not use your social security number as a general identification (ID), personal identification number (PIN), or password. Request to have your social security number removed from documents you receive in the mail and from ID cards for health insurance, driving, work, and so forth.

- **Check your credit report:** The best way to determine if someone has committed fraud against you is to check your credit report with all three credit bureaus at least once per year. Visit www.annualcreditreport.com to obtain a free yearly credit report. You can also make a request to have a fraud alert placed on your credit report.

- **Report suspected fraud:** Contact local law enforcement if you know of or suspect fraud and ask to file a report. Check and/or close accounts you believe have been tampered. File a report with the Federal Trade Commission at 877-ID-THEFT (43-84338) and the Social Security Administration Fraud Hotline at 800-269-0271. File copies of police reports with credit bureaus.

- **Protect information you give out:** Never give any identifying information over the phone or through e-mail or the internet unless you initiated the call or have verification that the website or e-mail communication is secure.

Other Helpful Websites

Privacy Rights Clearinghouse: Nonprofit Consumer Information and Advocacy Organization
Website: http://www.privacyrights.org

Identity Theft Resource Center
Website: http://www.idtheftcenter.org

Federal Trade Commission
Website: http://www.consumer.gov/idtheft

The National Center for Victims of Crime
Website: http://www.ncvc.org

U.S. Department of Justice
Website: http://www.usdoj.gov

Section 57.2

Applying for a New Social Security Number

"Social Security Information," © 2008 North Carolina Coalition Against Domestic Violence (www.nccadv.org). Reprinted with permission.

Social Security Information

Effective November 4, 1998, the Social Security Administration (SSA) changed its existing policy of assigning new Social Security numbers (SSN) to victims of harassment, abuse, or life endangerment, including victims of domestic violence, to make it easier to obtain new SSN. The change in policy was designed to make it easier for these individuals to elude their abusers and reduce the risk of further violence. Since its implementation, many questions and concerns have arisen about potential risks to individuals who may not be fully aware of the issues involved in obtaining a new Social Security number. This section will attempt to address those issues.

Potential Impact of Changing Identity or Social Security Numbers

Be aware: Changing the SSN should not be looked upon as the key to safety. Third-parties can cross-refer the new SSN with the old number, as allowed by their statutes, policies, and procedures. In addition, the victim may experience less freedom to travel (due to lack of documents), which can raise potential safety issues.

Remember: Getting a new Social Security number is only one part of a safety plan. It is recommended that when applying for a new Social Security number, the victim take evidence that shows a proactive intent and plan to evade the abuser. This evidence may include a safety plan which includes making a name change, getting an unlisted telephone number, moving to another address, changing jobs.

Advise the victim that changing identity, including the SSN, is a life-altering decision. It is important to keep in mind the potential impact of these changes, such as:

- the inability to get a passport or other federal documentation due to the lack of having a birth certificate under the new identity;

- the loss of previous work history resulting in the victim having to accept positions for which he/she is overqualified or positions in which he/she has no experience;

- difficulties or delays in receiving federal or state benefits, such as welfare, disability, social security income (SSI);

- difficulty trying to prove past abuse if past medical records and court papers are in a different name.

Social Security Administration (SSA) does not invalidate or destroy the original SSN when a new SSN is assigned. The original and new SSN are cross-referred in SSA records to make sure that the individual gets credit for all earnings and to ensure the integrity of Social Security's programs. SSA maintains the confidentiality of all its records and will not disclose information about an individual's SSN without the individual's consent, unless required by law to do so. SSA requires that each individual requesting information about himself or herself properly identify himself or herself as the subject of the record. An individual requesting information in person must present

503

documentary evidence. An individual requesting information over the phone must provide six pieces of identifying information which SSA can verify from its records.

Note: SSA has added an extra layer of security when an SSN has been assigned based on harassment, abuse, or life endangerment. SSA has implemented procedures to prevent inappropriate or erroneous disclosure of SSN information over the phone when a new number has been assigned in these situations, which includes domestic violence. The caller will be advised to go to the local field office for an in-person interview and properly identify himself or herself as the subject of the record before SSN information will be disclosed.

SSA's Cross-Referral and Disclosure Policies

SSA, as required by law, must disclose the new SSN information to other government agencies such as:

- law enforcement agencies to investigate violation of Social Security laws;

- government agencies administering entitlement, heath and welfare programs such as Medicaid, Medicare, veterans benefits, military pension, and civil service annuities, black lung, housing, student loans, railroad retirement benefits, and food stamps;

- Internal Revenue Service (IRS) for federal tax administration;

- Department of Justice, Immigration and Naturalization Service to identify and locate aliens in the U.S.;

- Selective Service System for draft registration;

- Department of Health and Human Services for child support enforcement purposes;

- state motor vehicles agencies that use the number in issuing drivers' licenses to verify the Social Security numbers, as authorized by the Social Security Act; and,

- Congressional representatives if they request information to answer questions you ask them.

Information provided to SSA may be used to match records by computer. Matching programs, which are allowed by law, compare SSA records with those of other federal, state, or local government agencies to determine whether a person qualifies for benefits paid by the federal government.

Third Party Cross-Referral and Disclosure Policies

Important note: Credit bureaus and other third parties also have the ability to cross-refer SSN in their data bases. Third parties also share information maintained in their data bases. SSA has no control over what uses third parties make of an individual's SSN. Therefore, it is important to take steps to protect the new number.

Applying for a New SSN

Advise your client to take the following steps to apply for a new SSN:

* Make an appointment to be interviewed in person at an SSA field office by calling 800-772-1213 (voice), or 800-325-0778 (TTY), or go directly to an SSA field office for the in-person interview.

* If the SSA representative at the Social Security office is not aware of the current policy for assigning new SSN in harassment, abuse, or life endangerment situations, refer the representative to Program Operations Manual System (POMS) Chapter RM 00205. If there are any problems applying for the new SSN, ask to speak with a supervisor or the field office manager.

* Be prepared to complete a statement explaining the need for a new number and a Form SS-5 (Application for a Social Security Card).

* Take evidence of age, identity, and U.S. citizenship or lawful alien status, such as a birth certificate and driver's license.

* If the client has a new name, take one or more documents identifying him or her by both the old name on SSA's records and the new name.

* A single document, such as a court order for a name change could be used to show both the old and new name.

* Two separate documents, such as a drivers license, employer ID card, passport, insurance policy, military record, divorce record, school ID card could be used to show the old and new names. (A birth certificate is not an identity document.)

505

- Take original documents or copies certified by the custodian of the record. Photocopies and notarized copies of documents are not acceptable.

- If your client wants new SSN for his or her children, take evidence showing he or she has legal custody of the children. SSA will not assign one parent a new SSN to deny the other parent court-ordered visitation privileges or otherwise assist one parent from hiding the child from the other parent. The parent requesting the new SSN needs to consider whether a new SSN will help him or her elude the harasser or abuser if the harasser or abuser is the other parent with visitation rights.

- Take all evidence documenting the harassment or abuse. SSA will assist him or her in obtaining any additional corroborating evidence, if needed.

- The best evidence of abuse comes from third parties, such as police, medical facilities, or doctors, and describes the nature and extent of the domestic violence.

- Other evidence might include court restraining orders; letters from shelters; and letters and/or affidavits from family members, friends, counselors, or others with knowledge of the domestic violence.

Protecting the New SSN

If the application is approved and a new number is assigned, SSA will keep the new number and records confidential. SSA will not furnish the number to unauthorized third parties. (Note that SSA is authorized to provide the new SSN to agencies and organizations listed under the "SSA's Cross Referral and Disclosure Policies" section of this chapter.) Therefore, victims of harassment, abuse, or life endangerment must be careful about sharing the new number with those who ask for it. Be careful to minimize the number of organizations that will have access to the new SSN.

Employers and financial institutions will likely need the SSN for wage and tax reporting purposes. Other private businesses may need the SSN to do a credit check, such as when applying for a car loan. Sometimes, however, they simply want the SSN for general record keeping. It is not necessary to give a business the SSN just because they ask for it. However, a business may not provide the service or benefit if a SSN is not provided. These questions will help the individual decide whether sharing the SSN with the business is worth the service or benefit. If someone asks for the SSN, ask the following questions:

- Why do you need my SSN?

- How will my SSN be used?

- What law requires me to give you my SSN?

- What will happen if I don't give you my SSN?

- Before revealing any personally identifying information, find out how it will be used and whether it will be shared by others. Ask if there is a choice about the use of personal information: can it be kept confidential?

- Do not give out personal information on the phone, through the mail, or over the internet unless the contact was self-initiated or you know who you are dealing with.

- Keep items with personal information in a safe place. Tear or shred copies of credit applications or any documents that contain identity information before discarding them.

- Find out who has access to your personal information at work and verify that the record is kept in a secure location.

- Give your SSN only when absolutely necessary. Ask to use other types of identifiers when possible.

- Do not carry your SSN card; keep it in a secure place to prevent loss or theft.

This list contains only a few suggestions on how to keep one's identity and SSN safe. Keep in mind that people can be located in many other ways. These include being tracked by bank or credit records and telephone records of family and friends still in contact with the victim. Emphasize to all victims the importance of keeping their records documenting domestic abuse with them so that their safety will not be compromised because they must go back to their former lives to obtain sufficient documentation of abuse to support an application for a new SSN.

Frequently Asked Questions with Answers Provided by SSA

Who should you contact if the SSA representative at the local office is not aware of the current policy for assigning a new SSN in harassment, abuse, or life endangerment situations which include domestic violence?

If the SSA representative at the Social Security office is not aware of the current policy for assigning a new SSN in harassment, abuse, or life endangerment situations, first refer the representative to SSA instructions in Program Operations Manual System (POMS) Chapter RM 00205. If there are any problems applying for the new SSN, ask to speak with a supervisor or the field office manager.

Should a person change his or her name before contacting SSA for a new number?

Changing one's name is one of the important steps a victim needs to take for personal protection. But, changing one's name and SSN are just two steps in a person's safety plan. We encourage other steps to be taken as well, such as changing addresses, changing schools, and/or changing jobs.

Since SSA assigns a SSN based on the name shown on the identity document submitted with the application for a new number, it is best that the applicant have a document identifying him or her by the new name when applying for the new number. SSA will not assign a third number just because the individual later changes his or her name. Rather, the records will be updated and a corrected card will be issued showing the new name and the current SSN.

What protections does SSA have in place so that third parties cannot access the new Social Security Number?

SSA has added an extra layer of security when an SSN has been assigned based on harassment, abuse, or life endangerment. SSA has implemented procedures to prevent inappropriate or erroneous disclosure of SSN information over the phone when a new number has been assigned in these situations, which includes domestic violence. The caller will be advised to go to the local field office for an in-person interview and properly identify himself or herself as the subject of the record before SSN information will be disclosed.

How accessible is the new number from the old number and vice versa?

SSA employees with proper clearances have access to cross-reference information, regardless of the reason why an individual has more than one SSN. This information is necessary to conduct SSA business. This is important information to share with your client so that he or she can make the most educated decision about their safety needs and options.

Section 57.3

Address Confidentiality Programs: Frequently Asked Questions

"Address Confidentiality Program: Frequently Asked Questions" © 2008 New Hampshire Department of Justice (www.doj.nh.gov). Reprinted with permission. Also included is "Address Confidentiality Programs," © 2007 National Coalition Against Domestic Violence (www.ncadv.org). All rights reserved. Reprinted with permission.

Persons attempting to escape from domestic violence, sexual assault, or stalking situations frequently establish new addresses in order to prevent their assailants from finding them. The address confidentiality program (ACP) will allow victims who move to a new location the opportunity to keep that address confidential.

What services does the program provide?

The program allows its participants to use the ACP substitute address whenever they obtain state and local services (a driver's license, food stamps, Medicaid, car registration, and so forth). Participants can also use the address to have other first class mail (with the exception of packages) forwarded to them from the substitute address to their actual, confidential, location.

The program will also allow participants, who are otherwise eligible to vote, to apply to vote as an absentee voter. Additionally, neither the participant's name nor address shall appear on any list of registered voters made available to the public.

Eligibility Guidelines

The ACP is intended to help victims who have permanently left abusive situations and are living in a location unknown to their abuser.

509

This means that the victim should have recently moved or is planning on moving in the near future. Additionally, the victim should not have created any local or state records using the new address they wish to keep confidential. ACP services are not retroactive and cannot provide confidentiality or protection if records have already been created with the new address.

Any adult person, a parent or guardian acting on behalf of a minor, or guardian acting on behalf of an incapacitated person, may apply to the program if they are a victim of domestic violence, sexual assault, or stalking, and meet the eligibility guidelines. Having a restraining order, criminal charges pending, or even reporting the abuse to law enforcement are not required in order to participate in the ACP.

Am I eligible?

Here are a few questions you should ask yourself if you think the ACP might be an appropriate program for you:

- Are you a victim or parent/guardian of a victim of domestic violence, sexual assault, or stalking?

- Do you live in the state where you are applying?

- Have you recently moved to a permanent location where your abuser or assailant does not know where you live? If not, are you planning on relocating n the next few weeks?

- Do you work where the abuser or assailant knows? (ACP won't work if the abuser/assailant knows where the victim goes to school or work and has a way to track them down)

- Have you created any state or local government documents (driver's license, car registration, food stamps, state assistance, registered to vote, and so forth) using your current residential address? If so, are you planning on moving to a new address in a few weeks?

- Are you willing to make the ACP your agent to receive mail and legal documents? This means you cannot evade your legal responsibilities (subpoena, divorce or custody orders, arrest warrant, and so forth). This also means that the ACP must always know how to reach you by mail and phone.

- Can you manage if your mail (including state assistance checks or child support) is delayed by as much as 5–7 days?

- Will the ACP substitute address actually help minimize a particular danger or risk?

If you answered "no" to any of these questions then the ACP may not be appropriate for you.

What must I do?

Since the ACP is only one piece of an overall safety plan, state laws vary in application requirements. For example, New Hampshire mandates that anyone interested in applying for the program access one of the 14 crisis centers in New Hampshire for consultation and assistance. It is very important that the applicants have the opportunity to discuss their situation with a trained domestic violence, stalking, and/or sexual assault advocate to explain all of the options and services available to them.

The services provided by crisis centers are free, confidential, and available regardless of age, race, gender, or sexual orientation. Some of the services include the following:

- Safety planning

- 24-hour hotline access

- Emergency shelter and transportation

- Legal advocacy in obtaining restraining order

- Hospital and court accompaniment

- Information and referrals to other service agencies

- Information on obtaining a legal name or social security number change

Address Confidentiality Programs: Why It Matters

Domestic violence is a pattern of behaviors involving physical, sexual, and emotional abuse by an intimate partner for the purpose of establishing and maintaining power and control over the other partner.[1] Violence frequently escalates when batterers believe that they are losing control of their victims, thus exposing victims to the greatest risk of serious injury or death when victims attempt to flee violent relationships.[2] Because many states allow information from voter registration and drivers' licenses to be accessible by the public, batterers often search public records to obtain their victims' physical addresses in order to stalk them. State-operated address confidentiality programs (ACP) provide victims of domestic violence—and in some states, stalking and sexual assault—with a legal substitute address to prevent their perpetrators from using public records to track them down.[3]

What do address confidentiality programs do?

* ACP provide victims with a substitute address, often the Secretary of State's address or a P.O. box on public records, thereby retaining confidentiality of their location.

* The Secretary of State's office or other government agency serves as an agent that collects and forwards all first class mail to victims.

* There are narrowly statutorily specified circumstances in which the actual address may be disclosed to:

  * law enforcement officials;

  * government officials, upon a showing of a bona fide statutory or administrative requirement for the physical address; or,

  * other third parties pursuant to a court order.

Why are ACPs important?

* One in four women will experience domestic violence during her lifetime.[4]

* 81% of women who are stalked by a current or former intimate partner are physically assaulted by that partner and 31% are sexually assaulted.[5]

Address Confidentiality Programs by State

* Twenty-four states currently operate address confidentiality programs and thirteen states offer confidential voter registration.

* Two states offer confidential motor vehicle registration, one state offers health insurance confidentiality, one state offers confidentiality for public utilities and government entities, one state offers confidentiality for child support and economic assistance

programs, one state offers jury duty exemptions, and three states have pending legislation with similar programs.

• One state opens their program to victims of domestic violence, sexual assault, stalking, and/or human trafficking; and nineteen states open their programs to victims of domestic violence, sexual assault, and stalking.

• One state opens their program to victims of domestic violence and sexual assault only, one state to victims of domestic violence and stalking only, and eight states only allow victims of domestic violence to apply.

Registration Requirements

• Many states require victims to apply for a confidential address through an enrolling agency, such as a domestic violence shelter/program, sexual assault crisis program, state or local agency, law enforcement office, certified advocate groups or victim assistance programs, or through an enrolling agent such as an application assistant or trained advocate.

• While some states require victims to report the abuse to law enforcement or to have obtained an order of protection, others only require eligibility to apply for a restraining order. Most states require that they have left the abuser and live at an unknown address.

• Although a few states require that the perpetrator be an intimate partner or family member, most states allow ACP registration for those who are victims of domestic violence, sexual assault, or stalking.

• A few states require victims to register a post office box, as opposed to a government agency, as their substitute address.

Real ID Act of 2005

• The passage of the Real ID Act in 2005 endangers victims of domestic violence, sexual assault, and stalking by jeopardizing their confidentiality.

  • Section 206(b)(6) of the Act requires that all applicants for drivers licenses or state identification cards must furnish their principal residence address to obtain a federally valid license or ID card.

- Section 827 of the Violence Against Women Act of 2005 includes a requirement for Department of Homeland Security (DHS) to give special consideration to victims of domestic abuse, sexual assault, stalking, or trafficking who are entitled to enroll in state ACP when the agency is "developing regulations or guidance with regard to identification documents, including drivers licenses." These groups include domestic violence and sexual assault victims.[6]

- The DHS draft regulations of March 2007 provided an exemption for those individuals enrolled in a state ACP (pg. 18) and proposed an exemption for individuals who are entitled to enroll in state ACP (pg. 36).[7]

Address Confidentiality Programs in Your State (as of June 30, 2007)

- Arizona: A.R.S. § 16-153
- Arkansas: A.C.A. §27-16-811
- California: West's Ann. Cal. Gov. Code §6206
- Colorado: HB 1350; C.R.S.A. § 24-21-201 (West 2007)
- Connecticut: C.G.S.A. § 54-240
- Delaware: 15 Del. C §1303; 21 Del. C §305
- Florida: F.S.A. § 741.465
- Illinois: 750 ILCS 61/1
- Indiana: IC 5-26.5-2-1
- Kansas: K.S.A. 75-451 through 75-458
- Louisiana: LSA-R.S. 44:52
- Maine: 5 M.R.S.A. § 90-B
- Maryland: MD Code, Family Law §4-519 through 4-530
- Massachusetts: 950 CMR 130
- Minnesota:* M.S.A. §5B.03
- Missouri: HB 610, SB 366, and SB 372**
- Montana: MCA 40-15-115 through 40-15-120
- Nebraska: Neb. Rev. St. §42-1201 through 42-1210
- Nevada: N.R.S.217.462

- New Hampshire: N.H. Rev. Stat. § 743
- New Jersey: N.J.S.A. 474-4
- New Mexico: HB 216*
- New York: Chapter 246 A. 1377-C; Stringer I S.936-B Balboni
- North Carolina: N.C.G.S.A. § 15C-3
- Oklahoma: 22 Okl. St. Ann. § 60.14
- Oregon: O.R.S. § 192.820 to 192.86
- Pennsylvania: 23 Pa.C.S.A. § 6703
- Rhode Island: RI ST § 17-28-3
- Tennessee: T.C.A. 10-7-504
- Texas: SB 74 and HB 569 *
- Vermont: 15 V.S.A. §1150-1160
- Virginia: Va. Code Ann. § 24.2-418
- Washington: West's RCW 40.24.030
- Wisconsin: W.S.A. 6.47

* Recently signed into law

**Pending legislation

For More Information or to Get Help

National Domestic Violence Hotline
P.O. Box 161810
Austin, TX 78716
Toll-Free Hotline: 800-799-SAFE (7233)
Toll-Free TTY: 800-787-3224
Website: http://www.ndvh.org

National Sexual Assault Hotline
Rape, Abuse & Incest National Network (RAINN)
2000 L Street, NW, Suite 406
Washington, DC 20036
Toll-Free: 800-656-HOPE (4673)
Phone: 202-544-3064
Fax: 202-544-3556
Website: http://www.rainn.org
E-mail: info@rainn.org

Sources

1. Pirro, Jeanine Ferris, Westchestser County DA (1997) *Commission on Domestic Violence Fatalities Report to the Governor*. Retrieved June 27, 2007 from New York State Office for the Prevention of Domestic Violence Website: http://www.opdv .state.ny.us/publications/fatality/part3.html.

2. Farr, KA (2002). Battered Women Who Were 'Being Killed and Survived It': Straight Talk from Survivors. *Violence & Victims*, 17, 267–281.

3. (2003) *Address Confidentiality Program for Victims Fleeing Violence*. Retrieved June 27, 2007 from Pennsylvania Coalition Against Domestic Violence Website: http://www.pcadv.org/ publications/AddConf.faxable.pdf.

4. Thoennes, N., and Tjaden, P. (2000). *Extent, Nature and Consequences of Intimate Partner Violence*. National Institute of Justice and Centers for Disease Control and Prevention, 5.

5. Thoennes, N., and Tjaden, P. (1998). *Stalking in America: Findings from the National Violence Against Women Survey*. National Institute of Justice and Centers for Disease Control and Prevention, 2.

6. Title VII, Subtitle C, Sec. 827 (Pub. L. 109–162, 119 Stat. 2960, 3066, Jan. 5, 2006).

7. "Minimum Standards for Driver's Licenses and Identification Cards Acceptable by Federal Agencies for Official Purposes; Notice of Proposed Rulemaking" *72 Federal Register 46* (9 March 2007) pp. 18, pp. 36.

Section 57.4

Internet Safety

Warning: Taking all of the listed actions may not prevent an abuser from discovering your e-mail and internet activity. The safest way to find information on the internet is to go to a safer computer. Some suggestions would be your local library, a friend's house, or your workplace. Other safety suggestions: Change your password often, do not pick obvious words or numbers for your password, and make sure to include a combination of letters and numbers for your password.

How an Abuser Can Track Your Activities

E-mail

If an abuser has access to your e-mail account, he or she may be able to read your incoming and outgoing mail. Even if you believe your account is secure, make sure you choose a password he or she will not be able to guess.

If an abuser sends you threatening or harassing e-mail messages, you can print and save them as evidence of this abuse. These messages may also constitute a federal offense. For more information on this issue, contact your local United States Attorney's Office.

Erasing Your Tracks

History/Cache File

If an abuser knows how to read your computer's history or cache file (automatically saved web pages and graphics), he or she may be able to see information you have viewed on the internet. You can clear your history or empty your cache file in your browser's settings.

Netscape: Pull down Edit menu, select Preferences. Click on Navigator or choose Clear History. Click on Advanced then select Cache. Click on Clear Disk Cache.

Internet Explorer: Pull down Tools menu, select Internet Options. On General page under Temporary Internet Files, click on Delete Files. If asked, check the box to delete all offline content. Still within the Temporary Internet Files section, click on Setting (This step may make it harder to navigate pages where you would like your information to be remembered, but these remaining cookies do show website pages you have visited. Therefore, use your own judgment as to whether or not to take this next step). Click on View Files, manually highlight all the files (cookies) shown, then hit Delete. Close that window, then on General page under History section, click on Clear History.

AOL: Pull down Members menu, select Preferences. Click on WWW icon. Then select Advanced. Purge Cache.

Additionally, you need to make sure that the Use Inline Autocomplete box is not checked. This function will complete partial web addresses while typing location in the address bar at the top of the browser.

If you are using Internet Explorer, this box can be found on the MS Internet Explorer Page by clicking on Tools at the top of the screen, then Internet Options and then the Advanced tab. About halfway down there is a Use Inline Autocomplete box that can be checked or unchecked by clicking on it. Uncheck the box to disable the feature that automatically completes an internet address when you start typing in the internet address box.

Important: This information may not completely hide your tracks. Many browser types have features that display recently visited sites. The safest way to find information on the internet would be at a local library, a friend's house, or at work.

For More Information

Survivors and Technology CD
National Network to End Domestic Violence
2001 S Street, NW, Suite 400
Washington, DC 20009
Phone: 202-543-5566
Fax: 202-543-5626
Website: http://www.nnedv.org

NNEDV offers a CD that educates victims, survivors, and advocates about how abusers may employ technology to tract their victims and teaches victims how to use technology to their advantage.

Chapter 58

Temporary Assistance for Needy Families (TANF) and the Family Violence Option

Family Assistance

The Office of Family Assistance administers the Temporary Assistance for Needy Families (TANF) program. TANF provides assistance and work opportunities to needy families by granting states the federal funds and wide flexibility to develop and implement their own welfare programs.

What is the Temporary Assistance for Needy Families Program (TANF)?

TANF is a block grant program to help move recipients into work and turn welfare into a program of temporary assistance. Under the welfare reform legislation of 1996, TANF replaced the old welfare programs known as Aid to Families with Dependent Children (AFDC), the Job Opportunities and Basic Skills Training (JOBS) program and the Emergency Assistance (EA) program. The law ended federal entitlement to assistance and instead created TANF as a block grant that provides states and tribes federal funds each year. These funds cover benefits, administrative expenses, and services targeted to needy families.

This chapter includes text from "Fact Sheet: Office of Family Assistance," reviewed December 5, 2008, U.S. Department of Health and Human Services (HHS); and an excerpt from "Reauthorization of the Temporary Assistance for Needy Families (TANF) Program," *Federal Register: February 5, 2008* (Volume 73, Number 24), HHS.

Congress passed, and President Bush signed into law, legislation that reauthorized the Temporary Assistance for Needy Families (TANF) program of 1996. The Deficit Reduction Act of 2005 reauthorized the TANF program through fiscal year (FY) 2010 with a renewed focus on work, program integrity, and strengthening families through healthy marriage promotion and responsible fatherhood.

Major Goals

The four purposes of TANF are:

- assisting needy families so that children can be cared for in their own homes;
- reducing the dependency of needy parents by promoting job preparation, work, and marriage;
- preventing out-of-wedlock pregnancies; and
- encouraging the formation and maintenance of two-parent families.

Highlights of TANF

Work requirements:

- Recipients (with few exceptions) must work as soon as they are job ready or no later than two years after coming on assistance.
- Single parents are required to participate in work activities for at least 30 hours per week. Two-parent families must participate in work activities 35 or 55 hours a week, depending upon circumstances.
- Failure to participate in work requirements can result in a reduction or termination of benefits to the family.
- States cannot penalize single parents with a child under six for failing to meet work requirements if they cannot find adequate childcare.
- States have to ensure that 50 percent of all families and 90 percent of two-parent families are participating in work activities. If a state reduces its caseload below the FY 2005 level, without restricting eligibility, it can receive a caseload reduction credit. This credit reduces the minimum participation rates the state must achieve.

Work activities that count toward a state's participation rates (some restrictions may apply) include the following:

- unsubsidized or subsidized employment
- on-the-job training
- work experience
- community service
- job search—not to exceed six total weeks and no more than four consecutive weeks
- vocational training—not to exceed 12 months
- job skills training related to work
- satisfactory secondary school attendance
- providing child care services to individuals who are participating in community service

Five-year time limit:

- Families with an adult who has received federally funded assistance for a total of five years (or less at state option) are not eligible for cash aid under the TANF program.
- States may extend assistance beyond 60 months to not more than 20 percent of their caseload. They may also elect to provide assistance to families beyond 60 months using state-only funds or social services block grants.

Reauthorization of the Temporary Assistance for Needy Families (TANF) Program

This final rule implements changes to the Temporary Assistance for Needy Families (TANF) program required by the Deficit Reduction Act of 2005 (DRA) (Pub. L. 109-171). The DRA reauthorized the TANF program through fiscal year (FY) 2010 with a renewed focus on work, program integrity, and strengthening families through healthy marriage promotion and responsible fatherhood.

Family Violence Option for Domestic Violence

Effective on October 1, 2008, existing provisions in the law address work participation rate issues for states dealing with victims of domestic

521

violence. A state that elects the Family Violence Option under Section 402(a)(7) of the Social Security Act must screen and identify victims of domestic violence, refer such individuals to services, and, if needed, waive participation and other program requirements for as long as necessary to escape domestic violence. The rules at Part 260, Subpart B allow states to grant good cause domestic violence waivers to victims of domestic violence that waive various program requirements, including work requirements. States have broad flexibility in determining which program requirements to waive and for how long. Although these recipients remain in the work participation rate calculation, there may be some activities that meet one of the work activity definitions that would make them countable toward the participation rate. If a state fails to meet a work participation rate, the federal government will determine that it had reasonable cause if the state can demonstrate that it failed to meet the rate due to granting federally recognized good cause domestic violence waivers. In this circumstance, the federal government would recalculate the work participation rate taking out any families in which individuals received a federally recognized good cause domestic violence waiver of work participation requirements.

Chapter 59

Assistance for Immigrant Victims of Domestic Violence

Chapter Contents

Section 59.1

Options and Help for Immigrant or Refugee Women

Domestic violence can be fatal. Thirty percent of women who are murdered in this country die at the hands of their husbands or partners. Abusers use violence in their relationships as a way to exert power and control their intimate partners and the family. Domestic violence takes many forms: It includes verbal, physical, economic, emotional, and sexual abuse.

If your partner has used any of the following forms of abuse, you may be in a violent and abusive relationship.

- He has hit, shoved, kicked, punched, choked, or used any other type of physical abuse.

- He has forced you to have sex when you didn't want to.

- He has used or threatened you with knives, guns, or other objects.

- He has humiliated, or insulted you, sometimes in front of others.

- He doesn't let you study or work outside the home.

- He's threatened to withdraw his support to help you obtain permanent residence status (green card) or United States citizenship.

- He has threatened to call immigration to have you deported.

- He is overly jealous.

- He has threatened to take away the children.

- He doesn't allow you to see your family or your friends.

- He controls the finances and does not give you access to money for the home.

- He controls where you go, who you speak with, and what you can do.

- He tells you that the violence is your fault.

You Are Not Alone

Unfortunately, many women are in relationships where there is abuse and violence. Sometimes these behaviors cause women to be intimidated and scared and they do not dare to seek help for fear of the consequences.

What can I do?

There are several services and options available to help you stop violence in your home:

- Community services, including domestic violence programs

- Legal assistance (protection orders, custody, child support, divorce)

- Shelters, safe houses

- Police intervention and assistance

- Medical assistance at hospitals, clinics, or local medical centers

- The National Domestic Violence Hotline

Almost all services are free of charge and provide assistance regardless of legal status.

Should I leave the home if I am in danger?

Absolutely. The first thing you should do if you are in danger of being beaten is to leave and go to a safe place as soon as possible. If you have children, take them with you wherever you go. Go to a friend's house or a shelter for women and children where you will feel safe and secure. Once you are there, you can obtain services you may need or information about what options and community services are available to you.

If you leave your home, be sure to take important documents with you. For example: passports, visas, work authorization card, birth and marriage certificates, tax returns, police reports, and medical reports. Keep copies of these documents in a safe place.

What is a protection order?

A protection order prohibits the abuser from coming near, attacking, or contacting you or your children. Through a protection order, in many states, you may also ask for custody of the children and for child support. You can also prevent the abuser from returning to the home, prevent him from interfering with your immigration status, and you can establish a visitation arrangement.

These are your rights, regardless of your immigration status. If you are thinking of requesting a protection order, first speak to a counselor in a domestic violence program to ask for relevant information.

If I am an immigrant woman and I call the police, what can happen?

If you call the police, they can help you find a safe place and accompany you there. It is possible your partner may be arrested because domestic violence is a crime. However, it is possible he may be freed in a few hours.

Ask the police to complete a report about the incident and give you a copy. Be aware that the police should not ask you for your immigration status or report you to the Immigration and Naturalization Service (INS). Their duty is protect you and your children.

Can I get lawful permanent residency without my husband's help?

Domestic violence is against the law and you have the right to be protected. There are laws to protect immigrant women who are victims of abuse. Depending on your situation, it is possible you can apply for permanent residence or a visa.

It is important to know that the only agency that can deport you is the INS. No one else can do that. Do not proceed without consulting with a domestic violence or immigration agency or a lawyer.

Self-petition: You can ask for permanent residence for yourself and your children in the following situations:

- You are married or were married to the abuser in good faith.
- Your husband or former husband is a permanent resident or citizen of the United States.
- You have not had legal problems.

- You have been or are being abused by your husband. Keep proof of abuse (medical or police reports, photos of bruises or injuries, notes taken by staff at a domestic violence program or by your social worker).

- If you have gotten a divorce or became a widow and have proof this happened during the two years prior to the petition. Once the petition has been approved, you can request a work permit and can become eligible for certain public benefits.

Cancellation of removal: Likewise, if you have been arrested, detained, or notified by the Immigration and Naturalization Service that you will be deported for not having proper documentation, you can request that the immigration court waive your deportation and grant you residency.

Other options and services: There are other ways of becoming a permanent resident or getting a visa. It would be beneficial for you to request help from programs that work with domestic violence or with immigrant women and that may have access to qualified lawyers. They can help you understand your situation and explain your legal rights.

- **Asylum:** For immigrants who are scared of returning to their countries for fear of being killed and do not qualify for self-petitioned residency because they are not married to permanent residents or to U.S. citizens.

- **U and T visas:** For immigrants who are victims of domestic violence crimes or of illegal human trafficking and are helping the legal system with the prosecution.

- **Family based option:** For women who have adult relatives who are U.S. citizens.

You must know that the options presented here are complex and should not be pursued without the assistance of an immigration lawyer or of an organization that is well informed about new immigration laws. It is recommended that you do not place yourself at risk by going to the Immigration and Naturalization Service by yourself.

There are many places that offer help 24-hour support, emergency shelters, legal services, and information about safe options for yourself or your friends.

Section 59.2

Legal Protections for Battered Immigrants

"Immigration Issues and Domestic Violence,"
© 2008 AARDVARC.org, Inc. Reprinted with permission.
For additional information, visit www.aardvarc.org.

Immigration Issues and Domestic Violence

How do I apply for immigration benefits as a battered spouse or child?

Generally, U.S. citizens (USC) and lawful permanent residents (LPR) file an immigrant visa petition with the U.S. Citizenship and Immigration Services (USCIS) on behalf of a spouse or child, so that these family members may emigrate to or remain in the United States. USCIS Form I-130, Petition for Alien Relative is filed by the USC/LPR, the petitioner, on behalf of the family member who is the beneficiary. The petitioner controls when or if the petition is filed. Unfortunately, some U.S. citizens and LPR misuse their control of this process to abuse their family members, or by threatening to report them to the USCIS. As a result, most battered immigrants are afraid to report the abuse to the police or other authorities.

Under the Violence Against Women Act (VAWA) passed by Congress in 1994, the spouses and children of United States citizens or lawful permanent residents may self-petition to obtain lawful permanent residency. The immigration provisions of VAWA allow certain battered immigrants to file for immigration relief without the abuser's assistance or knowledge, in order to seek safety and independence from the abuser. Victims of domestic violence should know that help is available to them through the National Domestic Violence hotline at 800-799-7233 or 800-787-3224 (TDD) for information about shelters, mental health care, legal advice, and other types of assistance, including information about self-petitioning for immigration status.

What is the Legal Foundation?

The Immigration and Nationality Act (INA) is the law that governs immigration in the United States. The Violence Against Women

Act (VAWA) provisions relating to immigration are codified in section 204(a) of the INA. Rules published in the *Federal Register* explain the eligibility requirements and procedures for filing a self-petition under the VAWA provisions. These rules can be found in the Code of Federal Regulations at 8 CFR&204. The Battered Immigrant Women Protection Act of 2000 (BIWPA) made significant amendments to section 204(a) of the INA. Self-petitions may be filed according to the amended requirements.

Who is Eligible?

To be eligible to file a self-petition (an application that you file for yourself for immigration benefits) you must qualify under one of the following categories:

- **Spouse:** You may self-petition if you are a battered spouse married to a U.S. citizen or lawful permanent resident. Unmarried children under the age of 21, who have not filed their own self-petition, may be included on your petition as derivative beneficiaries.

  1. The self-petitioning spouse must be legally married to the U.S. citizen or LPR batterer. A self-petition may be filed if the marriage was terminated by the death of the abusive spouse within the two years prior to filing. A self-petition may also be filed if the marriage to the abusive spouse was terminated, within the two years prior to filing, by divorce related to the abuse.

  2. The self-petitioning spouse must have been battered in the United States, unless the abusive spouse is an employee of the United States government or a U.S. military member.

  3. The self-petitioning spouse must have been battered or subjected to extreme cruelty during the marriage, or must be the parent of a child who was battered or subjected to extreme cruelty by the U.S. citizen or lawful permanent resident spouse during the marriage.

  4. The self-petitioning spouse is required to be a person of good moral character. This doesn't mean that you cannot have ever done anything wrong. Victims in abusive relationships often are forced or coerced into doing things they normally would not do, or must do things in order to survive. Authorities understand this, and will evaluate your case based on the total circumstances.

5. The self-petitioning spouse must have entered into the marriage in good faith, not solely for the purpose of obtaining immigration benefits.

*   **Parent:** You may self-petition if you are the parent of a child who has been abused by your U.S. citizen or lawful permanent resident spouse. Your children (under 21 years of age and unmarried), including those who may not have been abused, may be included on your petition as derivative beneficiaries, if they have not filed their own self-petition.

*   **Child:** You may self-petition if you are a battered child (under 21 years of age and unmarried) who has been abused by your U.S. citizen or lawful permanent resident parent. Your children (under 21 years of age and unmarried), including those who may not have been abused, may be included on your petition as derivative beneficiaries. They must qualify as the child of the abuser as child is defined in the INA for immigration purposes. Any relevant credible evidence that can prove the relationship with the parent will be considered.

How do I apply for benefits?

To self-petition, you must complete and file USCIS Form I-360 (Petition for Amerasian, Widow(er), or Special Immigrant) and include all supporting documentation. Self-petitions should be sent by certified return receipt mail (or any other method providing assurance of receipt). You should keep a copy of everything you submit, including the application and all accompanying documents, in addition to the proof of mailing.

Forms are available in person at a USCIS office, by calling 800-870-3676, or through the INS website at http://www.uscis.gov. Please see the USCIS Field Office locator for more information on USCIS service centers. It is available online at https://egov.uscis.gov/crisgwi/go?action=offices.type&OfficeLocator.office_type=LO.

What is the process?

Notice of receipt: You should receive an acknowledgement or Notice of Receipt within a few weeks after mailing the application and fee to the USCIS.

***Prima facie* determination:** Battered immigrants filing self-petitions who can establish a *prima facie* case are considered qualified aliens for the purpose of eligibility for public benefits (Section 501 of the Illegal Immigrant Responsibility and Immigration Reform Act [IIRIRA]). The USCIS reviews each petition initially to determine whether the self-petitioner has addressed each of the requirements listed and has provided some supporting evidence. This may be in the form of a statement that addresses each requirement. This is called a *prima facie* determination.

If the Service makes a *prima facie* determination, the self-petitioner will receive a Notice of *Prima Facie* Determination valid for 150 days. The notice may be presented to state and federal agencies that provide public benefits.

Approved self-petition: If the I-360 self-petition is approved, the Service may exercise the administrative option of placing the self-petitioner in deferred action, if the self-petitioner does not have legal immigration status in the United States. Deferred action means that the Service will not initiate removal (deportation) proceedings against the self-petitioner. States have the authority to grant appropriate extensions of deferred action beyond initial time periods upon receipt of a request for extension from the self-petitioner.

Employment authorization: Self-petitioners and their derivative children who have an approved Form I-360 and are placed in deferred action are also eligible for an Employment Authorization Card. To apply, USCIS Form I-765 (Application for Employment Authorization) should be filed. Applicants should indicate that they are seeking employment authorization pursuant to 8 CFR 274a.12(c)(14). The Form I-765 must be filed with a copy of the self-petitioner's USCIS Form I-360 approval notice.

Adjustment to permanent resident status: Self-petitioners who qualify as immediate relatives of U.S. citizens (spouses and unmarried children under the age of 21) do not have to wait for an immigrant visa number to become available. They may file USCIS Form I-485 (Application to Register Permanent Residence or Adjust Status) with their local USCIS office. Self-petitioners who require a visa number to adjust must wait for a visa number to be available before filing the Form I-485. The wait for visa numbers can be anywhere from 2–10 years.

How do I file an appeal if my application is denied?

If your application is denied, the denial letter will tell you how to appeal.

Can anyone help me?

If advice is needed, you may contact the USCIS district office near your home for a list of community-based, non-profit organizations that may be able to assist you in applying for an immigration benefit. Please see the USCIS field offices website for more information on contacting USCIS offices. In addition, please see the INS information on finding legal advice.

Victims of domestic violence should know that help is also available to them through the National Domestic Violence Hotline at 800-799-7233 or 800-787-3224 [TDD] for information about shelters, mental health care, legal advice, and other types of assistance, including information about self-petitioning for immigration status.

Can a man file a self-petition under the Violence Against Women Act?

Yes. Although the self-petitioning provisions for victims of domestic violence are contained in the Violence Against Women Act, they apply equally to victims of either sex.

Must the self-petitioner remain married to the abusive spouse until the self-petition is approved?

The regulations only require that the self-petitioning spouse be married at the time of filing. After the self-petition has been filed, legal termination of the marriage will not usually affect the self-petition, but you may want to seek advice from an immigration attorney or legal advocate. Statutory changes, effective October 28, 2000, allow for the marriage to have been terminated (there are some restrictions) within two years prior to the date of filing.

Can a divorced spouse seek relief through self-petitioning?

Statutory changes, effective October 28, 2000, allow for the marriage to have been terminated (there are some restrictions) within two years prior to the date of filing. A battered spouse who does not meet these restrictions may be eligible for cancellation of removal. This is provided for under Section 240A(b)(2) of the INA. To qualify he or she must meet the other requirements that would be necessary for approval of a self-petition and must have been physically present in the U.S. for three years immediately preceding the filing of the application for cancellation of removal. A self-petition will also be denied if the self-petitioner remarries before filing or after filing and before the self-petition is approved. Remarriage after the self-petition has been approved will not affect the validity of the approved I-360 self-petition.

What if the abusive U.S. citizen/LPR already filed a Form I-130 petition on behalf of the victim, and it is either still pending or the abuser withdrew it?

A self-petitioner who is the beneficiary of a Form I-130 petition filed by the abusive spouse will be able to transfer the priority date of the Form I-130 petition to the I-360 self-petition. This is extremely important for self-petitioners who must wait for a visa number as an earlier priority date will result in a shorter waiting time.

For More Information

U. S. Citizenship and Immigration Services (USCIS)
Toll-Free: 800-375-5283
Toll-Free TTY: 800-767-1833
Website: http://www.uscis.gov/portal/site/uscis

Chapter 60

Child Custody and Visitation Decisions in Domestic Violence

Chapter Contents

Section 60.1

Legal Trends, Risk Factors, and Safety Concerns

This section includes text from: Saunders, D. (2007, October). *Child custody and visitation decisions in domestic violence cases: Legal trends, risk factors, and safety concerns.* Harrisburg, PA: VAWnet (www.vawnet.org), a project of the National Resource Center on Domestic Violence/Pennsylvania Coalition Against Domestic Violence, © 2007. Reprinted with permission. To view the full report, visit http://new.vawnet.org/category/Main_Doc.php?docid=1134.

It may be hard to believe that an abusive partner can ever make good on his threat to gain custody of the children from his victim. After all, he has a history of violent behavior and she almost never does. Unfortunately, a surprising number of battered women lose custody of their children (Saccuzzo and Johnson, 2004). This section describes how this can happen through uninformed and biased courts, court staff, evaluators, and attorneys and how the very act of protecting ones' children can lead to their loss. It also describes the major legal and social trends surrounding custody and visitation decisions and the social science evidence supporting the need to consider domestic violence in these decisions. It ends with some recommendations for custody and visitation in domestic violence cases.

Legal Trends

Over the past 200 years, the bases for child custody decisions have changed considerably. The patriarchal doctrine of fathers' ownership of children gave way in the 1920s and 1930s to little formal preference for one parent or the other to obtain custody. When given such broad discretion, judges tended to award custody to mothers, especially of young children. The mother-child bond during the early, "tender years" was considered essential for children's development. In the 1970s, "the best interests of the children" became the predominant guideline, although it remains somewhat ambiguous (Fine and Fine, 1994). It was presumably neutral regarding parental rights. Little was known then about the negative impact of domestic violence on women and children, and domestic violence was not originally included in the list of factors used to determine the child's best interest.

States more recently came to recognize that domestic violence needs to be considered in custody decisions (Dunford-Jackson, 2004; Cahn, 1991; Hart, 1992). Every state now lists domestic violence as a factor to be considered, but does not necessarily give it special weight. However, since the mid-1990s, states have increasingly adopted the custody and visitation section of the Model Code on Domestic and Family Violence developed by the National Council of Juvenile and Family Court Judges (NCJFCJ, 1994), increasing from ten states using the code in 1995 to 24 in 2006 (NCJFCJ, 1995a; 2007). These statutes use the model's wording, or similar wording, that there is a "rebuttable presumption that it is detrimental to the child and not in the best interest of the child to be placed in sole custody, joint legal custody, or joint physical custody with the perpetrator of family violence" (p. 33).[1] Although statutes have become increasingly precise regarding definitions of domestic violence, they may leave children vulnerable to psychological abuse when it is not included in the definition (Dunford-Jackson, 2004).

Statutes also address other issues about custody and visitation, such as standards for supervised visitation and similar safeguards (Girdner and Hoff, 1996; Hart, 1990; Jaffe, Lemon, and Poisson, 2003), exempting battered women from mandated mediation (Dunford-Jackson, 2004; Girdner, 1996),[2] protecting battered women from charges of "child abandonment" if they flee for safety without their children (Cahn, 1991), and enabling a parent to learn if a person involved in a custody proceeding has been charged with certain crimes (see Pennsylvania's Jen and Dave Program on the web at http://www.jendaveprogram.us). Some recent statutes make it easier for victims to relocate if needed for safety reasons (Jaffe, et al., 2003; NCJFCJ, 1995a; 1999; see Zorza, 2000).

Other legal protections are also available. For example, in one state (Tennessee), if a parent alleges that a child is exposed to domestic violence, such allegations cannot be used against the parent bringing the allegation (NCJFCJ, 2004). In another state (Texas), a mediated agreement can be declined by the court if domestic violence affected the victim's ability to make the agreement (NCJFCJ, 2005). Some states (Massachusetts, Ohio) now make the presumption that custody or visitation should not be granted to anyone who is found guilty of murdering the other parent (for a more complete review of the above trends, including legal reforms in Australia, Canada, and New Zealand, see Jaffe, et al. 2003).

Unfortunately, courts and the mental health professionals advising them (Johnson, Saccuzzo, and Koen, 2005; Fields, in press) and lawyers (Fields, 2006) may pressure women to stay tied to their abusers. In addition, "friendly parent" provisions in statutes or policies create another factor for courts to assess in custody decisions, favoring the parent who will encourage frequent and continuing contact with the other parent or foster a better relationship between the child and the other parent (Zorza, 1992). Despite a reasonable reluctance to co-parent out of fear of harm to themselves or their children, battered women may end up being labeled "unfriendly," thereby increasing the risk of losing their children (American Psychological Association [APA], 1996).

Along with legal changes, training and resource manuals for judges and court managers are available, including guidelines for selecting custody evaluators and guardians *ad litem* (Dalton, Drozd, and Wong, 2006; Maxwell and Oehme, 2001; Goelman, Lehrman, and Valente, 1996; Lemon, Jaffe, and Ganley, 1995; NCJFCJ, 1995b; NCJFCJ, 2006; National Center for State Courts, 1997). One bench-book covers cultural considerations for diverse populations (Ramos and Runner, 1999). A recent trend is the use of "parenting coordinators" or "special masters," a mental health or legal professional with mediation training who focuses on the children's needs and helps the parents resolve disputes. With the approval of the parties and/or the court, they can make decisions within the bounds of the court order. The Association of Family and Conciliation Courts provide guidelines for parenting coordinators and a discussion of implementation issues (AFCC, 2006; Coates, et al., 2004). The guidelines require that parenting coordinators have training on domestic violence and caution that "the parenting coordinator's role may be inappropriate and potentially exploited by perpetrators of domestic violence who have exhibited patterns of violence, threat, intimidation, and coercive control over their co-parent" (AFCC, 2006, p. 165). When one parent seeks to maintain dominance over another, the parenting coordinator may need to act primarily as an enforcer of the court order.

Another legal trend is the ordering of "virtual visitation" (Flango, 2003; Shefts, 2002). Web cams and video conferencing can supplement face-to-face visits or replace face-to-face visits in more dangerous cases. Parents can read and play games with their children and help them with homework. The practice may loosen restrictions on parents moving to different communities. In one court case, the judge ordered each parent to purchase and install computer equipment that would allow video-conferencing (Flango, 2003). In 2004, Utah passed a law stating that virtual visitation should be permitted and encouraged if

538

available. In some states, prisons provide virtual visitation services (Pennsylvania Department of Corrections, http://www.cor.state.pa.us/ dallas/site/default.asp). Virtual visits are untested in domestic violence cases and are likely to require the same type of monitoring that occurs with telephone and in-person visits.

Despite the above trends for improved protections, some parents and children believe the legal system has failed them. They may form grassroots support and advocacy groups, such as networks in Arizona (http://www.azppn.com) and California (http://www.protectiveparents .com), that conduct court watches and help parents share common court experiences, especially when they lose custody when trying to protect children and themselves from abuse. The Courageous Kids Network in California makes suggestions to other children who are forced to live with an abuser or molester when professionals do not believe them. They describe themselves as "a growing group of young people whose childhood was shattered by biased and inhumane court rulings, which forced us to live with our abusive parents while restricting or sometimes completely eliminating contact with our loving and protective parent. We know how horrible it is to be forced into the arms of an abuser" (http://www.courageouskids.net). A national organization, Kourts for Kids, works to better protect abused children in the family courts by increasing awareness and education for judges, attorneys, guardians *ad litem*, social workers, officers of the law, legislators, and advocates (http://www.kourtsforkids.org/index.php?option =com_frontpage&Itemid=1). In 2007, ten mothers and a victimized child (now an adult) and national and state organizations filed suit against the United States with the Inter-American Commission on Human Rights. They claimed that the human rights of abused mothers and children were not protected because custody was awarded to abusers and child molesters (Klein, 2007; Stop Family Violence: http:// www.stopfamilyviolence.org/ocean/host.php?folder=3).

In summary, courts in all states must now consider domestic violence in custody and visitation decisions, but only about half of them make it the primary consideration. Legal innovations include protections for survivors who need to relocate due to safety concerns and exemptions from mandated mediation. Many states still have "friendly parent" statutes that do not recognize battered women's realistic reluctance to co-parent. Domestic violence training materials and guidelines are increasingly available for judges, court managers, custody evaluators, and parenting coordinators. Recent trends include the use of "virtual visitation" and the development of grass roots protective parent and advocacy organizations.

Parent Most at Risk for Physically and Emotionally Abusing the Children

Social science evidence can help establish which parent is most at risk to harm their children. The most convincing evidence that men who batter their partners are also likely to batter their children comes from a nationally representative survey (Straus, 1983). Half the men who battered their wives also abused their children. Abuse was defined as violence more severe than a slap or a spanking. Battered women were half as likely as men to abuse their children. Several non-representative surveys show similar results (reviewed in Saunders, 1994, and Edleson, 2001). When battered women are not in a violent relationship, there is some evidence that they are much less likely to direct anger toward their children (Walker, 1984). As expected, time away from the abuser seems to benefit battered mothers and their children (Rossman, 2001).

Emotional abuse of children by men who batter is even more likely than physical abuse because nearly all of these men's children are exposed to domestic violence (Wolfe, Crooks, McIntyre-Smith, and Jaffe, 2004). This exposure to domestic abuse by their fathers often constitutes a severe form of child abuse. The serious problems associated with witnessing abuse are now clearly documented (Edleson, 1999; Graham-Bermann and Edleson, 2002; Kitzmann, Gaylord, Holt, and Kenny, 2003; Wolfe, Crooks, McIntyre-Smith, and Jaffe, 2004). These include short- and long-term negative emotional and behavioral consequences for both boys and girls. However, one must be cautious about generalizing these findings to most or all children since many children find resources that buffer the ill effects of the violence (Edleson, 2006). Parents may not realize that their children can be affected, even if they do not see the violence. For example, children may be hiding in their bedrooms listening to repeated threats, blows, and breaking objects. They may be afraid their mother will be injured or killed and in many cases they intervene physically (Edleson, Mbilinyi, Beeman, and Hagemeister, 2003). However, they may have other reactions, such as divided loyalties toward their parents, guilt about not being able to intervene effectively, and anger at their mother for not leaving (Margolin, 1998; Saunders, 1994). If mothers cannot find safety, their fears and depression may reduce their ability to nurture and support their children as they normally would (Jaffe and Crooks, 2005).

As a result of children's exposure to domestic violence, mothers may be unjustly blamed for harming their children in cases where evaluators and practitioners do not understand the dynamics of abuse (Edleson,

1999). Cases are sometimes labeled as a "failure to protect" since mothers are supposedly capable of protecting their children from the physical and emotional abuse of their partners (Enos, 1996). Battered women may even face criminal charges (Kaufman Kantor and Little, 2003; Sierra, 1997) or removal of their children into foster care (Edleson, Gassman-Pines, and Hill, 2006). However, battered women's actions usually come from their desire to care for and protect their children. They may not leave because of financial needs, family pressures, believing the children need a father, or the fear that he will make good on threats to harm the children or gain custody (Hardesty and Chung, 2006; Hardesty and Ganong, 2006). They often leave the relationship when they recognize the impact of violence on their children, only to return when threatened with even greater violence or out of economic necessity (Anderson and Saunders, 2003, 2007). Innovative programs have been developed to address these concerns by helping to coordinate the actions of child protection, domestic violence, and family court systems. The "Greenbook Initiative" sponsored by the federal government is a notable example (Dunford-Jackson, 2004; for information see: http://www.thegreenbook.info). On a policy level, a few states allow evidence to show that the non-abusive spouse feared retaliation from her partner and thus could not reasonably prevent abuse to the child. However, most of these states impose restrictions on how quickly the protective parent must provide this evidence and how it must be done (Jaffe, et al., 2003).

Factors Related to Risk of Child Abuse

In a given custody case, a number of factors may correctly or incorrectly be attributed to the risk of child abuse and exposure to domestic violence. Several of these factors—parental separation, childhood victimization of the parents, the parents' psychological characteristics, and abuser interventions—are discussed next.

Parental Separation

Parental separation or divorce does not prevent abuse to children or their mothers. On the contrary, physical abuse, harassment, and stalking of women continue at fairly high rates after separation and divorce and sometimes only begin or greatly escalate after separation (Hardesty and Chung, 2006). Homicidal threats, stalking, and harassment affect as many as 25%–35% of survivors (Bachman and Saltzman, 1995; Leighton, 1989; Thoennes and Tjaden, 2000). In addition, up to a fourth of battered women report that their ex-partner threatened to hurt the children or kidnap them (Liss and Stahly, 1993), and children may witness violence more often after separation than before (Hardesty and Chung, 2006). Separation is a time of increased risk of homicide for battered women (Saunders and Browne, 2000), and these homicides sometimes occur in relation to custody hearings and visitation exchanges.

Many abusers appear to use the legal system to maintain contact and harass their ex-partners (Bancroft and Silverman, 2002; Hardesty and Ganong, 2006), at times using extensive and lengthy litigation (Jaffe, et al., 2003). Children may also be harmed if the abuser undermines their mothers' authority, disparages her character in front of the children, and attempts to use the children to control the mother (Bancroft and Silverman, 2004); this appears to occur more often after separation by the most severe abusers (Beeble, Bybee, and Sullivan, 2007). Children are also likely to be exposed to renewed violence if their fathers become involved with another woman. Over half of men who batter go on to abuse another woman (Wofford, Elliot, and Menard, 1994). As a result, judges should not necessarily consider the remarriage of the father as a sign of stability and maturity.

Parents' Characteristics

Evaluators may look to childhood risk factors of each parent to assess their child abuse potential. The link between being abused in childhood and becoming a child abuser is not as strong as was once thought, with about 30% of child abuse victims becoming child abusers (Kaufman and Zigler, 1987). Some evidence suggests that this link with child abuse is stronger in men than in women (Miller and Challas, 1981). Neither parent is likely to have severe and chronic mental disorders (for example, schizophrenia or bipolar disorder) (Gleason, 1997; Golding, 1999). Personality disorders, as distinct from mental disorders, are much more likely to appear on the psychological tests of the parents. However, the parents' personality traits and psychological disorders are generally poor predictors of child abuse (Wolfe, 1985). In addition, great care must be taken when interpreting parents' behaviors and psychological tests. Men who batter often have the types of personality disorders—such as anti-social, dependent, and narcissistic (Holtzworth-Munroe, Meehan, Herron, Rehman, and Stuart, 2000)—that may keep childhood traumas and other problems hidden from evaluators and judges.

To the extent that psychological disorders continue to be used to describe battered women, they can be placed at a serious disadvantage.

Compared with the chronic problems of her partner, a battered woman's psychological problems, primarily depression and posttraumatic stress disorder, appear to be reactions to the violence. These problems seem to decrease as victims become safer (Erickson, 2006). Many battered women may seem very unstable, nervous, and angry (APA, 1996; Erickson, 2006; Crites and Coker, 1988). Others may speak with a flat affect and appear indifferent to the violence they describe (Meier, 1993). These women probably suffer from the numbing symptoms of traumatic stress. The psychological test scores of some battered women may appear to indicate severe personality disorders and mental illness. However, their behaviors and test scores must be interpreted in the context of the traumas they faced or continue to face (Dalton, Drozd, and Wong, 2006; Dutton, 1992; Rosewater, 1987). For example, psychological test findings of borderline and paranoid traits can be misleading when the impact of domestic violence is not considered (Erickson, 2006). The psychological tactics used by abusers parallel those used against prisoners of war and include threats of violence, forced isolation, degradation, attempts to distort reality, and methods to increase psychological dependence (Stark, 2007). Severe depression and traumatic stress symptoms are the likely results (Golding, 1999). When women fear losing custody of children to an abusive partner, the stress can be overwhelming (Erickson, 2006; Bancroft and Silverman, 2004).

Interventions for the Abuser

Although there are numerous treatment programs around the country for abusive partners and parents, successful completion of a batterer intervention program does not mean that the risks of child and woman abuse are eliminated. The evaluation of programs for men who batter is in its infancy, including programs for men of color (Gondolf, in press; Saunders and Hammill, 2003). A substantial proportion of women (35% on average across a number of studies) report that physical abuse by their partners recurs within 6–12 months after treatment and psychological abuse often remains at high levels. In controlled studies, the recidivism rates average only 5% lower for the "treated" groups than the control groups (Babcock, Green, and Robie, 2004). These results are less optimistic than those implied in the section of the Model State Statute on Domestic and Family Violence (NCJFCJ, 1994) that recommends the successful completion of abuser treatment as a condition for visitation.

Only two studies of programs for men who batter investigated the reduction of actual or potential violence toward the children (Myers,

1984; Stacey and Shupe, 1984). Both of these studies showed promising results but did not specifically focus on parenting issues. Special parenting programs for men who batter have developed in recent years, either as modules within existing intervention programs or as stand-alone programs (Edleson, Mbilinyi, and Shetty, 2003; Edleson and Williams, 2007).

In summary, contrary to what one would expect, separation is a time of increased risk of violence, abusers' chronic problems may not be apparent, and the trauma from violence and continuing, intense fears may make battered women appear crazy. Furthermore, successful completion of an abuser intervention program does substantially reduce the risk of re-abuse on average.

Factors that Compromise Safety of Children and Survivors

Negative outcomes for domestic violence victims and their children include: (1) dangerous offenders in contact with ex-partners and children due to unsupervised or poorly supervised visitation; (2) sole or joint custody of children awarded to a violent parent, rather than a non-violent one; and, (3) urging or mandating mediation that compromises victims' rights or places them in more danger. Such negative outcomes are likely to be compounded for women of color, lesbian mothers, survivors whose English is not proficient, and/or immigrant women with little or no knowledge of the U.S. legal system (Barnsley, Goldsmith, Taylor, 1996; Ramos and Runner, 1999).

Joint custody can be quite beneficial for children of non-violent, low-conflict couples.[3] However, joint custody—in particular, joint physical custody or shared parenting—can obviously increase the opportunities for abusers to maintain control and to continue or to escalate abuse toward both women and children. Enthusiasm for joint custody[4] in the early 1980s was fueled by studies of couples who were highly motivated to "make it work" (Johnston, 1995). This enthusiasm has waned in recent years, in part because of social science findings. Solid evidence about the impact of divorce and custody arrangements is difficult to find because most data are gathered at one point in time, and thus statements about cause and effect are not possible (Bender, 1994). There is increasing evidence, however, that children of divorce have more problems because of the conflict between the parents before the divorce and not because of the divorce itself (Kelly, 1993). Johnston (1995) concluded from her review of research that "highly conflictual parents" (not necessarily violent) had a poor prognosis for becoming cooperative parents. In a study by Kelly (1993), more frequent transitions between high-conflict parents were related to more emotional and behavioral problems of the children. If exposure to high conflict parents is damaging to children, then they are even more likely to be damaged by exposure to domestic violence. We now have evidence that a high percentage of couples labeled high conflict are experiencing domestic violence, and thus attempts to detect domestic violence within high conflict families are crucial (for further review, see Jaffe and Crooks, 2007).

In general, domestic violence is often not detected or not documented in custody/visitation proceedings (Johnson, Saccuzzo and Koen, 2005; Kernic, Monary-Ernsdorff, Koepsell, and Holt, 2005). In one study that interviewed survivors with documented abuse, there were frequent failures to consider documentation of domestic abuse and/or child abuse in the custody decision; unsupervised visitation or custody was often recommended or granted to men who used violence against their partners and/or children (Silverman, Mesh, Cuthbert, Slote, and Bancroft, 2004). One study found that battered and non-battered women were equally likely to be awarded custody; in addition, offenders were just as likely as non-offenders to be ordered to supervised visits (Kernic, et al., 2005). Similarly, in a random sample of court cases, only minor differences existed between the custody evaluation process and custody recommendations for domestic violence versus non-domestic violence cases (Logan, Walker, Jordan, and Horvath, 2002). Most fathers with protection orders against them were not awarded custody (Rosen and O'Sullivan, 2005); however, this was not the case when mothers withdrew their petitions, which may have been from pressure from their abusers. Mediators in one study were about equally likely to recommend joint legal and physical custody for both domestic violence and non-domestic violence cases; rates of supervised and unsupervised visitation also did not differ between violent and non-violent cases (Johnson et al., 2005). Similarly, O'Sullivan and her colleagues report two studies showing that a history of domestic violence has little impact on courts' decisions regarding visitation (O'Sullivan, 2000; O'Sullivan, King, Levin-Russell, and Horowitz, 2006). (For further review, see Jaffe and Crooks, 2007.)

A number of reports from state and local commissions on gender bias in the courts have documented negative outcomes. For example, negative stereotypes about women, especially about their credibility, seem to encourage judges to disbelieve women's allegations about child abuse (Danforth and Welling, 1996; Meier, 2003; Zorza, 1996). A lack of understanding about domestic violence leads to accusations of lying, blaming the victim for the violence, and trivializing the violence (Abrams and Greaney, 1989). When the abuse is properly taken into account, court decisions that awarded abusive fathers custody are often reversed on appeal (Meier, 2003). Research evidence is now growing that allegations of domestic violence are generally not more common in disputed custody cases; and one study shows that mothers are more likely to have their abuse allegations substantiated than fathers (Johnston, Lee, Oleson, and Walters, 2005).

The influence of fathers' rights groups on evaluators and judges is unknown, but some groups tend to lobby for the presumption of joint custody and co-parenting and doubt the validity of domestic violence allegations (Williams, Boggess, and Carter, 2004). For example, the National Fathers' Resource Center (NFRC) and Fathers for Equal Rights, "demands that society acknowledge that false claims of domestic violence" are used to "gain unfair advantage in custody and divorce cases" (NFRC, 2007). They state, "Fathers' organizations now estimate that up to 80% of domestic violence allegations against men are false allegations." Consistent with what might be expected from the gender bias reports, female judges in one study showed more knowledge of domestic violence and greater support for victim protections (Morrill, Dai, Dunn, Sung, and Smith, 2005). Women of color and immigrant women can expect to be placed in double jeopardy, as many states report racial and ethnic bias in the courts, in addition to gender bias (Ramos and Runner, 1999).

Research is also illuminating the negative impact of friendly parent provisions. Zorza (1996; in press) notes that friendly parent statutes and policies work against battered women because any concerns they voice about father-child contact or safety for themselves are usually interpreted as a lack of cooperation and thus the father is more likely to gain custody. A woman might refuse to give her address or consent to unsupervised visitation (APA, 1996). Parents who raise concerns about child sexual abuse can be severely sanctioned for doing so. The sanctions include loss of custody to the alleged offender, restricted visitation, and being told not to report further abuse or take the child to a therapist (Faller and DeVoe, 1995; Neustein and Goetting, 1999; Neustein and Lesher, 2005). Even in jurisdictions with a presumption that custody should be awarded to the non-abusive parent, a friendly parent provision tends to override this presumption (Morrill, et al., 2005). At least 32 states have statutes with friendly parent provisions (Zorza, in press). "Unfriendly behaviors" generally include only those of the custodial parents and not behaviors of noncustodial parents, like nonpayment of child support (Zorza, in press).

The beliefs and training of custody evaluators and judges in relation to outcomes have received very little attention. Evaluators and judges may need more information on the continued safety risks to children from abusive fathers, the likelihood of post-separation violence, risks of mediation, the inadmissibility of parent alienation syndrome (Dalton, Drozd, and Wong, 2006), false allegations, and the limits of criminal justice and treatment interventions (Jaffe, Lemon, and Poisson, 2003; Saunders, 1994). Ackerman and Ackerman (1996) found that psychologists who conducted child custody evaluations did not consider domestic violence to be a major factor in making a recommendation. However, three-fourths of them recommended against sole or joint custody to a parent who "alienates the child from the other parent by negatively interpreting the other parent's behavior." In a more recent study of evaluators, Bow and Boxer (2003) found that many sources of information were used in evaluations, but evaluators did not tend to use domestic violence screening instruments— only 30% administered specialized questionnaires, instruments, or tests pertaining to domestic violence. When domestic violence was detected, it weighed heavily in their recommendations. In one study of judges, those with domestic violence education and more knowledge of domestic violence were more likely to grant sole custody to abused mothers (Morrill, et al., 2005). Some states require initial and/or continuing domestic violence education for judges,[5] custody evaluators, and mediators, which is essential to close the gap between professional standards and their implementation (Jaffe and Crooks, 2005).

Recommendations for Custody and Visitation

Some recommendations can be made based on practice experience and the growing body of research reviewed. The past and potential behavior of men who batter means that joint custody or sole custody to him is rarely the best option for the safety and well-being of the children. In addition to their propensity for continued violence toward children and adult partners, these men are likely to abuse alcohol (Bennett and Williams, 2003), be poor role models (Jaffe, Lemon, and Poisson, 2003), and communicate in a hostile, manipulative manner (Holtzworth-Munroe, et al., 2000). As noted earlier, the Model Code State Statute of the National Council of Juvenile and Family Court Judges states that there should be a presumption that it is detrimental to the child to be placed in sole or joint custody with a perpetrator of family violence (NCJFCJ, 1994). The model statute emphasizes that the safety and well-being of the child and the parent-survivor must be primary. In addition, states should repeal friendly parent provisions or, at a minimum, say that they have no weight in cases where domestic or family violence has occurred.

The perpetrator's history of causing fear and physical harm, as well as the potential for future harm to the mother or child, should be considered. A parent's relocation in an attempt to escape violence should not be used as a factor to determine custody. Courts sometimes label battered women as impulsive or uncooperative if they leave suddenly to find safety in another city or state. The model statute specifies that it is in the best interest of the child to reside with the non-violent parent and that this parent should be able to choose the location of the residence, even if it is in another state. The non-custodial parent may also be denied access to the child's medical and educational records if such information could be used to locate the custodial parent.

The model statute (NCJFCJ, 1994) states that visitation should be granted to the perpetrator only if adequate safety provisions for the child and adult victim can be made. Orders of visitation can specify, among other things, the exchange of the child in a protected setting, supervised visitation by a specific person or agency, completion by the perpetrator of a program of intervention for perpetrators, and no overnight visitation (NCJFCJ, 1994). If the court allows a family member to supervise the visitation, the court must set the conditions to be followed during visitation (O'Sullivan, et al., 2006). For example, an order might specify that the father not use alcohol prior to or during a visit and that the child be allowed to call the mother at any time (see Bancroft and Silverman, 2002, for a description of different levels of supervision).

Unsupervised visitation should be allowed only after the abuser completes a specialized program for men who batter (APA, 1996) and does not threaten or become violent for a substantial period of time. Practitioners need to be aware of the strong likelihood that men who batter will become violent in a new relationship and that they often use non-violent tactics that can harm the children. Visitation should be suspended if there are repeated violations of the terms of visitation, the child is severely distressed in response to visitation, or there are clear indications that the violent parent has threatened to harm or flee with the child. Even with unsupervised visitation, it is best to have telephone contact between parents only at scheduled times, to maintain restraining orders to keep the offender away from the victim, and to transfer the child in a neutral, safe place with the help of a third party (Johnston, 1992). Hart (1990) describes a number of safety planning strategies that can be taught to children in these situations.

In response to the need for safe visitation, supervised visitation and exchange programs are expanding rapidly across North America. Many programs follow the standards of the Supervised Visitation Network, an international organization. The standards include a special section on domestic violence that requires policies and procedures designed to increase safety for domestic abuse survivors and their children (http://www.svnetwork.net/Standards.html). In addition, a number of authors and programs have described the special features needed at these programs to increase the safety of domestic abuse survivors, including heightened security, staff knowledge of domestic violence, and special court reviews (Maxwell and Oehme, 2001; Sheeran and Hampton, 1999). Close coordination with family courts, lethality assessment prior to referral, and recognition of common abuser behaviors are some of the ingredients needed for effective operation of these programs (Maxwell and Oehme, 2001). Programs also need to be aware of the risks of keeping detailed intake, observation, and other records because currently they cannot be kept confidential in family court proceedings (Stern and Oehme, 2002, 2007). The evaluation of visitation programs has occurred only on a small scale thus far (Tutty, Weaver-Dunlop, Barlow, and Jesso, 2006). Finding promising practices is complicated by the growing recognition that not all men who batter are alike and that interventions need to be tailored to different types of abusers, with variations occurring by levels of dangerousness and the motivation to control. A think tank of advocates and legal and mental health professionals met in 2007 to explore the implications of such differences for custody and visitation decisions (Dunford-Jackson and Salem, 2007).

In 2003, the Office on Violence Against Women of the U.S. Department of Justice began the Safe Havens program in order to increase awareness of visitation/exchange programs and their community collaborators of the special needs of domestic violence cases. Safety audit reports from four demonstration sites are available, covering the role of visitation/exchange centers in domestic violence cases, how to increase culturally sensitive practices, centers' relationships with courts, and many other topics related to the infusion of domestic violence knowledge and awareness into programming (http://www.usdoj .gov/ovw/safehavens.htm).

Finally, termination of access needs to be considered more seriously than in the past. Those with a history of severe abuse and who have engaged in high levels of antisocial behavior may never be able to provide the safety and nurturing that their children need (Jaffe and Crooks, 2005; Stover, Van Horn, Turner, Cooper, and Lieberman, 2003).

In conclusion, although there is a need for much more practice experience and research, our current knowledge of risk factors for continued abuse of women and children means that decision-makers must exercise great caution in awarding custody or visitation to perpetrators of domestic violence. If visitation is granted, coordination with the courts, careful safety planning, and specific conditions attached to the court order are crucial for lowering the risk of harm to children and their mothers.

Endnotes

1. A few states set specific standards for meeting the definition of domestic violence; for example, "conviction of domestic abuse" and "convicted of a felony of the third degree or higher involving domestic violence."

2. The term mediation can cover many different practices and is not easily defined. Although many regard it as always unsafe for battered women, this view is not universally held, especially if risk assessment is done properly (Ellis and Stuckless, 2006).

3. Recently, however, concerns have been raised about how well joint custody works in general (Wallerstein, 2000).

4. Generally, joint physical custody is being referred to here rather than joint legal custody. There is a trend toward the term "shared parental rights" instead of joint custody.

5. As of October 2006, 18 states required education on domestic violence for judges (from a document obtained from the National Council of Juvenile and Family Court Judges: "State Legislation: Mandatory Domestic Violence Training for Judges").

Section 60.2

Supervised Visitation Information for Mothers Who Have Experienced Abuse

What are supervised visitation programs?

There are many different kinds of visitation programs. Some simply try to provide a safe place for children to visit with a parent. For most programs, a safe place means that a staff person watches the visit to make sure that the child is not abused during the visit. Some supervised visitation programs go beyond that to try to teach the visiting adult how to be a better parent. Other programs may offer a therapeutic approach during visits to try to establish or rebuild a damaged relationship between the parent and child. Some programs also provide a safe place for parents to drop off and pick up children for visitation, a service called visitation exchange or supervised exchange.

There are programs specifically designed to supervise visits when one parent has abused the other parent. Sometimes this abuse is called domestic violence. In these families, both the child and a parent may be in danger. So, these programs try to provide supervised visitation that is safe for the child and the parent. You can ask the visitation center in your area if it runs a specialized domestic violence program.

What should I be able to expect from supervised visitation program staff?

Each supervised visitation program is different, but all should work to keep your children and you safe. Staff will have different styles and approaches. Some will have a lot of experience and knowledge about children and abuse in families, and some will have very little. The following is a list of the things you should look for in any visitation program:

- Staff try to set up rules and procedures for the visitation that keep you and your children safe. They also do what they can to make the visitation a positive experience for your children.

- Staff listen to you, talk to you about the risks you and your children face, and explain what they will do to help you and your children.

- Staff understand how abuse affects a family. They are experienced enough to understand how you and your children might feel about visitation. They are also experienced enough to know that some fathers might try to use visitation to continue the abuse.

- Staff are able to connect you and your children to advocacy and other services in the community.

- Staff value the background and culture of your family. They understand that each family is different and do their best to make visitation work for your family.

How do programs provide a safe environment for visitation?

Most programs use three kinds of safety strategies:

1. **Rules and procedures:** For example, one parent is scheduled to arrive after the other parent in order to keep them from having contact.

2. **Building set-up and physical protections:** For example, metal detectors to scan for weapons, different entrances for each parent to prevent contact, a security person on site, or quick access to police response.

3. **Staff supervision of the visitation:** For example, staff are trained to know how an abusive parent might try to use visitation to continue the threats and control, they do not let an abusive parent use the visitation to get information from the children about the other parent, and they regularly check with parents to assess whether the safety strategies being used are adequate or should be changed.

Keep in mind that your program may not use the options that are listed in these examples and may offer other ways to keep you and your children safe. Every program will be different, so it is important that you talk with staff about your concerns and work with them to make the best use of the strategies that your program offers.

How do children react to supervised visitation?

Every child's experience is unique and will be affected by his or her age, experience, and parents' behavior. Even children from the same family can have different reactions to a visit. In general, most children know that supervised visitation is an artificial or fake setting and that most families don't have to go to a program to see each other.

Often children have mixed feelings. For example, a child might look forward to seeing her father, but be afraid that he will be angry with her. Some children just try to make one or both parents happy and say whatever they think a parent wants to hear. Others are unsure of what they think or feel. For some children, the supervised setting gives them the security and confidence to challenge or test the visiting parent. There are also children who are afraid of the unfamiliar setting, of seeing a parent, or of being rejected by a parent. It is common for children to worry about what may happen during or after the visit.

Whatever your children's reactions, you can be a very important source of support and guidance to them as they go through this experience.

How can I know if a program will work for me and my children?

Talk to the staff about the program and your family's needs. As you talk to the staff you'll know right away if they are willing to listen to you and will take your concerns seriously. You'll also get an idea of how they will try to provide a safe environment for you and your children during the visitation. If the information and options they are offering do not meet your needs or concerns, then the program might not be the best for you and your children. Trust your own judgment. If you're not sure, you may want to give the program a try or ask for more information.

Will the program help me with my court case?

Most programs are not very involved, but some work directly with the court. Ask the staff how their program handles court involvement.

Do they try to stay completely out of a court case? Or, do they write reports for the court or make recommendations? Do they charge a fee? Remember that sometimes an attorney or judge will order (subpoena) a program to come to court and bring its records, even if the program doesn't want to be involved. If you are in a legal fight about custody or visitation, what happens at the program and how it is documented—whether you're visiting or bringing the children to visit—might be very important to your case. Therefore, it is important to know what files the program is keeping and what type of information is recorded in those files. A knowledgeable attorney can help you think about how the program's records may help or hurt your court case.

Information on How to Prepare For and Use Visitation Services

What can I do to prepare myself if I'm bringing my children to visit with their father?

If you are concerned about safety, you can talk with program staff to find out what options and resources they have to help. For example, what would the staff do if your children's father left a threatening note on your windshield when your car was parked in the program's lot? The staff should work with you to develop a safety strategy based on your particular needs. You can also talk with your attorney or advocate.

You might want to think about where you'll wait during the visit and plan something to do while it's happening. Ask the program staff if there is a place where you can wait and if they offer any activities. Take some time to think about what you need. This visitation process might be hard for you, and it can be difficult to keep your children's needs and experiences separate from your own. For example, your daughter might really want to see her father while you dread it, or you may want your children to have a relationship with their father and they don't. You deserve and need support, too. Try to find people who understand what you've been through, and who will listen to and support you. Use the visitation time to do something nurturing for you.

How can I help prepare my children for visits with their father?

You can start by explaining the visitation process and answering their questions. You might tell them where and when you'll drop them off, where they'll go afterwards, where their father will be, and when you'll pick them up. You can tell them the staff person's name and explain what the staff person's role will be during the visit. Trust your own judgment about your children. You'll know how much information to provide, how to say it in a way that they'll understand, and what their concerns might be. You can also ask the staff for ideas about ways you can help your children get ready for the visit.

Most programs offer some kind of orientation that can be very reassuring to children. At the orientation, your children can see where they'll be dropped off, where they'll visit, and what toys and activities are there. They'll also get a chance to meet the people who work at the program.

Part of your preparation should be listening to your children talk about their ideas and concerns and answering their questions. It is important to support their feelings, whether those feelings are positive or negative. Try to make the visit seem like a regular family activity and explain that other children visit their dads there too. Help them plan activities or think about what items they might bring with them to the visit. You can also ask your children about what they think their father will say or do during the visit, and what they would like to say or do when they see him. If they haven't seen their father in a while, it might be helpful for them to see a photo of him.

Some children really look forward to visiting. It is important to try to stay positive, even if you don't feel that way. If your children's father was, or still is, abusive, then there are good reasons for you to be wary and protective of your children. It is understandably hard to balance those concerns with the chance for your children to have a safe and positive relationship with their father. It can be helpful to talk to a trusted friend, family member, counselor, or advocate as you decide on the best approach.

If your children have concerns or fears about the visits, talk to them about their options and let them know the people at the program are there to help. For example, if your child is afraid that his father will get mad and start yelling at him, you can explain how staff might take a break or end the visitation for that day. The staff might also arrange for a code word for your children to use if they need a break or want to talk with staff.

What if my children don't want to visit their father?

Encourage them to tell you why they don't want to go. Understanding their concerns will help you to guide them. Answer their questions and try to be positive and encouraging. For example, you might say, "I know it might be scary at first, but you know Sarah (the staff person) will be there the whole time. How about giving it a try?"

It's not easy to bring children to visitation when they don't want to see their father or to know what to say that's positive. It's even harder if he's been abusive. You might need help from a trusted friend, advocate, counselor, or family member to figure out what is best. You can talk with the staff about your children's concerns and work with them to come up with a plan that supports your children. Find out the program's policy when children don't want to visit and how the program staff will approach these situations.

You might be worried about your children, thinking that even if the staff keeps them physically safe, the visits with their father will hurt them emotionally. It's okay to give your children age-appropriate options, such as, "You can talk with the staff about the visits or ask them for a break if you want one." Make sure your kids know they can always count on you for support.

If you're in a legal fight over custody or visitation, keep in mind that your children's father might try to argue that the children don't want to go because you are "turning your children against him." It may be helpful to have legal advice from an attorney if you think this might happen in your case. Also, keep in mind that the program staff is not the problem or the reason there is conflict in your family. Just like you, they're trying to look out for your children and follow court orders.

What should I do for my children after they visit with their father?

Be available in whatever way your children may need you. Some children will want to tell you about their experiences visiting, just like they do when they come home from school or come in from playing. Even though it may be hard to hear, it is very important to listen. Let them offer what information they choose and try to be supportive and positive. Some children may not want to talk about the visit at all. This can be difficult, especially if you're concerned about the visit and want to know what happened. Be patient. When your children are ready to talk, they'll let you know.

It can be helpful to have a routine after visits, something that your children can rely on. If you need help figuring what to say to your children when they raise tough issues or fears, ask the program staff or another trusted person for advice.

How much information about the visits will the staff share with parents?

Programs differ, but most do not share information about the visits with the other parent. Programs try to keep the children out of the middle and protecting information about what happens during the visit is one way of doing this. This policy can also help the children feel free to say and do what they want with the parent they are visiting and not have to worry that it will get back to the other parent.

There may be exceptions to this policy and it can help you plan for your safety and the protection of your children if you know what the rules are. For example, will staff warn you if, during the visitation, your children's father threatens to hurt them or you? Will they tell you if something happened during the visit that upset your child? Or, if you are visiting your children, will they report back something that might endanger you or make things harder for your children? You can talk to the staff about what information would help you to protect yourself and your children.

Is it really okay for children to visit with their father, even though he's been violent?

Every child is different. Whether it is harmful for your child will depend on his or her father's behavior and your child's own temperament, personality, and support system. You can help make it easier by supporting your child and reassuring him or her that you'll continue that support no matter what happens with visitation. You can talk with a trusted counselor, therapist, advocate, or attorney to help you make sure you have as accurate a view as possible of any risks to your child. They can also help you plan how best to support your child.

If your child's father follows the program's rules and guidelines, then the visitation should be safe. It will give your child the chance to learn about his or her father in a protected setting. Sometimes children have unrealistic views or fantasies about their fathers. Visits can help children form a more accurate picture. Also, some children really want to see their fathers and enjoy visiting. If your child's father can act appropriately, visits may benefit your child. If your child's father says something hurtful or does something that is scary to your child, work with the program staff to help your child understand what happened and to feel safe again.

If your children are ordered by a judge to visit, then you may have little choice but to bring them to the program. An attorney can help explain your responsibilities and options.

Will the program change my children's father so that he is no longer controlling or violent?

Most programs are not designed for that purpose. They provide a protected environment for visitation, not an intervention to change a person's behavior. The staff will try to provide a safe visit for your children and a safe drop-off and pick-up for you. Safe visitation doesn't mean that your children's father will stop his violence, threats, intimidation, or attempts to control or scare you—or your children. However, there are some fathers who see how much they've hurt their children and do use the experience to try to become better parents.

If you are afraid or concerned about what he might do, you can talk with program staff. They should take your concerns seriously and work with you to develop a strategy to keep you and your children safe. Trust your own instincts and judgment about what will work. You can also ask for help from an advocate or attorney.

What should I do if I'm worried he'll manipulate or fool the staff (like he does everyone else)?

The first step is to understand the program's rules and guidelines and meet with the staff. Knowing how the program works will help you decide if he is truly fooling anyone. For example, when your child meets with the staff for orientation, they might seem very upbeat about the visitation. You might see this as the staff taking his side and believing his stories, when really they are just trying to make the visitation a positive experience for your child.

Trust your own level of comfort with staff. For example, did you feel that they took the time to understand your situation and the seriousness of your concerns? If you still have concerns you can talk to a staff supervisor. You can also contact an advocate or attorney.

What can I do to prepare for the end of supervised visitation?

If you don't already know, try to find out when visitation at the program will end and what will happen next. For example, will visitation take place without supervision? What will the schedule be? Will you have to have contact with your children's father? Or, will the case go back to court for the judge to decide what happens next? Once you have some idea, you'll be able to make plans for your safety and the safety of your children. You'll also be able to give your children accurate information about what to expect.

What can I do to prepare myself if I'm visiting my children at the program?

Try to stay positive. You have the chance for a fresh start with your children, to spend time with them in a place that is safe for you and full of new toys and activities for them. You'll also have the opportunity to get support around the challenges of parenting.

A consistent routine for every visit is important for children. Think about what routine your children might like. For example, you could read part of a book, draw a picture, ask about what happened in school that week, or talk about what to do at your next visit. Another way to prepare is to think through what questions your children might ask and plan what you'll say. Also, plan ahead to bring things your children might need or want, such as diapers or age appropriate toys, if you can afford them. You can always ask the staff for suggestions about what you can bring or what you might do or say. They can also guide you about potential difficult conversations or worries you may have. It is important that you understand the program's rules and follow them.

If you are concerned about safety, talk with program staff to find out what options and resources they may have to help. They can work with you to develop a safety strategy based on your particular needs. You can also talk with your attorney or advocate. Plan to do something to take care of you after each visit. It is not easy to see your children for a limited amount of time in an artificial setting and then leave without them, particularly if you're concerned about their safety. The visit might also raise issues. Sometimes children act in ways that are hurtful to a parent. Your children may say things that might hurt your feelings, such as repeating the same harmful words they have heard their father say to you. They may also be reluctant to see you. Try to stay calm and steady.

You deserve and need support. Try to find people who understand what you've been through, and who will listen to you and help you through difficult times.

How can I help prepare my children if I'm coming to visit them?

It is important to keep in mind that you'll need to follow any court orders, program rules, or limits placed on your contact with the children.

If you are allowed to write or talk on the phone, you can let your children know ahead of time how much you're looking forward to the visit. Otherwise, you might need to wait for the first visit. Think about things your children might want to do during the visit and ask them what they'd like to do. For example, you might talk to them about what games they'd like to play, or what book they'd like you to read to them, or whether they'd like to draw a picture or kick a soccer ball around. If the visit can include a meal, you might ask them what food they'd like you to bring. During your visit, you and your children can plan together what you'll do at the next visit. You can also ask the staff how you can help your children get ready for visits.

Chapter 61

Mental Health Concerns
for Victims of Violent Crime

As a survivor of violent crime, you may face a wide range of emotional and physical struggles, along with some difficult questions that often surface: Why did this happen to me? How will I ever heal from this? Why can't I connect with others the way I did before? When will I start to feel normal again? While the answers may be different for each individual, there are some striking similarities in how trauma affects nearly all victims. Understanding the nature and impact of violent trauma can be essential to the healing process. This chapter is intended as a guide to help you along the path to healing and to avoid some of the common pitfalls along the way.

What is posttraumatic stress disorder (PTSD)?

PTSD is a mental health condition that can be caused by experiencing or observing virtually any kind of deep emotional trauma, especially one that is unexpected. Millions of people in the United States suffer from PTSD, resulting from many different types of trauma— from enduring years of domestic violence to a single violent attack that lasts but a few seconds. PTSD is characterized by both emotional and physical suffering; many afflicted by it find themselves unintentionally revisiting their trauma through flashbacks or nightmares. PTSD can make you feel isolated, disconnected, and different from

"Answers in the Aftermath," National Mental Health Information Center, Substance Abuse and Mental Health Services Administration (SAMHSA), SMA 05–4027, April 2005.

other people—and it can even begin to affect the most routine activities of everyday life. PTSD is a potentially serious condition that should not be taken lightly.

Why is substance abuse common following a traumatic event?

Since violent trauma can bring about so many changes, questions, and uncertainties, many survivors turn to alcohol and illicit drugs in an attempt to get some relief from their almost round-the-clock emotional turmoil and suffering. Substance abuse and mental health problems often accompany violent trauma. All survivors of trauma manage their experiences in different ways. Substance abuse, however, is not only an ineffective tool in healing from trauma, but it also can present a host of additional problems that make the healing process even more difficult.

What can I do if I am experiencing PTSD or if substance abuse becomes a problem for me?

According to a recent study conducted by the Substance Abuse and Mental Health Services Administration (SAMHSA), the most effective way to combat trauma, substance abuse, and mental health problems is through an integrated, holistic approach, taking into account how each individual problem affects the others. To begin, it can help to share your experiences and concerns with a service provider (for example: counselor, physician, victim witness coordinator) who can assist in developing a plan to address all of your struggles comprehensively. Psychologists and counselors with experience treating trauma survivors can be very helpful in working through PTSD, and there are prescription drugs available to help ease PTSD symptoms.

PTSD can make you feel isolated, disconnected, and different from other people—and it can even begin to affect the most routine activities of everyday life.

What can I do to begin the healing process?

There are some positive steps that you can take right away to begin healing. Here are some suggestions:

- Recognize your loss.
- Establish personal safety.

- Respect the way you feel and your right to feel that way.
- Talk about your feelings with those you trust.
- Connect with other survivors of violence, many of whom experience similar difficulties.
- Do not be afraid to seek professional help.
- Try to recognize triggers that may take you back to the memory and fear of your trauma.
- Try to be patient and avoid making rash decisions—it can take time to figure out where you are, where you want to be, and how to get there.
- Take care of yourself—exercise, eat right, and take a deep breath when you feel tense.
- Try to turn your negative experience into something positive—volunteer, donate, or do something else to constructively channel your energy and emotions.
- Do not abandon hope—believe that healing can and will take place.

The healing process takes time, and many questions, hurdles, and frustrations may surface along the way.

For More Information

SAMHSA National Mental Health Information Center
P.O. Box 2345
Rockville, MD 20847
Toll-Free: 800-789-2647
Toll-Free TDD: 866-889-2647
Fax: 240-221-4295
Website: http://mentalhealth.samhsa.gov

SAMHSA's Mental Health Services Locator
Website: http://www.mentalhealth.samhsa.gov/databases

Witness Justice
P.O. Box 475
Frederick, MD 21705-0475
Toll-Free: 800-4WJ-HELP (95-4357)
Phone: 301-846-9110

Fax: 301-846-9113
Website: http://www.wintessjustice.org

Witness Justice provides an opportunity to connect with other survivors and experts from a wide range of professional fields as well as access to timely and pertinent information about trauma, mental health, and the healing and criminal justice processes.

Chapter 62

Spirituality in the Lives of Domestic Violence Survivors

As women search for means of coping with living with or leaving an abusive partner, many of them turn to their religious institutions and religious family for strength, comfort, and support (Boehm, Golec, Krahn, and Smyth, 1999; Giesbrecht and Sevcik, 2000). Giesbrecht and Sevcik (2000) found that many survivors of domestic violence identified spirituality and their identity within their faith community as integral components of their identity and experience. As a result, the women viewed both their experience of abuse and recovery from abuse as occurring within the context of their faith. Not surprisingly, then, many of the women turned to their religious communities for support. Some of these communities have minimized, denied, or enabled the abuse, whereas others have provided much needed social support, practical assistance, and spiritual encouragement. Social support from religious institutions (churches, synagogues, mosques) has been found to be a key factor in many women's abilities to rebuild their lives and family relationships (Giesbrecht and Sevcik, 2000). Unconditional love and acceptance from their supreme being (God) and the desire for a loving religious family is an expressed need for many women. Those women with a welcoming, caring religious experience have reported feelings of hope for healing after such a distressing life event (an abusive relationship) (Giesbrecht and Sevcik, 2000).

Text in this chapter is excerpted from: Tameka L. Gillum, Cris M. Sullivan, and Deborah I. Bybee. The Importance of Spirituality in the Lives of Domestic Violence Survivors. VIOLENCE AGAINST WOMEN 12: 240–250, © 2006. Reprinted by Permission of SAGE Publications.

Kreidler (1995) has identified the need for and usefulness of spiritual healing groups for those who are survivors of family violence. She argues that the experience of being hurt by someone one believes should love, cherish, and protect causes a great deal of spiritual distress. This distress can manifest itself in various ways, including feelings of despair, belief that life is meaningless, or perceptions of oneself as powerless. Other researchers have concurred that, because of the importance of spirituality in the lives of many victims of family violence and the spiritual distress that can be caused by victimization, spiritual healing is necessary to restore one's sense of meaningfulness of and power over one's life (Dunbar and Jeannechild, 1996; Mattis, 2002; Spiegel, 1996). Boehm et al. (1999) also highlight that in their talks with women who have experienced intimate partner violence, women have expressed feelings of spiritual anguish in the midst of the abuse. They found that women expressed their desire to seek comfort from their faith communities and religious leaders but often found this support lacking. Abused women, especially those in closed religious or ethnic communities, are more likely to disclose their experience of violence within their religious communities, and some find that other women within these communities are the ones who discreetly and informally provide them with much-needed forms of support (Nason-Clark, 2000).

Researchers have also identified the importance of spirituality to one's psychological well-being in general. Fiala, Bjorck, and Gorsuch's (2002) study of adult Protestants found religious support to be related to lower depression and greater life satisfaction. The authors looked specifically at three identified dimensions of religious support: God support, congregational support, and church leader support. They found that God support in particular was positively related to social support and was related to less depression and more life satisfaction. This relationship held even after controlling for church attendance, congregational support, and church leader support. Congregational support was also positively related to social support, decreased depression, and increased life satisfaction after controlling for church attendance, general social support, God support, and church leader support. In addition, church leader support was also found to be related to lower depression and greater life satisfaction.

Research has also shown the importance of spirituality in overcoming other life traumas including coping with serious mental illness (Corrigan, McCorkle, Schell, and Kidder, 2003), loss of loved ones (Fry, 2001; Michael, Crowther, Schmid, and Allen, 2003; Oram, Bartholomew, and Landolt, 2004), and life-threatening physical illness (Beasler, Derlega, Winstead, and Barbee, 2003; Simoni, Martone, and Kerwin, 2002).

In addition, spirituality has been demonstrated to be of particular importance to the African American community. Research suggests that religious involvement is generally higher among African Americans than among Caucasians (Chatters, Taylor, and Lincoln, 1999; Levin, Taylor, and Chatters, 1994; Taylor, Chatters, Jayakody, and Levin, 1996) and is higher among African American women than among African American men (Chatters et al., 1999; Levin et al., 1994). African Americans use spirituality and religious involvement to cope with life stressors ranging from perceived discrimination to recovery from substance abuse (Brome, Owens, Allen, and Vevaina, 2000; Constantine, Wilton, Gainor, and Lewis, 2002; Scott, 2003).

In light of these findings, it appears important to investigate the extent to which the role of spirituality and religious involvement relates to the emotional and psychological well-being of domestic violence survivors. If in fact survivors do benefit from a belief in a higher power to the extent that this adherence facilitates their healing process, and if survivors benefit emotionally and psychologically from involvement in spiritual communities, then this factor should be taken into account by domestic violence agencies as they attempt to help survivors overcome their abusive experiences. This study, then, was designed to assess the extent to which battered women's involvement with spirituality and their faith communities affected their depression, quality of life, social support, and self-esteem.

Discussion

The findings support the contention that spirituality and religious involvement are significant aspects of many survivors' identities (Boehm et al., 1999; Giesbrecht and Sevcik, 2000; Kreidler, 1995). Also, religious involvement appears to promote greater psychological well-being for domestic violence survivors, including greater quality of life and decreased depression.

The finding that women's number of children was significantly correlated with both self-esteem and depression is worthy of mention. For women in this study, the greater the number of children they had, the greater their self-esteem and the lower their level of depression. This may suggest that survivors of domestic violence, who by virtue of their abusive relationships are not receiving positive reinforcement from their intimate relationships, may receive added psychological satisfaction from their responsibilities as mothers and the closeness of their relationships with their children.

The finding that race moderated the relationship between religious involvement and social support is worthy of mention and further investigation. Higher religious involvement was a predictor of greater social support for women of color but not for Caucasian women. This finding is consistent with other studies that have found church involvement to be related to greater social support for members of the African American community (Brodsky, 2000; McAdoo, 1995). Research has also shown that spirituality and religiosity affect the physical and psychological well-being of African Americans, highlighting its significance in the lives of African Americans (Blaine and Crocker, 1995; Handal, Black-Lopez, and Moergen, 1989; McAdoo, 1995). This does, however, leave unanswered questions for future research. What is it about religious institutions that serve communities of color that increase women's social support? What is it about the spiritual identity of women of color that facilitates the increased network of support that they receive by virtue of their involvement in a faith-based institution?

It is important to view the results of this study cautiously, as only three questions were used to address the issue of spirituality and religious involvement in women's lives. We did not ask women to identify their religious affiliations nor to provide information about how their religious communities had been supportive or unsupportive of them in the past. Much more extensive research is needed to examine the full extent of the role religion and spirituality play in the lives of domestic violence survivors. In spite of these limitations, these findings have a number of implications for domestic violence victim service programs. Currently, many domestic violence shelter staff distance themselves from discussions of spirituality with shelter residents. Reasons for this include lack of staff time and resources, the personal nature of spirituality, the diversity of religious or spiritual beliefs among individuals, and apprehension around creating misunderstanding or intruding on a woman's privacy (Boehm et al., 1999). The end result, however, is that the shelter provides a haven for physical safety but fails to provide an environment for spiritual healing. This is especially ironic considering that the first shelters were homes operated by women helping women, and they often worked in coalition with religious groups and other community agencies (Boehm et al., 1999).

The inclusion of a voluntary spirituality component in victim service programs may serve to greatly benefit some battered women. It may serve to lessen the depression that women in shelter tend to experience by virtue of being uprooted from their homes and having to stay in a shelter environment. For women of color specifically, it may serve to increase their social support network, which may give them the added emotional and practical support they need to cope with the abuse they have experienced and possibly remain free from their abusers. This spirituality component may consist of bringing in a religious leader from the community to hold spiritual support groups and activities at the shelter or simply providing transportation and free time for women to facilitate their attendance at church services. Others have suggested making available a quiet room for prayer or reflection (Boehm et al., 1999).

Finally, this research has implications for religious communities. It speaks to the need for faith communities to address the issue of domestic violence and offer services to members of their congregations and communities that are involved in abusive situations. A harsh reality is that many religious leaders are reluctant to deal with the fact that women in their own congregations are being abused, and sometimes this abuse is inflicted by the hands of men who are also involved in these communities. Our faith communities can no longer afford to ignore this reality as many women are suffering, some tragically, as a result of domestic violence. Possible responses of faith communities could include offering domestic violence support groups, individual counseling, emergency relief funds, and possibly shelter for women who must leave their abusers. Spiritual leaders should also attend domestic violence educational trainings to make them more aware of the frequency of abuse, the dynamics of abusive relationships, and the experiences and needs of domestic violence survivors. Many state domestic violence coalitions offer such trainings and many conferences are beginning to address clergy and their significance in recognizing and addressing the issue of domestic violence. All aspects of our communities, including spiritual leaders and congregation members, should be available for women to turn to for both emotional support and practical assistance when seeking help from abusive relationships.

Chapter 63

Supporting the Survivor of Violent Trauma

In the United States, your odds of falling victim to violence at some point in your lifetime are high. Even if you don't encounter violence directly, chances are that you know someone who has experienced, or will experience, trauma. While a victim copes with the direct impact of trauma, those close to the victim also struggle in the aftermath. What do I say? What do I do? Why does my loved one seem so distant? This chapter is intended to help you begin to understand what happens to many victims of violent crime, and what you might do to help them along the healing process.

How Trauma Affects Survivors

Victims of violence often face a wide range of struggles. They often question what has happened or what they might have done to cause or prevent it. Many wonder how they will heal and why they cannot connect with their loved ones as they once did. It is also common for survivors to feel anger or frustration as they ponder whether they will ever feel normal again. While every survivor's experience is unique, violent trauma is almost always a life-changing experience that can affect everything from one's ability to sleep to his or her ability to concentrate at work.

"Supporting the Survivor," National Mental Health Information Center, Substance Abuse and Mental Health Services Administration (SAMHSA), SMA 05–4027, April 2005.

Understanding the nature and impact of trauma can be a key to helping your loved one. Many survivors find themselves in unfamiliar and distressing psychological territory. It is common for them to endure intense feelings of isolation, insecurity, and fear, and their most treasured relationships often suffer as a result. Trauma can also lead to posttraumatic stress disorder (PTSD), which may include both substance abuse and mental health problems.

Violent Trauma, Substance Abuse, and Mental Health Concerns

Many victims turn to alcohol or other substances in an attempt to get some relief from their emotional turmoil and suffering. All trauma survivors manage their experiences in different ways. However, substance abuse is not only ineffective in healing from trauma, but it also can present a host of additional problems that make the healing process even more difficult.

Violence is also a widely recognized catalyst for mental health concerns such as PTSD, a condition that can be caused by experiencing or observing virtually any kind of deep emotional or physical trauma. Millions of people in the United States suffer from PTSD, resulting from many different types of trauma—from enduring years of domestic violence to a single violent attack that lasts but a few seconds. PTSD is characterized by both emotional and physical suffering; many afflicted by it find themselves unintentionally revisiting their trauma through flashbacks or nightmares. PTSD can make a survivor feel isolated, disconnected, and different from other people, and it can even begin to affect the most routine activities of everyday life. Psychologists and counselors with experience in treating trauma survivors can be very helpful in working through PTSD, and there are prescription drugs available to help ease PTSD symptoms. PTSD is a potentially serious condition that should not be taken lightly.

According to a study conducted by the U.S. Department of Health and Human Services, Substance Abuse and Mental Health Services Administration, the most effective way to combat trauma, substance abuse, and mental health problems is through an integrated, holistic approach, taking into account how each individual problem affects the others. To begin, it can be helpful for a survivor to share experiences and concerns with a service provider who can assist in developing a plan to address these struggles comprehensively. Many wonder how they will heal and why they cannot connect with their loved ones as they once did.

What Can I Do to Help My Loved One?

Since each individual's experience is unique, there is no "one size fits all" remedy for victimized loved ones. For those who care about a person who has experienced a violent trauma, finding ways to be helpful and maintaining a healthy relationship can be challenging. Following are some tips to help your loved one who has been victimized.

Listen: Talking about the experience, when the survivor is ready, will help acknowledge and validate what has happened to him or her and can reduce stress and feelings of isolation. Let your loved one take the lead, and try not to jump in with too many comments or questions right away.

Research: If the victim wants more information, would like to report a crime, or has other questions, you can help find answers and resources.

Reassure: As strange as it may sound, survivors often question whether an incident was their fault or what they could have done to prevent the crime against them. They may need to hear that it was not their fault and be assured that they are not alone.

Empower: Following trauma, victims can feel as though much of his or her life is beyond his or her control. Aiding your loved one in maintaining routines can be helpful, as can offering survivors options or possible solutions.

Be patient: Every journey through the healing process is unique. Try to understand that it will take time, and do what you can to be supportive. The healing process has no predetermined timeline.

Ask: Your loved one may need help with any number of things or have questions on many different topics. Even a favor as mundane as running a few errands or taking the dog for a walk can be a big help, so consider lending a hand.

Remember: The healing process takes time, and many questions, hurdles, and frustrations may surface along the way.

For More Information

SAMHSA National Mental Health Information Center
P.O. Box 2345
Rockville, MD 20847
Toll-Free: 800-789-2647
Toll-Free TDD: 866-889-2647
Fax: 240-221-4295
Website: http://mentalhealth.samhsa.gov

SAMHSA's Mental Health Services Locator
Website: http://www.mentalhealth.samhsa.gov/databases

Witness Justice
P.O. Box 475
Frederick, MD 21705-0475
Toll-Free: 800-4WJ-HELP (95-4357)
Phone: 301-846-9110
Fax: 301-846-9113
Website: http://www.witnessjustice.org

Witness Justice provides an opportunity to connect with other survivors and experts from a wide range of professional fields as well as access to timely and pertinent information about trauma, mental health, and the healing and criminal justice processes.

Part Eight

Additional Help
and Information

Chapter 64

Glossary of Terms Related to Domestic Violence

aggravated assault: An unlawful attack by one person upon another wherein the offender uses a weapon or displays it in a threatening manner, or the victim suffers obvious severe or aggravated bodily injury involving apparent broken bones, loss of teeth, possible internal injury, severe laceration, or loss of consciousness.[1]

alleged perpetrator report source: An individual who reports an alleged incident of abuse or neglect in which he or she caused or knowingly allowed the maltreatment.

alleged victim: Person about whom a report regarding maltreatment has been made to an agency.

alleged victim report source: A person who alleges to have been a victim of maltreatment and who makes a report of the allegation.

anonymous or unknown report source: An individual who reports a suspected incident of maltreatment without identifying himself or herself; or the type of reporter is unknown.

Terms in this chapter are excerpted from "Glossary: National Child Abuse and Neglect Data Systems (NCANDS)," U.S. Health and Human Services (HHS), May 11, 2006. Terms marked with a [1] are from "Easy Access to NIBRS: Victims of Domestic Violence, 2005," Office of Juvenile Justice and Delinquency Prevention, released April 14, 2008. Terms marked with a [2] are from "Definitions," Office on Violence Against Women (OVW), 2006. Terms marked with a [3] are from "About Domestic Violence," OVW, 2008.

assessment: A process by which an agency determines whether the persons involved in the report of alleged maltreatment are in need of services.

case management services: Activities for the arrangement, coordination, and monitoring of services to meet the needs of individuals and their families.

child: A person less than 18 years of age or considered to be a minor under state law.

child victim: A child for whom an incident of abuse or neglect has been substantiated or indicated by an investigation or assessment. A state may include some children with other dispositions as victims.

children/families in need of services: Disposition by a welfare agency after an assessment; individuals or families with this assessment are generally not considered to be victims of maltreatment.

closed without a finding: Disposition that does not conclude with a specific finding because the investigation could not be completed for such reasons as: the family moved out of the jurisdiction; the family could not be located; or necessary diagnostic or other reports were not received within required time limits.

counseling services: Beneficial activities that apply the therapeutic processes to personal, family, situational, or occupational problems in order to bring about a positive resolution of the problem or improved individual or family functioning or circumstances.

court action: Legal action initiated by a representative of an agency on behalf of the victim. It does not include criminal proceedings against a perpetrator.

court-appointed representative: A person required to be appointed by the court to represent a person in neglect or abuse proceedings. May be an attorney or a court-appointed special advocate (or both) and is often referred to as a guardian ad litem. This individual makes recommendations to the court concerning the best interests of the individual.

dating violence: Violence committed by a person who is or has been in a social relationship of a romantic or intimate nature with the victim.[2]

domestic violence: A pattern of abusive behavior in any relationship that is used by one partner to gain or maintain power and control over another intimate partner.[3]

economic abuse: Making or attempting to make an individual financially dependent by maintaining total control over financial resources, withholding one's access to money, or forbidding one's attendance at school or employment.[3]

emotional abuse: Undermining an individual's sense of self-worth and/or self-esteem. This may include, but is not limited to constant criticism, diminishing one's abilities, name-calling, or damaging one's relationship with his or her children.[3]

family: A group of two or more persons related by birth, marriage, adoption, or emotional ties.

family support services: Community-based preventative activities designed to alleviate stress and promote parental competencies and behaviors that will increase the ability of families to successfully nurture their children, enable families to use other resources and opportunities available in the community, and create supportive networks to enhance child-rearing abilities of parents.

home-based services: In-home activities provided to individuals or families to assist with household or personal care and improve or maintain adequate family well-being. These may include homemaker, chore, home maintenance, and household management services.

housing services: Beneficial activities designed to assist individuals or families in locating, obtaining or retaining suitable housing.

inadequate housing: A risk factor related to substandard, overcrowded, or unsafe housing conditions, including homelessness.

indicated or reason to suspect: An investigation disposition that concludes that maltreatment cannot be substantiated under state law or policy, but there is reason to suspect that the individual may have been maltreated or was at risk of maltreatment. This is applicable only to states that distinguish between substantiated and indicated dispositions.

information and referral services: Resources or activities designed to provide facts about services made available by public and private providers, after a brief assessment of client needs (but not a diagnosis and evaluation) to facilitate appropriate referral to these community resources.

initial investigation: Face-to-face contact with the alleged victim, when this is appropriate, or contact with another person who can provide information essential to the disposition of the investigation or assessment.

intimidation: To unlawfully place another person in reasonable fear of bodily harm through the use of threatening words and/or other conduct, but without displaying a weapon or subjecting the victim to actual physical attack.[1]

investigation: The gathering and assessment of objective information to determine if a child has been or is at risk of being maltreated. Generally includes face-to-face contact with the victim and results in a disposition as to whether the alleged report is substantiated or not.

legal services: Beneficial activities provided by a lawyer, or other person(s) under the supervision of a lawyer, to assist individuals in seeking or obtaining legal help in civil matters such as housing, divorce, child support, guardianship, paternity, and legal separation.

maltreatment: An act or failure to act by a parent, caretaker, or other person as defined under state law which results in physical abuse, neglect, medical neglect, sexual abuse, emotional abuse, or an act or failure to act which presents an imminent risk of serious harm.

maltreatment death: Death of a child as a result of abuse or neglect, because either: (a) an injury resulting from the abuse or neglect was the cause of death; or (b) abuse and/or neglect were contributing factors to the cause of death.

maltreatment type: A particular form of maltreatment determined by investigation to be substantiated or indicated under state law. Types include physical abuse, neglect or deprivation of necessities, sexual abuse, psychological or emotional maltreatment, and other forms included in state law.

medical neglect: A type of maltreatment caused by failure by the caretaker to provide for the appropriate health care of the child although financially able to do so, or offered financial or other means to do so.

neglect or deprivation of necessities: A type of maltreatment that refers to the failure by the caretaker to provide needed, age-appropriate care although financially able to do so, or offered financial or other means to do so.

not substantiated: Investigation disposition that determines that there is not sufficient evidence under state law or policy to conclude that the child has been maltreated or is at risk of being maltreated.

perpetrator: The person who has been determined to have caused or knowingly allowed the maltreatment of the individual.

perpetrator prior abuser: Perpetrator with previous substantiated or indicated incidents of domestic violence or child maltreatment.

perpetrator relationship: Primary role of the perpetrator with a victim of maltreatment.

physical abuse: Hitting, slapping, shoving, grabbing, pinching, biting, hair-pulling, biting, etc. Physical abuse also includes denying a partner medical care or forcing alcohol and/or drug use.[3]

preventive services: Beneficial activities aimed at preventing domestic violence. Such activities may be directed at specific populations identified as being at increased risk of becoming abusive and may be designed to increase the strength and stability of families.

protection order (or restraining order): Any injunction, restraining order, or any other order issued by a civil or criminal court for the purpose of preventing violent or threatening acts or harassment against, sexual violence or contact or communication with, or physical proximity to, another person, including any temporary or final orders issued by civil or criminal courts in response to a complaint, petition, or motion filed by or on behalf of a person seeking protection.[2]

psychological abuse: Causing fear by intimidation; threatening physical harm to self, partner, children, or partner's family or friends; destruction of pets and property; and forcing isolation from family, friends, or school and/or work.[3]

public assistance: Any one or combination of the following welfare or social services programs including: Aid to Families with Dependent Children (AFDC), General Assistance, Medicaid, Social Security Income (SSI), and food stamps.

receipt of report: The log-in of a call to the agency from a reporter alleging domestic violence or child maltreatment.

report: Notification to an agency of suspected maltreatment; can include adults or children.

service date: Date of the report disposition or a date decided by the state to be more appropriate. The service date for cases for which services were continued (or changed) as a result of the investigation disposition is the date of the most recent case opening prior to the receipt of the report.

services: Non-investigative public or private beneficial activities provided or continued as a result of an investigation or assessment. In general, such activities occur within 90 days of the report.

sexual abuse: Coercing or attempting to coerce any sexual contact or behavior without consent. Sexual abuse includes, but is certainly not limited to marital rape, attacks on sexual parts of the body, forcing sex after physical violence has occurred, or treating one in a sexually demeaning manner.[3]

simple assault: An unlawful physical attack by one person upon another where neither the offender displays a weapon, nor the victim suffers obvious severe or aggravated bodily injury involving apparent broken bones, loss of teeth, possible internal injury, severe laceration, or loss of consciousness.[1]

stalking: A course of conduct directed at a specific person that would cause a reasonable person to feel fear for his or her safety, the safety of others, or suffer substantial emotional distress.[2]

substance abuse services: Beneficial activities designed to deter, reduce, or eliminate substance abuse or chemical dependency.

substantiated: A type of investigation disposition that concludes that the allegation of maltreatment or risk of maltreatment was supported or founded by state law or state policy. This is the highest level of finding by a state agency.

victim(s) type: More than one domestic violence victim can be involved in a single incident. Demographic information is available on each. This information is used to determine whether the incident involved a lone victim (juvenile, adult) or multiple victimization (multiple adults, multiple juveniles, or a combination of juvenile(s) and adult(s)).[1]

Chapter 65

Legal Resources for Domestic Violence Victims

The following organizations are a place to begin research for legal resources. Your local domestic violence shelters and violence prevention agencies may also offer information about legal resources in your community.

American Bar Association
Commission on Domestic Violence
740 15th St. NW
Washington, DC 20005
Phone: 202-662-1000
Website: http://www.abanet.org/domviol/home.html

Delaware Coalition Against Domestic Violence
100 W. 10th St., #703
Wilmington, DE 19801
Toll-Free in DE: 800-701-0456
Phone: 302-658-2958, Fax: 302-658-5049
Website: http://www.dcadv.org

Delaware Coalition Against Domestic Violence offers victim assistance programs which may be reviewed online at http://www.dcadv.org/04resources/victim_programs.html.

Information in this chapter was compiled from many sources deemed accurate. All contact information was updated and verified in December 2008. Inclusion does not constitute endorsement.

Florida Coalition Against Domestic Violence
Legal Department
425 Office Plaza Dr.
Tallahassee, FL 32301
Toll-Free: 800-500-1119, press prompt #3
Phone: 850-425-2749, Fax: 850-425-3091
Website: http://www.fcadv.org/legal.php

Legal Momentum
395 Hudson St.
New York, NY 10014
Phone: 212-925-6635, Fax: 212-226-1066
Website: http://www.legalmomentum.org

Legal Momentum's Immigrant Women Program
1101 14ᵗʰ St., NW, Suite 300
Washington, DC 20005
Phone: 202-326-0040, Fax: 202-589-0511
Website: http://www.legalmomentum.org
E-mail: iwp@legalmomentum.org

Legal Services Corporation
3333 K Street, NW, 3ʳᵈ Floor
Washington, DC 20007
Phone: 202-295-1500, Fax: 202-337-6797
Website: http://www.lsc.gov
E-mail: info@lsc.gov

Legal Services Corporation was established by the U.S. Congress to provide access for low-income individuals to civil legal aid. To find the nearest program, visit the online directory at http://www.rin.lsc.gov/rinboard/rguide/pdir1.htm.

National Academy of Elder Law Attorneys
1604 N. Country Club Rd.
Tucson, AZ 85716
Website: http://www.naela.org

NAELA offers an online directory to assist persons seeking a certified and experienced elder law attorney at http://www.naela.org/MemberDiretory.

National Association of Counsel for Children
Attorney Referral
Toll-Free: 888-828-6222
Website: http://www.naccchildlaw.org/?page=ResourceRequest

National Clearinghouse for the Defense of Battered Women
125 S. 9th St.
Philadelphia, PA 19107
Toll-Free: 800-903-0111, ext. 3
Phone: 215-351-0010, Fax: 215-351-0779
Website: http://www.bwjp.org/menu.htm

National District Attorneys Association
American Prosecutors Research Institute
National Center for Prosecution of Child Abuse
44 Canal Center Plaza, Suite 110
Alexandria, VA 22314
Phone: 703-549-9222, Fax: 703-836-3195
Website: http://www.ndaa.org/apri/programs/ncpca/ncpca_home.html

National Senior Citizens Law Center
Washington, DC Office
1444 Eye St., NW, Suite 1100
Washington, DC 20005
Phone: 202-289-6976, Fax: 202-289-7224
Website: http://www.nsclc.org/index.html

Northwest Justice Project
Refugee Immigrant Advocacy
401 Second Ave. S., Suite 407
Seattle, WA 98104
Toll-Free: 888-201-1012
Toll-Free TDD: 888-201-9737
Phone: 206-464-1519, Fax: 206-624-7501
Website: http://www.nwjustice.org
E-mail: njp@nwjustice.org

WomensLaw.org
55 Washington St., Suite 641
Brooklyn, NY 11201

Fax: 718-534-7412
Website: http://www.womenslaw.org

WomensLaw.org offers contact information for finding help in your state online at http://www.womenslaw.org/simple.php?sitemap_id=46.

Chapter 66

State Domestic Violence Organizations

Alabama Coalition Against Domestic Violence
P.O. Box 4762
Montgomery, AL 36101
Toll-Free Hotline: 800-650-6522
Phone: 334-832-4842
Fax: 334-832-4803
Website: http://www.acadv.org
E-mail: info@acadv.org

Alaska Network on Domestic and Sexual Violence
130 Seward St., #214
Juneau, AK 99801
Phone: 907-586-3650
Fax: 907-586-3650
Website: http://www.andvsa.org

Arizona Coalition Against Domestic Violence
301 E. Bethany Home Rd.
Suite C194
Phoenix, AZ 85012
Toll-Free: 800-782-6400
Toll-Free Legal Advocacy
Hotline: 800-782-6400
Phone: 602-279-2900
TTY: 602-279-7270
Fax: 602-279-2980
Website: http://www.azcadv.org
E-mail: acadv@azcadv.org

Information in this chapter was compiled from sourced deemed accurate. All contact information was updated and verified in December 2008.

587

Arkansas Coalition Against Domestic Violence
1401 W. Capitol Ave., Suite 170
Little Rock, AR 72201
Toll-Free: 800-269-4668
Phone: 501-907-5612
Fax: 501-907-5618
Website: http://www
.domesticpeace.com
E-mail: acadv@domesticpeace
.com

California Partnership to End Domestic Violence
P.O. Box 1798
Sacramento, CA 95812
Toll-Free: 800-524-4765
Phone: 916-444-7163
Fax: 916-444-7165
Website: http://www.cpedv.org
E-mail: info@cpedv.org

Colorado Coalition Against Domestic Violence
1120 Lincoln Street, Suite 900
Denver, CO 80203
Toll-Free: 888-778-7091
Phone: 303-831-9632
Fax: 303-832-7067
Website: http://www.ccadv.org

Connecticut Coalition Against Domestic Violence
90 Pitkin Street
East Hartford, CT 06108
Toll-Free in State Domestic Violence Hotline: 800-281-1481
Phone: 860-282-7899
Fax: 860-282-7892
Website: http://www.ctcadv.org
E-mail: info@ctcadv.org

Delaware Coalition Against Domestic Violence
100 W. 10th St., #703
Wilmington, DE 19801
Phone: 302-658-2958
Fax: 302-658-5049
Website: http://www.dcadv.org
E-mail: dcadv@dcadv.org

DC Coalition Against Domestic Violence
5 Thomas Circle NW
Washington, DC 20005
Phone: 202-299-1181
Fax: 202-299-1193
Website: http://www.dccadv.org
E-mail: info@dccadv.org

Florida Coalition Against Domestic Violence
425 Office Plaza Dr.
Tallahassee, FL 32301
Toll-Free in State: 800-500-1119
TTY Hotline: 800-621-4202
Phone: 850-425-2749
Fax: 850-425-3091
TDD: 850-621-4202
Website: http://www.fcadv.org

Georgia Coalition Against Domestic Violence
114 New St., Suite B
Decatur, GA 30030
Toll-Free Crisis Line:
800-334-2836
Phone/TTY: 404-209-0280
Fax: 404-766-3800
Website: http://www.gcadv.org
E-mail: info@gcadv.org

Hawaii State Coalition Against Domestic Violence
716 Umi Street
Suite 210
Honolulu, HI 96819-2337
Crisis Hotline: 808-841-0822
Phone: 808-832-9316
Fax: 808-841-6028
Website: http://www.hscadv.org

Idaho Coalition Against Sexual and Domestic Violence
300 E. Mallard Drive
Suite 130
Boise, ID 83706
Toll-Free: 888-293-6118
Phone: 208-384-0419
Fax: 208-331-0687
Website: http://www.idvsa.org
E-mail: thecoalition@idvsa.org

Illinois Coalition Against Domestic Violence
801 S. 11th St.
Springfield, IL 62703
Toll-Free Hotline: 877-863-6338
Phone: 217-789-2830
Fax: 217-789-1939
TTY: 217-242-0376
Website: http://www.ilcadv.org
E-mail: ilcadv@ilcadv.org

Indiana Coalition Against Domestic Violence
1915 W. 18th St.
Suite B
Indianapolis, IN 46202
Toll-Free in State Crisis Line:
800-332-7385
Toll-Free: 800-538-3393
Phone: 317-917-3685
Fax: 317-917-3695
Website: http://www
.violenceresource.org
E-mail: icadv@violenceresource
.org

Iowa Coalition Against Domestic Violence
515 28th St.
Suite 104
Des Moines, IA 50312
Toll-Free in State Hotline:
800-942-0333
Phone: 515-244-8028
Fax: 515-244-7417
Website: http://www.icadv.org
E-mail: admin@icadv.org

Kansas Coalition Against Sexual and Domestic Violence
634 SW Harrison St.
Topeka, KS 66603
Toll-Free in State Hotline:
888-END-ABUSE (363-22873)
Phone/TTY: 785-232-9784
Fax: 785-266-1874
Website: http://www.kcsdv.org
E-mail: coalition@kcsdv.org

Kentucky Domestic Violence Association
P.O. Box 356
Frankfort, KY 40602
Phone: 502-209-5382
Fax: 502-226-5382
Website: http://www.kdva.org
E-mail: info@kdva.org

Louisiana Coalition Against Domestic Violence
P.O. Box 77308
Baton Rouge, LA 70879
Phone: 225-752-1296
Fax: 225-751-8927
Website: http://www.lcadv.org

Maine Coalition To End Domestic Violence
170 Park Street
Bangor, ME 04401
Statewide Toll-Free Domestic
Violence Hotline: 866-834-4357
Phone: 207-941-1194
Fax: 207-941-2327
Website: http://www.mcedv.org
E-mail: info@mcedv.org

Maryland Network Against Domestic Violence
6911 Laurel-Bowie Rd.
Suite 309
Bowie, MD 20715
Toll-Free: 800-634-3577
Phone: 301-352-4574
Fax: 301-809-0422
Website: http://www.mnadv.org
E-mail: info@mnadv.org

Jane Doe, Inc./Massachusetts Coalition Against Sexual Assault and Domestic Violence
14 Beacon Street
Suite 507
Boston, MA 02108
Toll-Free in State Hotline:
877-785-2020
Phone: 617-248-0922
Fax: 617-248-0902
TTY: 617-263-2200
Website: http://www.janedoe.org
E-mail: info@janedoe.org

Michigan Coalition Against Domestic and Sexual Violence
3893 Okemos Road
Suite B2
Okemos, MI 48864
Phone: 517-347-7000
Fax: 517-347-1377
TTY: 517-381-8470
Website: http://www.mcadsv.org

Minnesota Coalition For Battered Women
590 Park St.
Suite 410
St. Paul, MN 55103
Toll-Free Domestic Violence Crisis Line: 866-223-1111
Toll-Free: 800-289-6177
Phone: 651-646-6177
Fax: 651-646-1527
Website: http://www.mcbw.org
E-mail: mcbw@mcbw.org

Mississippi Coalition Against Domestic Violence
P.O. Box 4703
Jackson, MS 39296
Toll-Free: 800-898-3234
(8 a.m.–5 p.m.)
Toll-Free: 800-799-7233
(after hours)
Phone: 601-981-9196
Fax: 601-981-2501
Website: http://www.mcadv.org
E-mail: dvpolicy@mcadv.org

Missouri Coalition Against Domestic and Sexual Violence
217 Oscar Dr.
Suite A
Jefferson City, MO 65101
Phone: 573-634-4161
Website: http://www.mocadsv.org
E-mail: mocadsv@mocadsv.org

Montana Coalition Against Domestic & Sexual Violence
P.O. Box 818
Helena, MT 59624
Toll-Free: 888-404-7794
Phone: 406-443-7794
Fax: 406-443-7818
Website: http://www.mcadsv.com
E-mail: mcadsv@mt.net

Nebraska Domestic Violence Sexual Assault Coalition
1000 "O" Street
Suite 102
Lincoln, NE 68508
Toll-Free in State Hotline:
800-876-6238
Toll-Free Spanish Hotline:
877-215-0167
Phone: 402-476-6256
Website: http://www.ndvsac.org
E-mail: help@ndvsac.org

Nevada Network Against Domestic Violence
220 S. Rock Blvd.
Reno, NV 89502
Toll-Free in State Hotline:
800-500-1556
Toll-Free: 800-230-1955
Phone: 775-828-1115
Fax: 775-828-9911
Website: http://www.nnadv.org

New Hampshire Coalition Against Domestic and Sexual Violence
P.O. Box 353
Concord, NH 03302
Toll-Free Domestic Violence
Hotline: 866-644-3574
Toll-Free Sexual Assault
Hotline: 800-277-5570
Phone: 603-224-8893
Fax: 603-228-6096
Website: http://www.nhcadsv.org
NH Crisis Centers: http://www
.nhcadsv.org/crisis_centers.cfm

New Jersey Coalition for Battered Women
1670 Whitehorse-Hamilton Sq. Rd.
Trenton, NJ 08690
Toll-Free Statewide Hotline: 800-572-7233
Phone: 609-584-8107
Fax: 609-584-9750
TTY: 609-584-0027
Website: http://www.njcbw.org
E-mail: info@njcbw.org

New Mexico Coalition Against Domestic Violence
201 Coal Avenue SW
Albuquerque, NM 87102
Toll-Free in State: 800-773-3645
Phone: 505-246-9240
Fax: 505-246-9434
Website: http://www.nmcadv.org
E-mail: info@nmcadv.org

New York State Coalition Against Domestic Violence
350 New Scotland Ave.
Albany, NY 12208
Toll-Free English in State: 800-942-6906
Toll-Free English TTY: 800-818-0656
Toll-Free Spanish in State: 800-942-6908
Toll-Free Spanish TTY: 800-780-7660
Phone: 518-482-5465
Fax: 518-482-3807
Website: http://www.nyscadv.org
E-mail: nyscadv@nyscadv.org

North Carolina Coalition Against Domestic Violence
123 W. Main St., Suite 700
Durham, NC 27701
Toll-Free: 888-232-9124
Phone: 919-956-9124
Fax: 919-682-1449
Website: http://www.nccadv.org

North Dakota Council on Abused Women's Services
418 E. Rosser Ave., Suite 320
Bismark, ND 58501
Toll-Free: 888-255-6240
Phone: 701-255-6240
Fax: 701-255-1904
Website: http://www.ndcaws.org
E-mail: ndcaws@ndcaws.org

Action Ohio Coalition For Battered Women
5900 Roche Dr., Suite 445
Columbus, OH 43229
Toll-Free in State: 888-622-9315
Phone: 614-825-0551
Fax: 614-825-0673
Website: http://www.actionohio.org
E-mail: actionohio@sbcglobal.net

Ohio Domestic Violence Network
4807 Evanswood Dr., Suite 201
Columbus, OH 43229
Toll-Free: 800-934-9840
Phone: 614-781-9651
Fax: 614-781-9652
TTY: 614-781-9654
Website: http://www.odvn.org
E-mail: info@odvn.org

Oklahoma Coalition Against Domestic Violence and Sexual Assault
3815 N. Sante Fe Ave., Suite 124
Oklahoma City, OK 73118
Toll-Free: 800-522-7233
Phone: 405-524-0700
Fax: 405-524-0711
Website: http://www.ocadvsa.org
E-mail: info@ocadvsa.org

Oregon Coalition Against Domestic and Sexual Violence
380 SE Spokane St., Suite 100
Portland, OR 97202
Statewide Crisis Line:
888-235-5333
Toll-Free: 877-230-1951
Phone: 503-230-1951
Fax: 503-230-1973
Website: http://www.ocadsv.com

Pennsylvania Coalition Against Domestic Violence
6400 Flank Drive, Suite 1300
Harrisburg, PA 17112
Toll-Free: 800-932-4632
Toll-Free TTY: 800-553-2508
Toll-Free Legal: 888-235-3425
Phone: 717-545-6400
Fax: 717-671-8149
Website: http://www.pcadv.org

The Office of Women Advocates
Box 11382
Fernandez Juancus Station
Santurce, PR 00910
Phone: 787-721-7676
Fax: 787-725-9248

Rhode Island Coalition Against Domestic Violence
422 Post Road, Suite 202
Warwick, RI 02888
Toll-Free in State: 800-494-8100
Phone: 401-467-9940
Fax: 401-467-9943
Website: http://www.ricadv.org
E-mail: ricadv@ricadv.org

South Carolina Coalition Against Domestic Violence and Sexual Assault
P.O. Box 7776
Columbia, SC 29202
Toll-Free: 800-260-9293
Phone: 803-256-2900
Fax: 803-256-1030
Website: http://
www.sccadvasa.org

South Dakota Coalition Against Domestic Violence & Sexual Assault
P.O. Box 141
Pierre, SD 57501
Toll-Free: 800-572-9196
Phone: 605-945-0869
Fax: 605-945-0870
Website: http://
www.southdakotacoalition.org
E-mail: chris@sdcadvsa.org

Tennessee Coalition Against Domestic and Sexual Violence
2 International Plaza Dr.
Suite 425
Nashville, TN 37217
Toll-Free in State: 800-289-9018
Phone: 615-386-9406
Fax: 615-383-2967
Website: http://www.tcadsv.org
E-mail: webmistress@tcadsv.org

Texas Council On Family Violence
P.O. Box 161810
Austin, TX 78716
Toll-Free: 800-525-1978
Phone: 512-794-1133
Fax: 512-794-1199
Website: http://www.tcfv.org

Utah Domestic Violence Council
205 N. 400 West
Salt Lake City, UT 84103
Phone: 801-521-5544
Fax: 801-521-5548
Website: http://www.udvac.org

Vermont Network Against Domestic Violence and Sexual Assault
P.O. Box 405
Montpelier, VT 05601
Toll-Free Statewide Domestic Violence Hotline: 800-228-7395
Toll-Free Statewide Sexual Violence Hotline: 800-489-7273
Phone: 802-223-1302
Fax: 802-223-6943
TTY: 802-223-1115
Website: http://www.vtnetwork.org
E-mail: info@vtnetwork.org

Women's Coalition of St. Croix
Box 22-2734
Christiansted, VI 00822
Phone: 340-773-9272
Fax: 340-773-9062
Website: http://www.wcstx.com
E-mail: wcsc@pennswoods.net

Virginia Sexual and Domestic Violence Action Alliance
5008 Monument Ave, Suite A
Richmond, VA 23230
Toll-Free in State V/TTY: 800-838-8238
Phone: 804-377-0335
Fax: 804-377-0339
Website: http://www.vadv.org;
and http://www.vsdvalliance.org
E-mail: info@vsdvalliance.org

Washington State Coalition Against Domestic Violence/ Olympia
711 Capitol Way, Suite 702
Olympia, WA 98501
Toll-Free in State: 800-562-6025
Phone: 360-586-1022
Fax: 360-586-1024
TTY: 360-586-1029
Website: http://www.wscadv.org
E-mail: wscadv@wscadv.org

Washington State Coalition Against Domestic Violence/ Seattle
1402 Third Avenue, Suite 406
Seattle, WA 98101
Toll-Free in State: 800-562-6025
Phone: 206-389-2515
Fax: 206-389-2520
TTY: 206-389-2900
Website: http://www.wscadv.org
E-mail: wscadv@wscadv.org

Washington State Native American Coalition Against Domestic and Sexual Assault
P.O. Box 13260
Olympia, WA 98508
Toll-Free: 888-352-3120
Phone: 360-352-3120
Fax: 360-357-3858
Website: http://
www.womenspiritcoalition.org

West Virginia Coalition Against Domestic Violence
5004 Elk River Rd., South
Elkview, WV 25071
Phone: 304-965-3552
Fax: 304-965-3572
Website: http://www.wvcadv.org

Wisconsin Coalition Against Domestic Violence
307 S. Paterson St., Suite 1
Madison, WI 53703
Phone: 608-255-0539
Fax: 608-255-3560
Website: http://www.wcadv.org
E-mail: wcadv@wcadv.org

Wyoming Coalition Against Domestic Violence and Sexual Assault
409 S. Fourth St.
P.O. Box 236
Laramie, WY 82073
Toll-Free Crisis Line:
800-990-3877
Phone: 307-755-5481
Legal Staff: 307-755-0992
Fax: 307-755-5482
Website: http://www
.wyomingdvsa.org
E-mail:
info@mail.wyomingdvsa.org

Chapter 67

States That Have Address Confidentiality Programs

Arizona
Election Division
Secretary of State
1700 W. Washington St. 7th Floor
Phoenix, AZ 85007
Phone: 602-364-4700
Website: http://www.azsos.gov/
Info/Office.htm

California
Safe at Home Program
P.O. Box 846
Sacramento, CA 95812
Phone: 877-322-5227
Websites: http://www.sos.ca.gov/
safeathome

Colorado Address Confidentiality Program
1001 E. 62nd Avenue
Denver, CO 80216
Toll-Free: 888-341-0002
Toll-Free TTY: 800-659-2656
Phone: 303-869-4911
Fax: 303-869-4871
Website: http://
www.acp.colorado.gov
E-mail: acp@sos.state.co.us

Connecticut
Address Confidentiality Program
P.O. Box 150470
Hartford, CT 06115
Phone: 860-509-6006
Website: http://www.sots.ct.gov/
sots/cwp/view.asp?A=3177
&QUESTION_ID=391912
#theacpsubstituteaddress

Information in this chapter was compiled from sourced deemed accurate. All contact information was updated and verified in December 2008.

Florida
Address Confidentiality Program
Office of the Attorney General
The Capital PL-01
Tallahassee, FL 32399
Phone: 850-414-3300
Toll-Free: 800-226-6667

Idaho
Address Confidentiality Program
P.O. Box 83720
Boise, ID 83720
Phone: 208-334-2852
Fax: 208-334-2282
Website: http://www.idsos.state
.id.us/ACP/ACP.htm
E-mail: sosinfo@sos.idaho.gov

Indiana
Address Confidentiality Program
P.O. Box 6243
Indianapolis, IN 46206
Toll-Free: 800-321-1907
Website: http://www.in.gov/
attorneygeneral/legal/victim/
address_confidentiality.html
E-mail: confidential@atg
.state.in.us

Kansas
Safe at Home–Kansas
P.O. Box 798
Topeka, KS 66601
Phone: 785-296-3806
Website: http://www.kssos.org/
safeathome
E-mail: safeathome@kssos.org

Louisiana
Address Confidentiality Program
P.O. Box 91301
Baton Rouge, LA 70821
Toll-Free in Louisiana:
800-825-3805
Phone: 225-925-4792
Website: http://www.sos
.louisiana.gov/acp
E-mail: acp@sos.louisiana.gov

Maine
ACP Manager
148 Statehouse Station
Augusta, ME 04333
Phone: 207-626-8400
Website: http://www.maine.gov/
sos/acp
E-mail: acp.sos@maine.gov

Maryland
Safe at Home
P.O. Box 2995
Annapolis, MD 21404
Toll-Free: 800-633-9657 Ext. 3875
Phone: 410-260-3875
Website: http://www.marylandsos
.gov

Massachusetts
Address Confidentiality Program
P.O. Box 9120
Chelsea, MA 02150
Toll-Free: 866-Safe-ADD
(723-3233)
Phone: 617-727-3261
Website: http://www.sec.state
.ma.us/acp/acpidx.htm

Minnesota
Safe at Home
P.O. Box 17370
St. Paul, MN 55117
Toll-Free: 866-723-3035
Toll-Free TTY: 800-627-3529
Phone: 651-201-1399
Website: http://www.sos.state.mn
.us/home/index.asp?page=859
E-mail: Safe.athome@state.mn.us

Missouri
Safe At Home
P.O. Box 1409
Jefferson City, MO 65102
Toll-Free: 866-509-1409
Fax: 573-522-1525
Website: http://www.sos.mo.gov/
SafeAtHome
E-mail: SafeAtHome@sos.mo.gov

Montana
Address Confidentiality Program
P.O. Box 201410
Helena, MT 59620
Phone: 406-444-5803
Website: http://www.doj.mt.gov/
victims/domesticviolence.asp

Nebraska
Nebraska Address Confidentiality Program
P.O. Box 92921
Lincoln, NE 68501
Toll-Free: 866-227-6327
Phone: 402-471-3568
Website: http://www.sos.ne.gov/
business/acp_menu.html
E-mail: ACP@sos.ne.gov

Nevada
Confidential Address Program
P.O. Box 2743
Carson City, NV 89702
Toll-Free in Nevada:
888-432-6189
Phone: 775-684-5707
Fax: 775-684-5718
Website: http://sos.state.nv.us/
information/cap
E-mail:
nvcap@sosmail.state.nv.us

New Hampshire
Address Confidentiality Program
33 Capital St.
Concord, NH 03301
Toll-Free in New Hampshire:
800-300-4500
Phone: 603-271-1240
Website: http://doj.nh.gov/vic-
tim/address.html

New Jersey
Address Confidentiality Program
P.O. Box 207
Trenton, NJ 08625
Phone: 877-218-9133

New Mexico
Confidential Address Program
P.O. Box 53220
Albuquerque, NM 87153
Toll-Free: 888-432-5469
Fax: 505-827-8081
Website: http://
www.sos.state.nm.us
E-mail: CAP.sos@state.nm.us

North Carolina

Address Confidentiality Program
9099 Mail Service Center
Raleigh, NC 27699
Phone: 919-716-6785
Website: http://www.ncdoj.gov/
about/about_division_address
_confidentiality_program.jsp
E-mail: acp@ncdoj.gov

Oklahoma

Address Confidentiality Program
P.O. Box 60189
Oklahoma City, OK 73146
Toll-Free in Oklahoma:
866-227-7784
Phone: 405-557-1700
Fax: 405-557-1770
Website: http://www.sos.state.ok
.us/acp/acp_welcome.htm
E-mail: ACP@sos.state.ok.us

Oregon

Address Confidentiality Program
P.O. Box 1108
Salem, OR 97308
Toll-Free: 888-559-9090
Phone: 503-373-1323
Fax: 503-373-1340
Website: http://www.doj.state.or
.us/crimev/confidentiality.shtml
E-mail: acp@doj.state.or.us

Pennsylvania

Address Confidentiality Program
c/o Office of the Victim Advocate
1101 S. Front St. Suite 5200
Harrisburg, PA 17104
Toll-Free: 800-563-6399
Toll-Free TDD: 877-349-1064
Website: http://www.paacp.state
.pa.us

Texas

Address Confidentiality Program
P.O. Box 12199 MC069
Austin, TX 78711
Toll-Free: 888-832-2322
Phone: 512-936-1750
Website: http://www.oag.state.tx.
us/victims/acp.shtml
E-mail: Crimevictims@oag
.state.tx.us

Vermont

Safe at Home
P.O. Box 1568
Montpelier, VT 05601
Toll-Free in Vermont:
800-439-8683
Phone Voice/TTY: 802-828-0586
Fax: 802-828-2496
Website: http://www.sec.state.vt
.us/otherprg/safeathome/
safeathome.html
E-mail: safeathome@sec.state
.vt.us

Virginia

Address Confidentiality Program
900 East Main Street
Richmond, VA 23219
Toll-Free: 800-838-8238 (locate a
local VA domestic violence pro-
gram to apply for ACP)
Phone: 804-692-0952
Website: http://www.vaag.com/
KEY_ISSUES/DOMESTIC
_VIOLENCE/DV
_AddressConfidentiality.html

Washington

Address Confidentiality Program
P.O. Box 257
Olympia, WA 98507
Toll-Free in Washington:
800-822-1065
Toll-Free TTY: 800-664-9677
Phone: 360-753-2972
TTY: 360-664-0515
Website: http://
www.secstate.wa.gov/acp
E-mail: acp@secstate.wa.gov

West Virginia

Address Confidentiality Program
1900 Kanawha Blvd. East
Building 1, Suite 157K
Charleston, WV 25305-0009
Phone: 304-558-6000

Chapter 68

Hotlines for Victim Assistance

The following organizations offer hotlines for victims of domestic violence. If you, or someone you know, is a victim of domestic violence, sexual assault, stalking, or dating violence, please know that help is available. If you need immediate help, call 911.

Al-Anon Meeting Group Information Line
Toll-Free: 888-425-2666

Bureau of Indian Affairs Indian Country Child Abuse Hotline
Toll-Free: 800-633-5155

Childhelp USA National Child Abuse Hotline
Toll-Free: 800-4-A-CHILD (22-4453)

Covenant House Teen Crisis Line
Toll-Free: 800-999-9999

Eldercare Locator: Abuse of the Elderly
Toll-Free: 800-677-1116

Gay and Lesbian National Hotline
Toll-Free: 888-THE-GLNH (843-4564)

Girls and Boys Town National Hotline
Toll-Free: 800-448-3000
Toll-Free TDD: 800-448-1833

Information in this chapter was compiled from many sources deemed accurate. All contact information was updated and verified in December 2008. Inclusion does not constitute endorsement.

National Center for Victims of Crime
Toll-Free: 800-394-2255 (8:30 a.m.–5:30 p.m.)
Toll-Free TTY: 800-211-7996

National Domestic Violence Hotline
Toll-Free: 800-799-SAFE (7233)
Toll-Free TTY: 800-787-3224
Verizon Cell Phones: #HOPE (toll and airtime free)

National Hopeline Network
Toll-Free: 800-SUICIDE (784-2433)

National Organization for Victim Assistance
Toll-Free: 800-TRY-NOVA (879-6682)

National Runaway Switchboard
Toll-Free: 800-RUNAWAY (786-2929); or 800-621-4000

National Suicide Prevention Lifeline
Toll-Free: 800-273-8255

National Teen Dating Abuse Helpline
Toll-Free: 866-331-9474
Toll-Free TTY: 866-331-8453

National Youth Crisis Hotline
Toll-Free: 800-442-4673

Rape, Abuse, and Incest National Network (RAINN)
Toll-Free: 800-656-HOPE (4673)

Resource Center on Domestic Violence, Child Protection and Custody
Toll-Free: 800-527-3223

Trevor Project: Gay Teen Suicide Hotline
Toll-Free: 866-488-7386

Chapter 69

Resources for More Information about Domestic Violence

American Humane Association
63 Inverness Dr. East
Englewood, CO 80112
Toll-Free: 800-227-4645
Phone: 303-792-9900
Fax: 303-792-5333
Website: http://
www.americanhumane.org
E-mail:
info@americanhumane.org

Child Welfare Information Gateway
Children's Bureau/ACYF
1250 Maryland Ave., SW, 8th Floor
Washington, DC 20024
Toll-Free: 800-394-3366
Phone: 703-385-7565
Fax: 703-385-3206
Website: http://www.childwelfare
.gov
E-mail: info@childwelfare.gov

Corporate Alliance to End Partner Violence
2416 E. Washington St., Suite E
Bloomington, IL 61704
Phone: 309-664-0667
Fax: 309-664-0747
Website: http://www.caepv.org
E-mail: caepv@caepv.org

Information in this chapter was compiled from many sources deemed accurate. All contact information was updated and verified in December 2008. Inclusion does not constitute endorsement.

Eldercare Locator
Toll-Free Voice/TTY:
800-677-1116
Website: http://www.eldercare.gov
E-mail: eldercarelocator
@infospherix.com

Family Violence Prevention Fund
383 Rhode Island St., Suite #304
San Francisco, CA 94103-5133
Phone: 415-252-8900
Toll-Free TTY: 800-595-4889
Fax: 415-252-8991
Website: http://www.endabuse.org
E-mail: info@endabuse.org

Federal Bureau of Investigation (FBI)
J. Edgar Hoover Building
935 Pennsylvania Ave. NW
Washington, DC 20535
Phone: 202-324-3000
Website: http://www.fbi.gov

Guttmacher Institute
125 Maiden Lane, 7th Floor
New York, NY 10038
Toll-Free: 800-355-0244
Phone: 212-248-1111
Fax: 212-248-1951
Website: http://
www.guttmacher.org

INCITE! Women of Color Against Violence
P.O. Box 226
Redmond, WA 98073
Phone: 484-932-3166
Website: http://www
.incite-national.org
E-mail: incite_national-at-yahoo
.com

Institute on Domestic Violence in the African American Community
University of Minnesota School of Social Work
290 Peters Hall
1404 Gortner Ave.
St. Paul, MN 55108
Toll-Free: 877-643-8222
Website: http://
www.dvinstitute.org

LAMBDA GLBT Community Services
216 S. Ochoa St.
El Paso, TX 79901
Phone: 206-600-4297
Website: http://www.lambda.org
E-mail: admin.@lambda.org

Men Stopping Violence
533 W. Howard Ave.
Decatur, GA 30030
Toll-Free: 866-717-9317
Phone: 404-270-9894
Fax: 404-270-9895
Website: http://www
.menstoppingviolence.org/
index.php
E-mail:
msv@menstoppingviolence.org

National Center on Elder Abuse

c/o Center for Community
Research and Services
University of Delaware
297 Graham Hall
Newark, DE 19716
Phone: 302-831-3525
Fax: 302-831-4225
Website: http://www.ncea.aoa.gov
E-mail: ncea-info@aoa.hhs.gov

National Center for Victims of Crime

2000 M Street NW, Suite 480
Washington, DC 20036
Toll-Free: 800-394-2255
Toll-Free TTY: 800-211-7996
Phone: 202-467-8700
Fax: 202-467-8701
Website: http://www.ncvc.org
E-mail: gethelp@ncvc.org

National Child Abuse Hotline

15757 N. 78th St.
Scottsdale, AZ 85260
Toll-Free: 800-4-A-CHILD
(22-4453)
Toll-Free TDD: 800-222-4453
Phone: 480-922-8212
Fax: 480-922-7061
Website: http://www.region4wib
.org/ChildhelpUSA.htm
E-mail: info@childhelpusa.org

National Clearinghouse for the Defense of Battered Women

125 S. 9th St., Suite 302
Philadelphia, PA 19107
Toll-Free: 800-903-0111 ext. 3
Phone: 215-351-0010
Fax: 215-351-0779
Website: http://www.ncdbw.org

National Clearinghouse on Abuse in Later Life

307 S. Paterson St. #1
Madison, WI 53703
Phone: 608-255-0539
Fax: 608-255-3560
Website: http://www.ncall.us
E-mail: ncallspec@wcadv.org

National Coalition Against Domestic Violence

P.O. Box 18749
Denver, CO, 80218-0749
Phone: 303-839-1852
Fax: 303-831-9251
TTY: 303-839-1681
Website: http://www.ncadv.org

National Coalition for the Homeless

2201 P Street NW
Washington, DC 20037
Phone: 202-462-4822
Fax: 202-462-4823
Website: http://www
.nationalhomeless.org
E-mail:
info@nationalhomeless.org

National Domestic Violence Hotline

P.O. Box 161810
Austin, TX 78716
Toll-Free Hotline:
800-799-SAFE (7233)
Toll-Free TTY: 800-787-3224
Website: http://www.ndvh.org

National Latino Alliance for the Elimination of Domestic Violence

New Mexico Office
P.O. Box 4136
Espanola, NM 87533
Toll-Free: 800-342-9908
Phone: 505-692-6054
Toll-Free Fax: 800-216-2404
Fax: 505-692-6055
Website: http://www.dvalianza.org
E-mail: amedina@dvalianza.org

National Network to End Domestic Violence

2001 S Street, NW, Suite 400
Washington, DC 20009
Phone: 202-543-5566
Fax: 202-543-5626
Website: http://www.nnedv.org

National Organization for Victim Assistance

510 King St., Suite 424
Alexandria, VA 22314
Toll-Free 24-Hr. Helpline:
800-TRY-NOVA (879-6682)
Phone: 703-535-NOVA (6682)
Fax: 703-535-5500
Website: http://www.trynova.org
E-mail: nova@try-nova.org

National Resource Center on Domestic Violence

6400 Flank Dr., Suite 1300
Harrisburg, PA 17112
Toll-Free: 800-537-2238
Toll-Free TTY: 800-553-2508
Fax: 717-545-9456
Website: http://www.nrcdv.org

Office for Victims of Crime

U.S. Department of Justice
810 Seventh St. NW, 8th Floor
Washington, DC 20531
Phone: 202-307-5983
Fax: 202-514-6383
Website: http://www.ovc.gov

Office on Violence Against Women (OVW)

800 K Street, NW, Suite 920
Washington, DC 20530
Phone: 202-307-6026
Fax: 202-305-2589
TTY: 202-307-2277
Website: http://www.usdoj.gov/ovw

Rape, Abuse & Incest National Network (RAINN)

2000 L Street, NW, Suite 406
Washington, DC 20036
Toll-Free: 800-656-HOPE (4673)
Phone: 202-544-3064
Fax: 202-544-3556
Website: http://www.rainn.org
E-mail: info@rainn.org

Rural Assistance Center
School of Medicine and Health
Sciences, Rm. 4520
501 N. Columbia Rd., Stop 9037
Grand Forks, ND 58202-9037
Toll-Free: 800-270-1898
Fax: 800-270-1913
Website: http://www.raconline
.org
E-mail: info@raconline.org

Sacred Circle
National Resource Center to
End Violence Against Native
Women
722 St. Joseph St.
Rapid City, SC 57701
Toll-Free: 877-RED-ROAD
(733-7623)
Phone: 605-341-2050
Fax: 605-341-2472
Website: http://www.sacred-circle
.com
E-mail: scircle@sacred-circle.com

**SAMHSA National Mental
Health Information Center**
P.O. Box 2345
Rockville, MD 20847
Toll-Free: 800-789-2647
Toll-Free TDD: 866-889-2647
Fax: 240-221-4295
Website: http://mentalhealth
.samhsa.gov

**SAMHSA's Mental Health
Services Locator**
Website: http://www.mentalhealth
.samhsa.gov/databases

**Sport in Society, Mentors in
Violence Prevention**
Richards Hall Suite 350
360 Huntington Ave.
Boston MA 02115
Phone: 617-373-4025
Fax: 617-373-4566
Website: http://www
.sportinsociety.org/index.php
E-mail: sportinsociety@neu.edu

Stalking Resource Center
Toll-Free: 800-FYI-CALL
(394-2255)
Toll-Free TTY: 800-211-7996
Phone: 202-467-8700
Website: http://www.ncvc.org
E-mail: src@ncvc.org

**U. S. Citizenship and
Immigration Services
(USCIS)**
Toll-Free: 800-375-5283
Toll-Free TTY: 800-767-1833
Website: http://www.uscis.gov

Witness Justice
P.O. Box 475
Frederick, MD 21705-0475
Toll-Free: 800-4WJ-HELP
(95-4357)
Phone: 301-846-9110
Fax: 301-846-9113
Website: http://
www.wintessjustice.org

Index

Index

Page numbers followed by 'n' indicate a footnote. Page numbers in *italics* indicate a table or illustration.

A

State Department
  see US Department of State
"Statistical Brief #48: Violence-
  Related Stays in U.S. Hospitals,
  2005" (AHRQ) 36n
statistics
  animal cruelty 105–6
  Asian communities, domestic
    violence 242–52
  child maltreatment 301–3,
    309–13
  dating violence 328–31
  domestic violence, disaster
    aftermath 63–66
  domestic violence, military
    settings 269–70
  domestic violence, women 225–29
  domestic violence services 23–36
  domestic violence services by
    state *33–35*
  elder abuse 354–55
  family violence 18–22, 337
  homelessness 77–78
  homeless youth 81
  human trafficking 206–8
  intimate partner violence 114,
    117–29
  juvenile violent behavior
    342–48
  pregnancy, physical
    violence 57–59
  rural victims 263–64
  sexual assaults 92
  sexual violence 161–62
  stalking 174–76
  state courts, domestic
    violence 41–49
  tribal communities, domestic
    violence 257–62
  workplace, intimate partner
    violence 140–44
stress
  children 316
  elder abuse 371–75
students, violent behavior 337
substance abuse
  date rape 332
  male sexual trauma victims 167
  violent crime victims 562–63

Substance Abuse and Mental
  Health Services Administration
  (SAMHSA)
  Mental Health Information
    Center, contact
    information 563, 574, 609
  Mental Health Services Locator,
    website address 563, 574, 609
  publications
    alcohol abuse, domestic
      violence 87n
    childhood abuse recovery 452n,
      457n
    mental health concerns 561n
    survivor support 571n
substance abuse services,
  defined 582
substantiated, defined 582
suicide attempts, childhood
  stress 321
Sullivan, Chris M. 565n
super parent syndrome,
  described 285–86
"Supervised Visitation Programs:
  Information for Mothers
  Who Have Experienced Abuse"
  (Family Violence Prevention Fund)
  551n
support groups, elder abuse 378
"Supporting the Survivor"
  (SAMHSA) 571n
Survivors and Technology CD,
  contact information 518
syndromes, abuser tactics 285–88

T

TANF *see* Temporary Assistance
  for Needy Families
Taylor, Lauren R. 155n
technology
  disabled victims 200–201
  stalking 180–98
telephones
  disabled victims 201
  stalkers 184–85
Temporary Assistance for Needy
  Families (TANF) 69–70, 519–22

X

Health Reference Series

Complete Catalog

List price $93 per volume. School and library price $84 per volume.

Adolescent Health Sourcebook, 2nd Edition

Basic Consumer Health Information about the Physical, Mental, and Emotional Growth and Development of Adolescents, Including Medical Care, Nutritional and Physical Activity Requirements, Puberty, Sexual Activity, Acne, Tanning, Body Piercing, Common Physical Illnesses and Disorders, Eating Disorders, Attention Deficit Hyperactivity Disorder, Depression, Bullying, Hazing, and Adolescent Injuries Related to Sports, Driving, and Work

Along with Substance Abuse Information about Nicotine, Alcohol, and Drug Use, a Glossary, and Directory of Additional Resources

Edited by Joyce Brennfleck Shannon. 655 pages. 2007. 978-0-7808-0943-7.

"A particularly good resource for both parents and teens. The concise presentation of the material in brief and well-organized chapters creates an easy volume to browse."
—*School Library Journal, Jun '07*

"I don't believe there are any other books written in such easy to understand language that encompass such a breadth of topics. This is a complete revision of the book and is an excellent resource for parents and teens."
—*Doody's Review Service, 2007*

Adult Health Concerns Sourcebook

Basic Consumer Health Information about Medical and Mental Concerns of Adults, Including Facts about Choosing Healthcare Providers, Navigating Insurance Options, Maintaining Wellness, Preventing Cancer, Heart Disease, Stroke, Diabetes, and Osteoporosis, and Understanding Aging-Related Health Concerns, Including Menopause, Cognitive Changes, and Changes in the Coronary and Vascular Systems

Along with Tips on Caring for Aging Parents and Dealing with Health-Related Work and Travel Issues, a Glossary, and a Directory of Resources for Additional Help and Information

Edited by Sandra J. Judd. 648 pages. 2008. 978-0-7808-0999-4.

"Provides a thorough list of topics that are important to adult health and for caregivers."
—*CHOICE, Nov '08*

"Written in easy-to-understand language . . . the content is well-organized and is intended to aid adults in making health care-related decisions."
—*AORN Journal, Dec '08*

AIDS Sourcebook, 4th Edition

Basic Consumer Health Information about Human Immunodeficiency Virus (HIV) and Acquired Immunodeficiency Syndrome (AIDS), Featuring Updated Statistics and Facts about Risks, Prevention, Screening, Diagnosis, Treatments, Side Effects, and Complications, and Including a Section about the Impact of HIV/AIDS on the Health of Women, Children, and Adolescents

Along with Tips on Managing Life with AIDS, Reports on Current Research Initiatives and Clinical Trials, a Glossary of Related Terms, and Resource Directories for Further Help and Information

Edited by Ivy L. Alexander. 680 pages. 2008. 978-0-7808-0997-0.

SEE ALSO *Contagious Diseases Sourcebook, 2nd Edition*

Alcoholism Sourcebook, 2nd Edition

Basic Consumer Health Information about Alcohol Use, Abuse, and Dependence, Featuring Facts about the Physical, Mental, and Social Health Effects of Alcohol Addiction, Including Alcoholic Liver Disease, Pancreatic Disease, Cardiovascular Disease, Neurological Disorders, and the Effects of Drinking during Pregnancy

Along with Information about Alcohol Treatment, Medications, and Recovery Programs, in Addition to Tips for Reducing the Prevalence of Underage Drinking, Statistics about Alcohol Use, a Glossary of Related Terms, and Directories of Resources for More Help and Information

Edited by Amy L. Sutton. 625 pages. 2007. 978-0-7808-0942-0.

"A comprehensive look at the adverse effects of alcohol on people of all ages . . . It serves to whet the reader's appetite to continue learning using other resources. It is practical, easy to read, and enlightening, and is the first book a lay person should consult to learn about alcoholism."

—Doody's Review Service, 2007

"Should be a basic acquisition for any serious public or college-level library including health reference titles for general-interest readers."

—California Bookwatch, Feb '07

SEE ALSO Drug Abuse Sourcebook, 2nd Edition

Allergies Sourcebook, 3rd Edition

Basic Consumer Health Information about Allergic Disorders, Such as Anaphylaxis, Hives, Eczema, Rhinitis, Sinusitis, and Conjunctivitis, and Their Triggers, Including Pollen, Mold, Dust Mites, Animal Dander, Insects, Chemicals, Food, Food Additives, and Medications

Along with Advice about the Diagnosis and Treatment of Allergy Symptoms, a Glossary of Related Terms, a Directory of Resources for Help and Information, and Suggestions for Additional Reading

Edited by Amy L. Sutton. 588 pages. 2007. 978-0-7808-0950-5.

SEE ALSO Asthma Sourcebook, 2nd Edition

Alzheimer Disease Sourcebook, 4th Edition

Basic Consumer Health Information about Alzheimer Disease, Other Dementias, and Related Disorders, Including Multi-Infarct Dementia, Dementia with Lewy Bodies, Fronto-temporal Dementia (Pick Disease), Wernicke-Korsakoff Syndrome (Alcohol-Related Dementia), AIDS Dementia Complex, Huntington Disease, Creutzfeldt-Jacob Disease, and Delirium

Along with Information about Coping with Memory Loss and Forgetfulness, Maintaining

Skills, and Long-Term Planning for People with Dementia, and Suggestions Addressing Common Caregiver Concerns, Updated Information about Current Research Efforts, a Glossary of Related Terms, and Directories of Sources for Additional Help and Information

Edited by Karen Bellenir. 603 pages. 2008. 978-0-7808-1001-3.

"An invaluable resource for persons who have received a diagnosis, for caregivers, and for family members dealing with this insidious disease. It is recommended for public, community college, and ready-reference sections in academic libraries."

—ARBAonline, Jul '08

SEE ALSO Brain Disorders Sourcebook, 2nd Edition

Arthritis Sourcebook, 2nd Edition

Basic Consumer Health Information about Osteoarthritis, Rheumatoid Arthritis, Other Rheumatic Disorders, Infectious Forms of Arthritis, and Diseases with Symptoms Linked to Arthritis, Featuring Facts about Diagnosis, Pain Management, and Surgical Therapies

Along with Coping Strategies, Research Updates, a Glossary, and Resources for Additional Help and Information

Edited by Amy L. Sutton. 567 pages. 2004. 978-0-7808-0667-2.

"This easy-to-read volume is recommended for consumer health collections within public or academic libraries."

—E-Streams, May '05

"As expected, this updated edition continues the excellent reputation of this series in providing sound, usable health information. . . . Highly recommended."

—American Reference Books Annual, 2005

Asthma Sourcebook, 2nd Edition

Basic Consumer Health Information about the Causes, Symptoms, Diagnosis, and Treatment of Asthma in Infants, Children, Teenagers, and Adults, Including Facts about Different Types of Asthma, Common Co-Occurring Conditions, Asthma Management Plans, Triggers, Medications, and Medication Delivery Devices

Along with Asthma Statistics, Research Updates, a Glossary, a Directory of Asthma-Related Resources, and More

Edited by Karen Bellenir. 581 pages. 2006. 978-0-7808-0866-9.

Attention Deficit Disorder Sourcebook

Basic Consumer Health Information about Attention Deficit/Hyperactivity Disorder in Children and Adults, Including Facts about Causes, Symptoms, Diagnostic Criteria, and Treatment Options Such as Medications, Behavior Therapy, Coaching, and Homeopathy

Along with Reports on Current Research Initiatives, Legal Issues, and Government Regulations, and Featuring a Glossary of Related Terms, Internet Resources, and a List of Additional Reading Material

Edited by Dawn D. Matthews. 447 pages. 2002. 978-0-7808-0624-5.

"Recommended reference source."
—*Booklist, Jan '03*

SEE ALSO *Learning Disabilities Sourcebook, 3rd Edition*

Autism and Pervasive Developmental Disorders Sourcebook

Basic Consumer Health Information about Autism Spectrum and Pervasive Developmental Disorders, Such as Classical Autism, Asperger Syndrome, Rett Syndrome, and Childhood Disintegrative Disorder, Including Information about Related Genetic Disorders and Medical Problems and Facts about Causes, Screening Methods, Diagnostic Criteria, Treatments and Interventions, and Family and Education Issues

Along with a Glossary of Related Terms, Tips for Evaluating the Validity of Health Claims, and a Directory of Resources for Additional Help and Information

Edited by Sandra J. Judd. 603 pages. 2007. 978-0-7808-0953-6.

"Recommended for public libraries"
—*SciTech Book News, Mar '08*

SEE ALSO *Learning Disabilities Sourcebook, 3rd Edition*

Back and Neck Disorders Sourcebook, 2nd Edition

Basic Consumer Health Information about Spinal Pain, Spinal Cord Injuries, and Related Disorders, Such as Degenerative Disk Disease, Osteoarthritis, Scoliosis, Sciatica, Spina Bifida, and Spinal Stenosis, and Featuring Facts about Maintaining Spinal Health, Self-Care, Pain Management, Rehabilitative Care, Chiropractic Care, Spinal Surgeries, and Complementary Therapies

Along with Suggestions for Preventing Back and Neck Pain, a Glossary of Related Terms, and a Directory of Resources

Edited by Amy L. Sutton. 607 pages. 2004. 978-0-7808-0738-9.

"Recommended. ...An easy to use, comprehensive medical reference book."
—*E-Streams, Sep '05*

"For anyone who has back or neck problems, this book is ideal. Its easy-to-understand language and variety of topics makes this sourcebook a worthwhile read. The price...is reasonable for the amount of information contained in the book"
—*Occupational Therapy in Health Care, 2007*

Blood and Circulatory Disorders Sourcebook, 2nd Edition

Basic Consumer Health Information about the Blood and Circulatory System and Related Disorders, Such as Anemia and Other Hemoglobin Diseases, Cancer of the Blood and Associated Bone Marrow Disorders, Clotting and Bleeding Problems, and Conditions That Affect the Veins, Blood Vessels, and Arteries, Including Facts about the Donation and Transplantation of Bone Marrow, Stem Cells, and Blood and Tips for Keeping the Blood and Circulatory System Healthy

Along with a Glossary of Related Terms and Resources for Additional Help and Information

Edited by Amy L. Sutton. 634 pages. 2005. 978-0-7808-0746-4.

"Highly recommended pick for basic consumer health reference holdings at all levels."
—*The Bookwatch, Aug '05*

Brain Disorders Sourcebook, 2nd Edition

Basic Consumer Health Information about Acquired and Traumatic Brain Injuries, Infections of the Brain, Epilepsy and Seizure Disorders, Cerebral Palsy, and Degenerative Neurological Disorders, Including Amyotrophic Lateral Sclerosis (ALS), Dementias, Multiple Sclerosis, and More

Along with Information on the Brain's Structure and Function, Treatment and Rehabilitation Options, Reports on Current Research Initiatives, a Glossary of Terms Related to Brain Disorders and Injuries, and a Directory of Sources for Further Help and Information

Edited by Sandra J. Judd. 600 pages. 2005. 978-0-7808-0744-0.

"This easy-to-read volume provides up-to-date health information... Recommended for consumer health collections within public or academic libraries."

—*E-Streams, Feb '06*

SEE ALSO *Alzheimer Disease Sourcebook, 4th Edition*

Breast Cancer Sourcebook, 3rd Edition

Basic Consumer Health Information about Breast Health and Breast Cancer, Including Facts about Environmental, Genetic, and Other Risk Factors, Prevention Efforts, Screening and Diagnostic Methods, Surgical Treatment Options and Other Care Choices, Complementary and Alternative Therapies, and Post-Treatment Concerns

Along with Statistical Data, News about Research Advances, a Glossary of Related Terms, and Directories of Resources for Additional Information and Support

Edited by Karen Bellenir. 606 pages. 2009. 978-0-7808-1030-3.

SEE ALSO *Cancer Sourcebook for Women, 3rd Edition, Women's Health Concerns Sourcebook, 3rd Edition*

Breastfeeding Sourcebook

Basic Consumer Health Information about the Benefits of Breastmilk, Preparing to Breastfeed, Breastfeeding as a Baby Grows,

Nutrition, and More, Including Information on Special Situations and Concerns Such as Mastitis, Illness, Medications, Allergies, Multiple Births, Prematurity, Special Needs, and Adoption

Along with a Glossary and Resources for Additional Help and Information

Edited by Jenni Lynn Colson. 367 pages. 2002. 978-0-7808-0332-9.

SEE ALSO *Pregnancy and Birth Sourcebook, 2nd Edition*

Burns Sourcebook

Basic Consumer Health Information about Various Types of Burns and Scalds, Including Flame, Heat, Cold, Electrical, Chemical, and Sun Burns

Along with Information on Short-Term and Long-Term Treatments, Tissue Reconstruction, Plastic Surgery, Prevention Suggestions, and First Aid

Edited by Allan R. Cook. 604 pages. 1999. 978-0-7808-0204-9.

"This is an exceptional addition to the series and is highly recommended for all consumer health collections, hospital libraries, and academic medical centers."
—*E-Streams, Mar '00*

"This key reference guide is an invaluable addition to all health care and public libraries in confronting this ongoing health issue."
—*American Reference Books Annual, 2000*

SEE ALSO *Dermatological Disorders Sourcebook, 2nd Edition*

Cancer Sourcebook, 5th Edition

Basic Consumer Health Information about Major Forms and Stages of Cancer, Featuring Facts about Head and Neck Cancers, Lung Cancers, Gastrointestinal Cancers, Genitourinary Cancers, Lymphomas, Blood Cell Cancers, Endocrine Cancers, Skin Cancers, Bone Cancers, Metastatic Cancers, and More

Along with Facts about Cancer Treatments, Cancer Risks and Prevention, a Glossary of Related Terms, Statistical Data, and a Directory of Resources for Additional Information

Edited by Karen Bellenir. 1105 pages. 2007. 978-0-7808-0947-5.

"The 5th, updated edition of *Cancer Sourcebook* should be in every public and health lending library collection... An unparalleled discussion essential for any health collections considering an all-in-one basic general reference."

—*California Bookwatch, Aug '07*

SEE ALSO *Breast Cancer Sourcebook, 3rd Edition, Cancer Sourcebook for Women, 3rd Edition, Cancer Survivorship Sourcebook, Leukemia Sourcebook*

Cancer Sourcebook for Women, 3rd Edition

Basic Consumer Health Information about Leading Causes of Cancer in Women, Featuring Facts about Gynecologic Cancers and Related Concerns, Such as Breast Cancer, Cervical Cancer, Endometrial Cancer, Uterine Sarcoma, Vaginal Cancer, Vulvar Cancer, and Common Non-Cancerous Gynecologic Conditions, in Addition to Facts about Lung Cancer, Colorectal Cancer, and Thyroid Cancer in Women

Along with Information about Cancer Risk Factors, Screening and Prevention, Treatment Options, and Tips on Coping with Life after Cancer Treatment, a Glossary of Cancer Terms, and a Directory of Resources for Additional Help and Information

Edited by Amy L. Sutton. 687 pages. 2006. 978-0-7808-0867-6.

"This excellent book provides the general public with information compiled in a way that will help them to gain the knowledge they need. 4 Stars!"

—*Doody's Review Service, Dec '06*

"An indispensable reference for health consumers and cancer patients. Recommended for public libraries and academic libraries with a medical department."

—*E-Streams, Sep '08*

Cancer Survivorship Sourcebook

Basic Consumer Health Information about the Physical, Educational, Emotional, Social, and Financial Needs of Cancer Patients from Diagnosis, through Cancer Treatment, and Beyond, Including Facts about Researching Specific Types of Cancer and Learning about Clinical Trials and Treatment Options, and

Featuring Tips for Coping with the Side Effects of Cancer Treatments and Adjusting to Life after Cancer Treatment Concludes

Along with Suggestions for Caregivers, Friends, and Family Members of Cancer Patients, a Glossary of Cancer Care Terms, and Directories of Related Resources

Edited by Karen Bellenir. 633 pages. 2007. 978-0-7808-0985-7.

"Well organized and comprehensive in coverage, the book speaks to issues encountered both during and after cancer treatment. Recommended for consumer health and public libraries."

—*Library Journal, Aug 1 '07*

"*Cancer Survivorship Sourcebook* will be useful to anyone who has a friend or loved one with a cancer diagnosis."

—*American Reference Books Annual, 2008*

SEE ALSO *Cancer Sourcebook, 5th Edition*

Cardiovascular Diseases and Disorders Sourcebook, 3rd Edition

Basic Consumer Health Information about Heart and Vascular Diseases and Disorders, Such as Angina, Heart Attacks, Arrhythmias, Cardiomyopathy, Valve Disease, Atherosclerosis, and Aneurysms, with Information about Managing Cardiovascular Risk Factors and Maintaining Heart Health, Medications and Procedures Used to Treat Cardiovascular Disorders, and Concerns of Special Significance to Women

Along with Reports on Current Research Initiatives, a Glossary of Related Medical Terms, and a Directory of Sources for Further Help and Information

Edited by Sandra J. Judd. 687 pages. 2005. 978-0-7808-0739-6.

"This updated sourcebook is still the best first stop for comprehensive introductory information on cardiovascular diseases."

—*American Reference Books Annual, 2006*

"Recommended for public libraries and libraries supporting health care professionals."

—*E-Streams, Sep '05*

Caregiving Sourcebook

Basic Consumer Health Information for Caregivers, Including a Profile of Caregivers, Caregiving Responsibilities and Concerns, Tips for Specific Conditions, Care Environments, and the Effects of Caregiving

Along with Facts about Legal Issues, Financial Information, and Future Planning, a Glossary, and a Listing of Additional Resources

Edited by Joyce Brennfleck Shannon. 583 pages. 2001. 978-0-7808-0331-2.

"Essential for most collections."
— *Library Journal, Apr 1 '02*

"An ideal addition to the reference collection of any public library. Health sciences information professionals may also want to acquire the *Caregiving Sourcebook* for their hospital or academic library for use as a ready reference tool by health care workers interested in aging and caregiving."
— *E-Streams, Jan '02*

Child Abuse Sourcebook, 2nd Edition

Basic Consumer Health Information about the Physical, Sexual, and Emotional Abuse of Children, Neglect, Münchhausen Syndrome by Proxy (MSBP), and Shaken Baby Syndrome, and Featuring Facts about Withholding Medical Care, Corporal Punishment, Child Maltreatment in Youth Sports, and Parental Substance Abuse

Along with Information about Child Protective Services, Foster Care, Adoption, Parenting Challenges, Abuse Prevention Programs, and Intervention, Treatment, and Recovery Guidelines, a Glossary of Related Terms, and Resources for Additional Help and Information

Edited by Joyce Brennfleck Shannon. 600 pages. 2009. 978-0-7808-1037-2.

SEE ALSO Domestic Violence Sourcebook, 3rd Edition

Childhood Diseases and Disorders Sourcebook, 2nd Edition

Basic Consumer Health Information about the Physical, Mental, and Developmental Health of Pre-Adolescent Children, Including Facts about Infectious Diseases, Asthma, Allergies, Diabetes, and Other Acute and Chronic Conditions Affecting the Gastrointestinal Tract, Ears, Nose, Throat, Liver, Kidneys, Heart, Blood, Brain, Muscles, Bones, and Skin

Along with Reports on Recommended Childhood Vaccinations, Wellness Guidelines, a Glossary of Related Medical Terms, and a List of Resources for Parents

Edited by Sandra J. Judd. 694 pages. 2009. 978-0-7808-1031-0.

SEE ALSO Healthy Children Sourcebook

Colds, Flu and Other Common Ailments Sourcebook

Basic Consumer Health Information about Common Ailments and Injuries, Including Colds, Coughs, the Flu, Sinus Problems, Headaches, Fever, Nausea and Vomiting, Menstrual Cramps, Diarrhea, Constipation, Hemorrhoids, Back Pain, Dandruff, Dry and Itchy Skin, Cuts, Scrapes, Sprains, Bruises, and More

Along with Information about Prevention, Self-Care, Choosing a Doctor, Over-the-Counter Medications, Folk Remedies, and Alternative Therapies, and Including a Glossary of Important Terms and a Directory of Resources for Further Help and Information

Edited by Chad T. Kimball. 622 pages. 2001. 978-0-7808-0435-7.

"A good starting point for research on common illnesses. It will be a useful addition to public and consumer health library collections."
— *American Reference Books Annual, 2002*

"Will prove valuable to any library seeking to maintain a current, comprehensive reference collection of health resources. . . Excellent reference."
— *The Bookwatch, Aug '01*

Communication Disorders Sourcebook

Basic Information about Deafness and Hearing Loss, Speech and Language Disorders, Voice Disorders, Balance and Vestibular Disorders, and Disorders of Smell, Taste, and Touch

Edited by Linda M. Ross. 533 pages. 1996. 978-0-7808-0077-9.

640

"This is skillfully edited and is a welcome resource for the layperson. It should be found in every public and medical library."
—*Booklist Health Sciences Supplement, Oct '97*

■

Complementary and Alternative Medicine Sourcebook, 3rd Edition

Basic Consumer Health Information about Complementary and Alternative Medical Therapies, Including Acupuncture, Ayurveda, Traditional Chinese Medicine, Herbal Medicine, Homeopathy, Naturopathy, Biofeedback, Hypnotherapy, Yoga, Art Therapy, Aromatherapy, Clinical Nutrition, Vitamin and Mineral Supplements, Chiropractic, Massage, Reflexology, Crystal Therapy, Therapeutic Touch, and More

Along with Facts about Alternative and Complementary Treatments for Specific Conditions Such as Cancer, Diabetes, Osteoarthritis, Chronic Pain, Menopause, Gastrointestinal Disorders, Headaches, and Mental Illness, a Glossary, and a Resource List for Additional Help and Information

Edited by Sandra J. Judd. 630 pages. 2006. 978-0-7808-0864-5.

"A 'must' reference for any serious healthcare collection. Public library holdings, too, will welcome it as a popular reference."
—*California Bookwatch, Oct '06*

"Both basic and informative at the same time. . . a useful resource for health care professionals as well as consumers interested in learning more information about CAM therapies."
—*AORN Journal, Jan '08*

"A quality, indexed, referenced guideline for many alternative practices that are quite popular around the world...It is neatly organized to find facts quickly, is peer-reviewed, and stays current with the most recent advances."
—*Journal of Dental Hygiene, Jul '07*

■

Congenital Disorders Sourcebook, 2nd Edition

Basic Consumer Health Information about Non-hereditary Birth Defects and Disorders Related to Prematurity, Gestational Injuries, Congenital Infections, and Birth Complications, Including Heart Defects, Hydrocephalus, Spina Bifida, Cleft Lip and Palate, Cerebral Palsy, and More

Along with Facts about the Prevention of Birth Defects, Fetal Surgery and Other Treatment Options, Research Initiatives, a Glossary of Related Terms, and Resources for Additional Information and Support

Edited by Sandra J. Judd. 619 pages. 2007. 978-0-7808-0945-1.

"Congenital Disorders Sourcebook provides an excellent, non-technical overview of many aspects of pregnancy with the focus on congenital disorders."
—*American Reference Books Annual, 2008*

"An excellent readable reference aimed at the lay public for difficult to understand medical problems. An excellent starting point for the interested parent or family member who may then be motivated to seek more information."
—*Doody's Review Service, 2007*

SEE ALSO *Pregnancy and Birth Sourcebook, 2nd Edition*

■

Contagious Diseases Sourcebook, 2nd Edition

Basic Consumer Health Information about Diseases Spread from Person to Person through Direct Physical Contact, Airborne Transmissions, Sexual Contact, or Contact with Blood or Other Body Fluids, Including Pneumococcal, Staphylococcal, and Streptococcal Diseases, Colds, Influenza, Lice, Measles, Mumps, Tuberculosis, and Others

Along with Facts about Self-Care and Over-the-Counter Medications, Antibiotics and Drug Resistance, Disease Prevention, Vaccines, and Bioterrorism, a Glossary, and a Directory of Resources for More Information

Edited by Joyce Brennfleck Shannon. 600 pages. 2009. 978-0-7808-1075-4.

SEE ALSO *AIDS Sourcebook, 4th Edition, Hepatitis Sourcebook*

■

Cosmetic and Reconstructive Surgery Sourcebook, 2nd Edition

Basic Consumer Information about Plastic Surgery and Non-Surgical Appearance-Enhancing Procedures, Including Facts about Botulinum Toxin, Collagen Replacement, Dermabrasion,

Chemical Peels, Eyelid Surgery, Nose Reshaping, Lip Augmentation, Liposuction, Breast Enlargement and Reduction, Tummy Tucking, and Other Skin, Hair, Facial, and Body Shaping Procedures

Along with Information about Reconstructive Procedures for Congenital Disorders, Disfiguring Diseases, Burns, and Traumatic Injuries, a Glossary of Related Terms, and a Directory of Additional Resources

Edited by Karen Bellenir. 483 pages. 2007. 978-0-7808-0951-2.

"A practical guide for health care consumers and health care workers. . . . This easy-to-read reference guide would be useful for novice and veteran health care consumers, surgical technology students, nursing students, and perioperative nurses new to plastic and reconstructive surgery. It also may be helpful for medical-surgical nurses as a guide for patient teaching in their practices."

—*AORN Journal, Aug '08*

SEE ALSO *Surgery Sourcebook, 2nd Edition*

Death and Dying Sourcebook, 2nd Edition

Basic Consumer Health Information about End-of-Life Care and Related Perspectives and Ethical Issues, Including End-of-Life Symptoms and Treatments, Pain Management, Quality-of-Life Concerns, the Use of Life Support, Patients' Rights and Privacy Issues, Advance Directives, Physician-Assisted Suicide, Caregiving, Organ and Tissue Donation, Autopsies, Funeral Arrangements, and Grief

Along with Statistical Data, Information about the Leading Causes of Death, a Glossary, and Directories of Support Groups and Other Resources

Edited by Joyce Brennfleck Shannon. 626 pages. 2006. 978-0-7808-0871-3.

Dental Care and Oral Health Sourcebook, 3rd Edition

Basic Consumer Health Information about Dental Care and Oral Health Throughout the Lifespan, Including Facts about Cavities, Bad Breath, Cold and Canker Sores, Dry Mouth, Toothaches, Gum Disease, Malocclusion, Temporomandibular Joint and Muscle Disorders, Oral Cancers, and Dental Emergencies

Along with Information about Mouth Hygiene, Crowns, Bridges, Implants, and Fillings, Surgical, Orthodontic, and Cosmetic Dental Procedures, Pain Management, Health Conditions that Impact Oral Care, a Glossary of Related Terms, and a Directory of Additional Resources

Edited by Amy L. Sutton. 619 pages. 2008. 978-0-7808-1032-7.

Depression Sourcebook, 2nd Edition

Basic Consumer Health Information about Unipolar Depression, Bipolar Disorder, Dysthymia, Seasonal Affective Disorder, Postpartum Depression, and Other Depressive Disorders, Including Facts about Populations at Special Risk, Coexisting Medical Conditions, Symptoms, Treatment Options, and Suicide Prevention

Along with Statistical Data, a Glossary of Related Terms, and a Directory of Resources for Additional Help and Information

Edited by Sandra J. Judd. 646 pages. 2008. 978-0-7808-1003-7.

"Recommended for public libraries."
—*ARBAonline, Nov '08*

SEE ALSO *Mental Health Disorders Sourcebook, 4th Edition*

Dermatological Disorders Sourcebook, 2nd Edition

Basic Consumer Health Information about Conditions and Disorders Affecting the Skin, Hair, and Nails, Such as Acne, Rosacea, Rashes, Dermatitis, Pigmentation Disorders, Birthmarks, Skin Cancer, Skin Injuries, Psoriasis, Scleroderma, and Hair Loss, Including Facts about Medications and Treatments for Dermatological Disorders and Tips for Maintaining Healthy Skin, Hair, and Nails

Along with Information about How Aging Affects the Skin, a Glossary of Related Terms, and a Directory of Resources for Additional Help and Information

Edited by Amy L. Sutton. 617 pages. 2006. 978-0-7808-0795-2.

SEE ALSO *Burns Sourcebook*

▩

Diabetes Sourcebook, 4th Edition

Basic Consumer Health Information about Type 1 and Type 2 Diabetes Mellitus, Gestational Diabetes, Monogenic Forms of Diabetes, and Insulin Resistance, with Guidelines for Lifestyle Modifications and the Medical Management of Diabetes, Including Facts about Insulin, Insulin Delivery Devices, Oral Diabetes Medications, Self-Monitoring of Blood Glucose, Meal Planning, Physical Activity Recommendations, Foot Care, and Treatment Options for People with Kidney Failure

Along with a Section about Diabetes Complications and Co-Occurring Conditions, a Glossary of Related Terms, and Directories of Resources for Additional Help and Information

Edited by Karen Bellenir. 627 pages. 2008. 978-0-7808-1005-1.

SEE ALSO *Endocrine and Metabolic Disorders Sourcebook, 2nd Edition*

▩

Diet and Nutrition Sourcebook, 3rd Edition

Basic Consumer Health Information about Dietary Guidelines and the Food Guidance System, Recommended Daily Nutrient Intakes, Serving Proportions, Weight Control, Vitamins and Supplements, Nutrition Issues for Different Life Stages and Lifestyles, and the Needs of People with Specific Medical Concerns, Including Cancer, Celiac Disease, Diabetes, Eating Disorders, Food Allergies, and Cardiovascular Disease

Along with Facts about Federal Nutrition Support Programs, a Glossary of Nutrition and Dietary Terms, and Directories of Additional Resources for More Information about Nutrition

Edited by Joyce Brennfleck Shannon. 605 pages. 2006. 978-0-7808-0800-3.

SEE ALSO *Digestive Diseases and Disorders Sourcebook, Eating Disorders Sourcebook, 2nd Edition, Gastrointestinal Diseases and Disorders Sourcebook, 2nd Edition, Vegetarian Sourcebook*

▩

Digestive Diseases and Disorders Sourcebook

Basic Consumer Health Information about Diseases and Disorders that Impact the Upper and Lower Digestive System, Including Celiac Disease, Constipation, Crohn's Disease, Cyclic Vomiting Syndrome, Diarrhea, Diverticulosis and Diverticulitis, Gallstones, Heartburn, Hemorrhoids, Hernias, Indigestion (Dyspepsia), Irritable Bowel Syndrome, Lactose Intolerance, Ulcers, and More

Along with Information about Medications and Other Treatments, Tips for Maintaining a Healthy Digestive Tract, a Glossary, and Directory of Digestive Diseases Organizations

Edited by Karen Bellenir. 323 pages. 2000. 978-0-7808-0327-5.

SEE ALSO *Diet and Nutrition Sourcebook, 3rd Edition, Gastrointestinal Diseases and Disorders Sourcebook, 2nd Edition*

▩

Disabilities Sourcebook

Basic Consumer Health Information about Physical and Psychiatric Disabilities, Including Descriptions of Major Causes of Disability, Assistive and Adaptive Aids, Workplace Issues, and Accessibility Concerns

Along with Information about the Americans with Disabilities Act, a Glossary, and Resources for Additional Help and Information

Edited by Dawn D. Matthews. 602 pages. 2000. 978-0-7808-0389-3.

"A must for libraries with a consumer health section."
—*American Reference Books Annual, 2002*

"A much needed addition to the Omnigraphics *Health Reference Series*. A current reference work to provide people with disabilities, their families, caregivers or those who work with them, a broad range of information in one volume, has not been available until now. . . . It is recommended for all public and academic library reference collections."
—*E-Streams, May '01*

"An excellent source book in easy-to-read format covering many current topics; highly recommended for all libraries."
—*CHOICE, Jan '01*

Disease Management Sourcebook

Basic Consumer Health Information about Coping with Chronic and Serious Illnesses, Navigating the Health Care System, Communicating with Health Care Providers, Assessing Health Care Quality, and Making Informed Health Care Decisions, Including Facts about Second Opinions, Hospitalization, Surgery, and Medications

Along with a Section about Children with Chronic Conditions, Information about Legal, Financial, and Insurance Issues, a Glossary of Related Terms, and Directories of Additional Resources

Edited by Joyce Brennfleck Shannon. 621 pages. 2008. 978-0-7808-1002-0.

"Consumers need to know how to manage their health care the same way they manage anything else in their lives. The text is very readable and is written for the layperson and consumer. The cost is not prohibitive. This book should be in all collections of health care libraries and public libraries."
—*ARBAonline, Jul '08*

"The information is very current, and the selection of font and layout make the book easy to read. A hardback that will stand up to much usage, this is an excellent resource for

consumers. . . . Recommended. General readers."
—*CHOICE, Nov '08*

"Intended for lay readers, this resource clarifies the many confusing and overwhelming details associated with chronic disease care. Meticulous and clearly explained, the book even includes diagrams intended to ease comprehension of over-the-counter medication labels. An essential guide to navigating the health-care rapids."
—*Library Journal, Aug '08*

Domestic Violence Sourcebook, 3rd Edition

Basic Consumer Health Information about Warning Signs, Risk Factors, and Health Consequences of Intimate Partner Violence, Sexual Violence and Rape, Stalking, Human Trafficking, Child Maltreatment, Teen Dating Violence, and Elder Abuse

Along with Facts about Victims and Perpetrators, Strategies for Violence Prevention, and Emergency Interventions, Safety Plans, and Financial and Legal Tips for Victims, a Glossary of Related Terms, and Directories of Resources for Additional Information and Support

Edited by Joyce Brennfleck Shannon. 600 pages. 2009. 978-0-7808-1038-9.

SEE ALSO *Child Abuse Sourcebook, 2nd Edition*

Drug Abuse Sourcebook, 2nd Edition

Basic Consumer Health Information about Illicit Substances of Abuse and the Misuse of Prescription and Over-the-Counter Medications, Including Depressants, Hallucinogens, Inhalants, Marijuana, Stimulants, and Anabolic Steroids

Along with Facts about Related Health Risks, Treatment Programs, Prevention Programs, a Glossary of Abuse and Addiction Terms, a Glossary of Drug-Related Street Terms, and a Directory of Resources for More Information

Edited by Catherine Ginther. 581 pages. 2004. 978-0-7808-0740-2.

"Commendable for organizing useful, normally scattered government and association-produced data into a logical sequence."
—*American Reference Books Annual, 2006*

SEE ALSO *Alcoholism Sourcebook, 2nd Edition*

Ear, Nose, and Throat Disorders Sourcebook, 2nd Edition

Basic Consumer Health Information about Disorders of the Ears, Hearing Loss, Vestibular Disorders, Nasal and Sinus Problems, Throat and Vocal Cord Disorders, and Otolaryngologic Cancers, Including Facts about Ear Infections and Injuries, Genetic and Congenital Deafness, Sensorineural Hearing Disorders, Tinnitus, Vertigo, Ménière Disease, Rhinitis, Sinusitis, Snoring, Sore Throats, Hoarseness, and More

Along with Reports on Current Research Initiatives, a Glossary of Related Medical Terms, and a Directory of Sources for Further Help and Information

Edited by Sandra J. Judd. 631 pages. 2007. 978-0-7808-0872-0.

Eating Disorders Sourcebook, 2nd Edition

Basic Consumer Health Information about Anorexia Nervosa, Bulimia, Binge Eating, Compulsive Exercise, Female Athlete Triad, and Other Eating Disorders, Including Facts about Body Image and Other Cultural and Age-Related Risk Factors, Prevention Efforts, Adverse Health Effects, Treatment Options, and the Recovery Process

Along with Guidelines for Healthy Weight Control, a Glossary, and Directories of Additional Resources

Edited by Joyce Brennfleck Shannon. 557 pages. 2007. 978-0-7808-0948-2.

SEE ALSO *Diet and Nutrition Sourcebook, 3rd Edition, Mental Health Disorders Sourcebook, 4th Edition*

Emergency Medical Services Sourcebook

Basic Consumer Health Information about Preventing, Preparing for, and Managing Emergency Situations, When and Who to Call for Help, What to Expect in the Emergency Room, the Emergency Medical Team, Patient Issues, and Current Topics in Emergency Medicine

Along with Statistical Data, a Glossary, and Sources of Additional Help and Information

Edited by Jenni Lynn Colson. 472 pages. 2002. 978-0-7808-0420-3.

SEE ALSO *Injury and Trauma Sourcebook*

Endocrine and Metabolic Disorders Sourcebook, 2nd Edition

Basic Consumer Health Information about Hormonal and Metabolic Disorders that Affect the Body's Growth, Development, and Functioning, Including Disorders of the Pancreas, Ovaries and Testes, and Pituitary, Thyroid, Parathyroid, and Adrenal Glands, with Facts about *Growth Disorders, Addison Disease, Cushing Syndrome, Conn Syndrome, Diabetic Disorders, Multiple Endocrine Neoplasia, Inborn Errors of Metabolism, and More*

Along with Information about Endocrine Functioning, Diagnostic and Screening Tests, a Glossary of Related Terms, and Directories of Additional Resources

Edited by Joyce Brennfleck Shannon. 597 pages. 2007. 978-0-7808-0952-9.

SEE ALSO Diabetes Sourcebook, 4th Edition

Environmental Health Sourcebook, 2nd Edition

Basic Consumer Health Information about the Environment and Its Effect on Human Health, Including the Effects of Air Pollution, Water Pollution, Hazardous Chemicals, Food Hazards, Radiation Hazards, Biological Agents, Household Hazards, Such as Radon, Asbestos, Carbon Monoxide, and Mold, and Information about Associated Diseases and Disorders, Including Cancer, Allergies, Respiratory Problems, and Skin Disorders

Along with Information about Environmental Concerns for Specific Populations, a Glossary of Related Terms, and Resources for Further Help and Information

Edited by Dawn D. Matthews. 650 pages. 2003. 978-0-7808-0632-0.

"Recommended for teenage and adult students and readers, and for public and academic libraries, as well as any library focusing on consumer health."
—*E-Streams, May '04*

"This recently updated edition continues the level of quality and the reputation of the numerous other volumes in Omnigraphics' *Health Reference Series.*"
—*American Reference Books Annual, 2004*

Ethnic Diseases Sourcebook

Basic Consumer Health Information for Ethnic and Racial Minority Groups in the United States, Including General Health Indicators and Behaviors, Ethnic Diseases, Genetic Testing, the Impact of Chronic Diseases, Women's Health, Mental Health Issues, and Preventive Health Care Services

Along with a Glossary and a Listing of Additional Resources

Edited by Joyce Brennfleck Shannon. 648 pages. 2001. 978-0-7808-0336-7.

"Not many books have been written on this topic to date, and the *Ethnic Diseases Sourcebook* is a strong addition to the list. It will be an important introductory resource for health consumers, students, health care personnel, and social scientists. It is recommended for public, academic, and large hospital libraries."
—*American Reference Books Annual, 2002*

"Will prove valuable to any library seeking to maintain a current, comprehensive reference collection of health resources. . . . An excellent source of health information about genetic disorders which affect particular ethnic and racial minorities in the U.S."
—*The Bookwatch, Aug '01*

Eye Care Sourcebook, 3rd Edition

Basic Consumer Health Information about Eye Care and Eye Disorders, Including Facts about the Diagnosis, Prevention, and Treatment of Refractive Disorders, Cataracts, Glaucoma, Macular Degeneration, and Problems Affecting the Cornea, Retina, and Lacrimal Glands

Along with Advice about Preventing Eye Injuries and Tips for Living with Low Vision or Blindness, a Glossary of Related Terms, and Directories of Resources for More Help and Information

Edited by Amy L. Sutton. 646 pages. 2008. 978-0-7808-1000-6.

Family Planning Sourcebook

Basic Consumer Health Information about Planning for Pregnancy and Contraception, Including Traditional Methods, Barrier Methods, Hormonal Methods, Permanent Methods, Future Methods, Emergency Contraception, and Birth Control Choices for Women at Each Stage of Life

Along with Statistics, a Glossary, and Sources of Additional Information

Edited by Amy Marcaccio Keyzer. 503 pages. 2001. 978-0-7808-0379-4.

"Recommended for public, health, and undergraduate libraries as part of the circulating collection."
—*E-Streams, Mar '02*

"Will prove valuable to any library seeking to maintain a current, comprehensive reference collection of health resources. . . . Excellent reference."

—*The Bookwatch, Aug '01*

SEE ALSO *Pregnancy and Birth Sourcebook, 2nd Edition*

▪

Fitness and Exercise Sourcebook, 3rd Edition

Basic Consumer Health Information about the Physical and Mental Benefits of Fitness, Including Cardiorespiratory Endurance, Muscular Strength, Muscular Endurance, and Flexibility, with Facts about Sports Nutrition and Exercise-Related Injuries and Tips about Physical Activity and Exercises for People of All Ages and for People with Health Concerns

Along with Advice on Selecting and Using Exercise Equipment, Maintaining Exercise Motivation, a Glossary of Related Terms, and a Directory of Resources for More Help and Information

Edited by Amy L. Sutton. 635 pages. 2007. 978-0-7808-0946-8.

"Updates the consumer information on the physical and mental benefits of physical activity throughout the lifespan offered in earlier editions. . . . Recommended. All readers; all levels."

—*CHOICE, Oct '07*

"An exceptionally well-rounded coverage perfect for any concerned about developing and understanding a fitness program."

—*California Bookwatch, Jun '07*

SEE ALSO *Sports Injuries Sourcebook, 3rd Edition*

▪

Food Safety Sourcebook

Basic Consumer Health Information about the Safe Handling of Meat, Poultry, Seafood, Eggs, Fruit Juices, and Other Food Items, and Facts about Pesticides, Drinking Water, Food Safety Overseas, and the Onset, Duration, and Symptoms of Foodborne Illnesses, Including Types of Pathogenic Bacteria, Parasitic Protozoa, Worms, Viruses, and Natural Toxins

Along with the Role of the Consumer, the Food Handler, and the Government in Food Safety; a Glossary, and Resources for Additional Help and Information

Edited by Dawn D. Matthews. 327 pages. 1999. 978-0-7808-0326-8.

"Recommended reference source."

—*Booklist, May '00*

"This book takes the complex issues of food safety and foodborne pathogens and presents them in an easily understood manner. [It does] an excellent job of covering a large and often confusing topic."

— *American Reference Books Annual, 2000*

▪

Forensic Medicine Sourcebook

Basic Consumer Information for the Layperson about Forensic Medicine, Including Crime Scene Investigation, Evidence Collection and Analysis, Expert Testimony, Computer-Aided Criminal Identification, Digital Imaging in the Courtroom, DNA Profiling, Accident Reconstruction, Autopsies, Ballistics, Drugs and Explosives Detection, Latent Fingerprints, Product Tampering, and Questioned Document Examination

Along with Statistical Data, a Glossary of Forensics Terminology, and Listings of Sources for Further Help and Information

Edited by Annemarie S. Muth. 574 pages. 1999. 978-0-7808-0232-2.

"Given the expected widespread interest in its content and its easy to read style, this book is recommended for most public and all college and university libraries."

—*E-Streams, Feb '01*

"A wealth of information, useful statistics, references are up-to-date and extremely complete. This wonderful collection of data will help students who are interested in a career in any type of forensic field. It is a great resource for attorneys who need information about types of expert witnesses needed in a particular case. It also offers useful information for fiction and nonfiction writers whose work involves a crime. A fascinating compilation. All levels."

—*CHOICE, Jan '00*

"There are several items that make this book attractive to consumers who are seeking certain forensic data. . . . This is a useful current

source for those seeking general forensic medical answers."
—*American Reference Books Annual, 2000*

Gastrointestinal Diseases and Disorders Sourcebook, 2nd Edition

Basic Consumer Health Information about the Upper and Lower Gastrointestinal (GI) Tract, Including the Esophagus, Stomach, Intestines, Rectum, Liver, and Pancreas, with Facts about Gastroesophageal Reflux Disease, Gastritis, Hernias, Ulcers, Celiac Disease, Diverticulitis, Irritable Bowel Syndrome, Hemorrhoids, Gastrointestinal Cancers, and Other Diseases and Disorders Related to the Digestive Process

Along with Information about Commonly Used Diagnostic and Surgical Procedures, Statistics, Reports on Current Research Initiatives and Clinical Trials, a Glossary, and Resources for Additional Help and Information

Edited by Sandra J. Judd. 654 pages. 2006. 978-0-7808-0798-3.

"**The text is designed for the general reader seeking information on prevention, disease warning signs, diagnostic and therapeutic questions. . . . It is an excellent resource for the general reader to conveniently locate credible, coordinated and indexed information. . . . The sourcebook will prove very helpful for patients, caregivers and should be available in every physician waiting room."**
—*Doody's Review Service, 2006*

SEE ALSO *Diet and Nutrition Sourcebook, 3rd Edition, Digestive Diseases and Disorders Sourcebook*

Genetic Disorders Sourcebook, 4th Edition

Basic Consumer Health Information about Hereditary Diseases and Disorders, Including Facts about the Human Genome, Genetic Inheritance Patterns, Disorders Associated with Specific Genes, Such as Sickle Cell Disease, Hemophilia, and Cystic Fibrosis, Chromosome Disorders, Such as Down Syndrome, Fragile X Syndrome, and Turner Syndrome, and Complex Diseases and Disorders Resulting from the Interaction of Environmental and Genetic Factors, Such as Allergies, Cancer, and Obesity

Along with Facts about Genetic Testing, Suggestions for Parents of Children with Special Needs, Reports on Current Research Initiatives, a Glossary of Genetic Terminology, and Resources for Additional Help and Information

Edited by Sandra J. Judd. 600 pages. 2009. 978-0-7808-1076-1.

Head Trauma Sourcebook

Basic Information for the Layperson about Open-Head and Closed-Head Injuries, Treatment Advances, Recovery, and Rehabilitation

Along with Reports on Current Research Initiatives

Edited by Karen Bellenir. 414 pages. 1997. 978-0-7808-0208-7.

Headache Sourcebook

Basic Consumer Health Information about Migraine, Tension, Cluster, Rebound and Other Types of Headaches, with Facts about the Cause and Prevention of Headaches, the Effects of Stress and the Environment, Headaches during Pregnancy and Menopause, and Childhood Headaches

Along with a Glossary and Other Resources for Additional Help and Information

Edited by Dawn D. Matthews. 342 pages. 2002. 978-0-7808-0337-4.

"**Highly recommended for academic and medical reference collections."**
—*Library Bookwatch, Sep '02*

SEE ALSO *Pain Sourcebook, 3rd Edition*

Healthy Aging Sourcebook

Basic Consumer Health Information about Maintaining Health through the Aging Process, Including Advice on Nutrition, Exercise, and Sleep, Help in Making Decisions about Midlife Issues and Retirement, and Guidance Concerning Practical and Informed Choices in Health Consumerism

Along with Data Concerning the Theories of Aging, Different Experiences in Aging by Minority Groups, and Facts about Aging Now and Aging in the Future; and Featuring a Glossary, a Guide to Consumer Help, Additional Suggested Reading, and Practical Resource Directory

Edited by Jenifer Swanson. 537 pages. 1999. 978-0-7808-0390-9.

"Recommended reference source."
—*Booklist, Feb '00*

SEE ALSO *Physical and Mental Issues in Aging Sourcebook*

Healthy Children Sourcebook

Basic Consumer Health Information about the Physical and Mental Development of Children between the Ages of 3 and 12, Including Routine Health Care, Preventative Health Services, Safety and First Aid, Healthy Sleep, Dental Care, Nutrition, and Fitness, and Featuring Parenting Tips on Such Topics as Bedwetting, Choosing Day Care, Monitoring TV and Other Media, and Establishing a Foundation for Substance Abuse Prevention

Along with a Glossary of Commonly Used Pediatric Terms and Resources for Additional Help and Information.

Edited by Chad T. Kimball. 624 pages. 2003. 978-0-7808-0247-6.

"Should be required reading for parents and teachers."
—*E-Streams, Jun '04*

"It is hard to imagine that any other single resource exists that would provide such a comprehensive guide of timely information on health promotion and disease prevention for children aged 3 to 12."
—*American Reference Books Annual, 2004*

"This easy-to-read volume is a tremendous resource."
—*AORN Journal, May '05*

SEE ALSO *Childhood Diseases and Disorders Sourcebook, 2nd Edition*

Healthy Heart Sourcebook for Women

Basic Consumer Health Information about Cardiac Issues Specific to Women, Including Facts about Major Risk Factors and Prevention, Treatment and Control Strategies, and Important Dietary Issues

Along with a Special Section Regarding the Pros and Cons of Hormone Replacement Therapy and Its Impact on Heart Health, and Additional Help, Including Recipes, a Glossary, and a Directory of Resources

Edited by Dawn D. Matthews. 321 pages. 2000. 978-0-7808-0329-9.

"A good reference source and recommended for all public, academic, medical, and hospital libraries."
—*Medical Reference Services Quarterly, Summer '01*

"Contains very important information about coronary artery disease that all women should know. The information is current and presented in an easy-to-read format. The book will make a good addition to any library."
—*American Medical Writers Association Journal, Summer '00*

SEE ALSO *Cardiovascular Diseases and Disorders Sourcebook, 3rd Edition, Women's Health Concerns Sourcebook, 3rd Edition*

Hepatitis Sourcebook

Basic Consumer Health Information about Hepatitis A, Hepatitis B, Hepatitis C, and Other Forms of Hepatitis, Including Autoimmune Hepatitis, Alcoholic Hepatitis, Nonalcoholic Steatohepatitis, and Toxic Hepatitis, with Facts about Risk Factors, Screening Methods, Diagnostic Tests, and Treatment Options

Along with Information on Liver Health, Tips for People Living with Chronic Hepatitis, Reports on Current Research Initiatives, a Glossary of Terms Related to Hepatitis, and a Directory of Sources for Further Help and Information

Edited by Sandra J. Judd. 570 pages. 2006. 978-0-7808-0749-5.

"The breadth of information found in this one book would not be readily found in another source. Highly recommended."
—*American Reference Books Annual, 2006*

SEE ALSO *Contagious Diseases Sourcebook*

Household Safety Sourcebook

Basic Consumer Health Information about Household Safety, Including Information about Poisons, Chemicals, Fire, and Water Hazards in the Home

Along with Advice about the Safe Use of Home Maintenance Equipment, Choosing Toys and Nursery Furniture, Holiday and Recreation Safety, a Glossary, and Resources for Further Help and Information

Edited by Dawn D. Matthews. 587 pages. 2002. 978-0-7808-0338-1.

"As a sourcebook on household safety this book meets its mark. It is encyclopedic in scope and covers a wide range of safety issues that are commonly seen in the home."
—*E-Streams, Jul '02*

Hypertension Sourcebook

Basic Consumer Health Information about the Causes, Diagnosis, and Treatment of High Blood Pressure, with Facts about Consequences, Complications, and Co-Occurring Disorders, Such as Coronary Heart Disease, Diabetes, Stroke, Kidney Disease, and Hypertensive Retinopathy, and Issues in Blood Pressure Control, Including Dietary Choices, Stress Management, and Medications

Along with Reports on Current Research Initiatives and Clinical Trials, a Glossary, and Resources for Additional Help and Information

Edited by Dawn D. Matthews and Karen Bellenir. 588 pages. 2004. 978-0-7808-0674-0.

"Academic, public, and medical libraries will want to add the **Hypertension Sourcebook** to their collections."
—*E-Streams, Aug '05*

"The strength of this source is the wide range of information given about hypertension."
—*American Reference Books Annual, 2005*

SEE ALSO *Stroke Sourcebook, 2nd Edition*

Immune System Disorders Sourcebook, 2nd Edition

Basic Consumer Health Information about Disorders of the Immune System, Including Immune System Function and Response, Diagnosis of Immune Disorders, Information about Inherited Immune Disease, Acquired Immune Disease, and Autoimmune Diseases, Including Primary Immune Deficiency, Acquired Immunodeficiency Syndrome (AIDS), Lupus, Multiple Sclerosis, Type 1 Diabetes, Rheumatoid Arthritis, and Graves' Disease

Along with Treatments, Tips for Coping with Immune Disorders, a Glossary, and a Directory of Additional Resources

Edited by Joyce Brennfleck Shannon. 643 pages. 2005. 978-0-7808-0748-8.

"Highly recommended for academic and public libraries."
—*American Reference Books Annual, 2006*

"The updated second edition is a 'must' for any consumer health library seeking a solid resource covering the treatments, symptoms, and options for immune disorder sufferers. . . . An excellent guide."
—*MBR Bookwatch, Jan '06*

SEE ALSO *AIDS Sourcebook, 4th Edition, Arthritis Sourcebook, 2nd Edition*

Infant and Toddler Health Sourcebook

Basic Consumer Health Information about the Physical and Mental Development of Newborns, Infants, and Toddlers, Including Neonatal Concerns, Nutrition Recommendations, Immunization Schedules, Common Pediatric Disorders, Assessments and Milestones, Safety Tips, and Advice for Parents and Other Caregivers

Along with a Glossary of Terms and Resource Listings for Additional Help

Edited by Jenifer Swanson. 570 pages. 2000. 978-0-7808-0246-9.

"As a reference for the general public, this would be useful in any library."
—*E-Streams, May '01*

"Recommended reference source."
—*Booklist, Feb '01*

Infectious Diseases Sourcebook

Basic Consumer Health Information about Non-Contagious Bacterial, Viral, Prion, Fungal, and Parasitic Diseases Spread by Food and Water, Insects and Animals, or Environmental Contact, Including Botulism, E. Coli, Encephalitis, Legionnaires' Disease, Lyme Disease, Malaria, Plague, Rabies, Salmonella, Tetanus, and Others, and Facts about Newly Emerging Diseases, Such as Hantavirus, Mad Cow Disease, Monkeypox, and West Nile Virus

Along with Information about Preventing Disease Transmission, the Threat of Bioterrorism, and Current Research Initiatives, with a Glossary and Directory of Resources for More Information

Edited by Karen Bellenir. 610 pages. 2004. 978-0-7808-0675-7.

"This reference continues the excellent tradition of the *Health Reference Series* in consolidating a wealth of information on a selected topic into a format that is easy to use and accessible to the general public."
—*American Reference Books Annual, 2005*

"Recommended for public and academic libraries."
—*E-Streams, Jan '05*

Injury and Trauma Sourcebook

Basic Consumer Health Information about the Impact of Injury, the Diagnosis and Treatment of Common and Traumatic Injuries, Emergency Care, and Specific Injuries Related to Home, Community, Workplace, Transportation, and Recreation

Along with Guidelines for Injury Prevention, a Glossary, and a Directory of Additional Resources

Edited by Joyce Brennfleck Shannon. 675 pages. 2002. 978-0-7808-0421-0.

"Practitioners should be aware of guides such as this in order to facilitate their use by patients and their families."
—*Doody's Health Sciences Book Review Journal, Sep-Oct '02*

"Recommended reference source."
—*Booklist, Sep '02*

"Highly recommended for academic and medical reference collections."
—*Library Bookwatch, Sep '02*

SEE ALSO *Emergency Medical Services Sourcebook, Sports Injuries Sourcebook, 3rd Edition*

Learning Disabilities Sourcebook, 3rd Edition

Basic Consumer Health Information about Dyslexia, Auditory and Visual Processing Disorders, Communication Disorders, Dyscalculia, Dysgraphia, and Other Conditions That Impede Learning, Including Attention Deficit/Hyperactivity Disorder, Autism Spectrum Disorders, Hearing and Visual Impairments, Chromosome-Based Disorders, and Brain Injury

Along with Facts about Brain Function, Assessment, Therapy and Remediation, Accommodations, Assistive Technology, Legal Protections, and Tips about Family Life, School Transitions, and Employment Strategies, a Glossary of Related Terms, and Directories of Additional Resources

Edited by Joyce Brennfleck Shannon. 613 pages. 2009. 978-0-7808-1039-6.

SEE ALSO *Attention Deficit Disorder Sourcebook, Autism and Pervasive Developmental Disorders Sourcebook*

Leukemia Sourcebook

Basic Consumer Health Information about Adult and Childhood Leukemias, Including Acute Lymphocytic Leukemia (ALL), Chronic Lymphocytic Leukemia (CLL), Acute Myelogenous Leukemia (AML), Chronic Myelogenous Leukemia (CML), and Hairy Cell Leukemia, and Treatments Such as Chemotherapy, Radiation Therapy, Peripheral Blood Stem Cell and Marrow Transplantation, and Immunotherapy

Along with Tips for Life During and After Treatment, a Glossary, and Directories of Additional Resources

Edited by Joyce Brennfleck Shannon. 564 pages. 2003. 978-0-7808-0627-6.

"Unlike other medical books for the layperson, . . . the language does not talk down to the reader. . . . This volume is highly recommended for all libraries."
—*American Reference Books Annual, 2004*

"A fine title which ranges from diagnosis to alternative treatments, staging, and tips for life during and after diagnosis."
—*The Bookwatch, Dec '03*

SEE ALSO *Cancer Sourcebook, 5th Edition*

Liver Disorders Sourcebook

Basic Consumer Health Information about the Liver and How It Works; Liver Diseases, Including Cancer, Cirrhosis, Hepatitis, and Toxic and Drug Related Diseases; Tips for Maintaining a Healthy Liver; Laboratory Tests, Radiology Tests, and Facts about Liver Transplantation

Along with a Section on Support Groups, a Glossary, and Resource Listings

Edited by Joyce Brennfleck Shannon. 580 pages. 2000. 978-0-7808-0383-1.

"This title is recommended for health sciences and public libraries with consumer health collections."
—E-Streams, Oct '00

"Recommended reference source."
—Booklist, Jun '00

SEE ALSO Gastrointestinal Diseases and Disorders Sourcebook, 2nd Edition, Hepatitis Sourcebook

Lung Disorders Sourcebook

Basic Consumer Health Information about Emphysema, Pneumonia, Tuberculosis, Asthma, Cystic Fibrosis, and Other Lung Disorders, Including Facts about Diagnostic Procedures, Treatment Strategies, Disease Prevention Efforts, and Such Risk Factors as Smoking, Air Pollution, and Exposure to Asbestos, Radon, and Other Agents

Along with a Glossary and Resources for Additional Help and Information

Edited by Dawn D. Matthews. 657 pages. 2002. 978-0-7808-0339-8.

"Highly recommended for academic and medical reference collections."
—Library Bookwatch, Sep '02

SEE ALSO Respiratory Disorders Sourcebook, 2nd Edition

Medical Tests Sourcebook, 3rd Edition

Basic Consumer Health Information about X-Rays, Blood Tests, Stool and Urine Tests, Biopsies, Mammography, Endoscopic Procedures, Ultrasound Exams, Computed Tomography, Magnetic Resonance Imaging (MRI), Nuclear Medicine, Genetic Testing, Home-Use Tests, and More

Along with Facts about Preventive Care and Screening Test Guidelines, Screening and Assessment Tests Associated with Such Specific Concerns as Cancer, Heart Disease, Allergies, Diabetes, Thyroid Disfunction, and Infertility, a Glossary of Related Terms, and a Directory of Resources for Additional Help and Information

Edited by Karen Bellenir. 627 pages. 2008. 978-0-7808-1040-2

"This volume has a wide scope that makes it useful . . . Can be a valuable reference guide."
—ARBAonline, Nov '08

Men's Health Concerns Sourcebook, 3rd Edition

Basic Consumer Health Information about Wellness in Men and Gender-Related Differences in Health, With Facts about Heart Disease, Cancer, Traumatic Injury, and Other Leading Causes of Death in Men, Reproductive Concerns, Sexual Dysfunction, Disorders of the Prostate, Penis, and Testes, Sex-Linked Genetic Disorders, and Other Medical and Mental Concerns of Men

Along with Statistical Data, a Glossary of Related Terms, and a Directory of Resources for Additional Information

Edited by Sandra J. Judd. 600 pages. 2009. 978-0-7808-1033-4.

SEE ALSO Prostate and Urological Disorders Sourcebook

Mental Health Disorders Sourcebook, 4th Edition

Basic Consumer Health Information about the Causes and Symptoms of Mental Health Problems, Including Depression, Bipolar Disorder, Anxiety Disorders, Posttraumatic Stress Disorder, Obsessive-Compulsive Disorder, Eating Disorders, Addictions, and Personality and Psychotic Disorders

Along with Information about Medications and Treatments, Mental Health Concerns in Children, Adolescents, and Adults, Tips on Living with Mental Health Disorders, a Glossary of Related Terms, and a Directory of Resources for Additional Help and Information

Edited by Amy L. Sutton. 600 pages. 2009. 978-0-7808-1041-9.

SEE ALSO Depression Sourcebook, 2nd Edition, Stress-Related Disorders Sourcebook, 2nd Edition

Mental Retardation Sourcebook

Basic Consumer Health Information about Mental Retardation and Its Causes, Including

Down Syndrome, Fetal Alcohol Syndrome, Fragile X Syndrome, Genetic Conditions, Injury, and Environmental Sources

Along with Preventive Strategies, Parenting Issues, Educational Implications, Health Care Needs, Employment and Economic Matters, Legal Issues, a Glossary, and a Resource Listing for Additional Help and Information

Edited by Joyce Brennfleck Shannon. 627 pages. 2000. 978-0-7808-0377-0.

"Public libraries will find the book useful for reference and as a beginning research point for students, parents, and caregivers."
—American Reference Books Annual, 2001

"The strength of this work is that it compiles many basic fact sheets and addresses for further information in one volume. It is intended and suitable for the general public."
—E-Streams, Nov '00

"An invaluable overview."
—Reviewer's Bookwatch, Jul '00

Movement Disorders Sourcebook, 2nd Edition

Basic Consumer Health Information about the Symptoms and Causes of Movement Disorders, Including Parkinson Disease, Amyotrophic Lateral Sclerosis, Cerebral Palsy, Muscular Dystrophy, Multiple Sclerosis, Myasthenia, Myoclonus, Spina Bifida, Dystonia, Essential Tremor, Choreatic Disorders, Huntington Disease, Tourette Syndrome, and Other Disorders That Cause Slowed, Absent, or Excessive Movements

Along with Information about Surgical and Nonsurgical Interventions, Physical Therapies, Strategies for Independent Living, a Glossary of Related Terms, and a Directory of Resources for Additional Help and Information

Edited by Amy L. Sutton. 600 pages. 2009. 978-0-7808-1034-1.

SEE ALSO Multiple Sclerosis Sourcebook, Muscular Dystrophy Sourcebook

Multiple Sclerosis Sourcebook

Basic Consumer Health Information about Multiple Sclerosis (MS) and Its Effects on Mobility, Vision, Bladder Function, Speech,

Swallowing, and Cognition, Including Facts about Risk Factors, Causes, Diagnostic Procedures, Pain Management, Drug Treatments, and Physical and Occupational Therapies

Along with Guidelines for Nutrition and Exercise, Tips on Choosing Assistive Equipment, Information about Disability, Work, Financial, and Legal Issues, a Glossary of Related Terms, and a Directory of Additional Resources

Edited by Joyce Brennfleck Shannon. 553 pages. 2007. 978-0-7808-0998-7.

SEE ALSO Movement Disorders Sourcebook, 2nd Edition

Muscular Dystrophy Sourcebook

Basic Consumer Health Information about Congenital, Childhood-Onset, and Adult-Onset Forms of Muscular Dystrophy, Such as Duchenne, Becker, Emery-Dreifuss, Distal, Limb-Girdle, Facioscapulohumeral (FSHD), Myotonic, and Ophthalmoplegic Muscular Dystrophies, Including Facts about Diagnostic Tests, Medical and Physical Therapies, Management of Co-Occurring Conditions, and Parenting Guidelines

Along with Practical Tips for Home Care, a Glossary, and Directories of Additional Resources

Edited by Joyce Brennfleck Shannon. 552 pages. 2004. 978-0-7808-0676-4.

"This book is highly recommended for public and academic libraries as well as health care offices that support the information needs of patients and their families."
—E-Streams, Apr '05

"Excellent reference."
—The Bookwatch, Jan '05

SEE ALSO Movement Disorders Sourcebook, 2nd Edition

Obesity Sourcebook

Basic Consumer Health Information about Diseases and Other Problems Associated with Obesity, and Including Facts about Risk Factors, Prevention Issues, and Management Approaches

Along with Statistical and Demographic Data, Information about Special Populations,

Research Updates, a Glossary, and Source Listings for Further Help and Information

Edited by Wilma Caldwell and Chad T. Kimball. 360 pages. 2001. 978-0-7808-0333-6.

"The book synthesizes the reliable medical literature on obesity into one easy-to-read and useful resource for the general public."
—*American Reference Books Annual, 2002*

"Well suited for the health reference collection of a public library or an academic health science library that serves the general population."
—*E-Streams, Sep '01*

Osteoporosis Sourcebook

Basic Consumer Health Information about Primary and Secondary Osteoporosis and Juvenile Osteoporosis and Related Conditions, Including Fibrous Dysplasia, Gaucher Disease, Hyperthyroidism, Hypophosphatasia, Myeloma, Osteopetrosis, Osteogenesis Imperfecta, and Paget's Disease

Along with Information about Risk Factors, Treatments, Traditional and Non-Traditional Pain Management, a Glossary of Related Terms, and a Directory of Resources

Edited by Allan R. Cook. 568 pages. 2001. 978-0-7808-0239-1.

"This resource is recommended as a great reference source for public, health, and academic libraries, and is another triumph for the editors of Omnigraphics."
—*American Reference Books Annual, 2002*

"Will prove valuable to any library seeking to maintain a current, comprehensive reference collection of health resources. . . . From prevention to treatment and associated conditions, this provides an excellent survey."
—*The Bookwatch, Aug '01*

SEE ALSO Healthy Aging Sourcebook, Women's Health Concerns Sourcebook, 3rd Edition

Pain Sourcebook, 3rd Edition

Basic Consumer Health Information about Acute and Chronic Pain, Including Nerve Pain, Bone Pain, Muscle Pain, Cancer Pain, and Disorders Characterized by Pain, Such as Arthritis, Temporomandibular Muscle and Joint (TMJ) Disorder, Carpal Tunnel Syndrome,

Headaches, Heartburn, Sciatica, and Shingles, and Facts about Diagnostic Tests and Treatment Options for Pain, Including Over-the-Counter and Prescription Drugs, Physical Rehabilitation, Injection and Infusion Therapies, Implantable Technologies, and Complementary Medicine

Along with Tips for Living with Pain, a Glossary of Related Terms, and a Directory of Additional Resources

Edited by Joyce Brennfleck Shannon. 644 pages. 2008. 978-0-7808-1006-8.

"Excellent for ready-reference users and can be used for beginning students in health fields . . . appropriate for the consumer health collection in both public and academic libraries."
—*ARBAonline, Nov '08*

Pediatric Cancer Sourcebook

Basic Consumer Health Information about Leukemias, Brain Tumors, Sarcomas, Lymphomas, and Other Cancers in Infants, Children, and Adolescents, Including Descriptions of Cancers, Treatments, and Coping Strategies

Along with Suggestions for Parents, Caregivers, and Concerned Relatives, a Glossary of Cancer Terms, and Resource Listings

Edited by Edward J. Prucha. 575 pages. 1999. 978-0-7808-0245-2.

"An excellent source of information. Recommended for public, hospital, and health science libraries with consumer health collections."
—*E-Streams, Jun '00*

"A valuable addition to all libraries specializing in health services and many public libraries."
—*American Reference Books Annual, 2000*

SEE ALSO Childhood Diseases and Disorders Sourcebook, 2nd Edition, Healthy Children Sourcebook

Physical and Mental Issues in Aging Sourcebook

Basic Consumer Health Information on Physical and Mental Disorders Associated with the Aging Process, Including Concerns about Cardiovascular Disease, Pulmonary Disease, Oral Health, Digestive Disorders, Musculoskeletal and Skin Disorders, Metabolic

Changes, Sexual and Reproductive Issues, and Changes in Vision, Hearing, and Other Senses

Along with Data about Longevity and Causes of Death, Information on Acute and Chronic Pain, Descriptions of Mental Concerns, a Glossary of Terms, and Resource Listings for Additional Help

Edited by Jenifer Swanson. 660 pages. 1999. 978-0-7808-0233-9.

"This is a treasure of health information for the layperson."
—CHOICE Health Sciences Supplement, May '00

"Recommended for public libraries."
—American Reference Books Annual, 2000

SEE ALSO Healthy Aging Sourcebook

Podiatry Sourcebook, 2nd Edition

Basic Consumer Health Information about Disorders, Diseases, and Deformities that Affect the Foot and Ankle, Including Sprains, Corns, Calluses, Bunions, Plantar Warts, Plantar Fasciitis, Neuromas, Clubfoot, Flat Feet, Achilles Tendonitis, and Much More

Along with Information about Selecting a Foot Care Specialist, Foot Fitness, Shoes and Socks, Diagnostic Tests and Corrective Procedures, Financial Assistance for Corrective Devices, a Glossary of Related Terms, and a Directory of Resources for Additional Help and Information

Edited by Ivy L. Alexander. 516 pages. 2007. 978-0-7808-0944-4.

"An excellent resource. . . . Although there have been various types of 'foot books' published in the past, none are as comprehensive as this one. 5 Stars (out of 5)!"
—Doody's Review Service, 2007

"Perfect for both health libraries and general-interest lending collections."
—Internet Bookwatch, Jul '07

Pregnancy and Birth Sourcebook, 3rd Edition

Basic Consumer Health Information about Pregnancy and Fetal Development, Including Facts about Fertility and Conception, Physical and Emotional Changes during Pregnancy, Prenatal Care and Diagnostic Tests, High-Risk Pregnancies and Complications, Labor, Delivery, and the Postpartum Period

Along with Tips on Maintaining Health and Wellness during Pregnancy and Caring for Newborn Infants, a Glossary of Related Terms, and Directories of Resources for Additional Help and Information

Edited by Amy L. Sutton. 600 pages. 2009. 978-0-7808-1074-7.

SEE ALSO Breastfeeding Sourcebook, Congenital Disorders Sourcebook, 2nd Edition, Family Planning Sourcebook, Women's Health Concerns Sourcebook, 3rd Edition

Prostate and Urological Disorders Sourcebook

Basic Consumer Health Information about Urogenital and Sexual Disorders in Men, Including Prostate and Other Andrological Cancers, Prostatitis, Benign Prostatic Hyperplasia, Testicular and Penile Trauma, Cryptorchidism, Peyronie Disease, Erectile Dysfunction, and Male Factor Infertility, and Facts about Commonly Used Tests and Procedures, Such as Prostatectomy, Vasectomy, Vasectomy Reversal, Penile Implants, and Semen Analysis

Along with a Glossary of Andrological Terms and a Directory of Resources for Additional Information

Edited by Karen Bellenir. 604 pages. 2006. 978-0-7808-0797-6.

"Certain to be a popular pick among library reference holdings. . . . No prior knowledge is assumed for any of the conditions or terms herein, making it a most accessible general-interest reference."
—California Bookwatch, Apr '06

SEE ALSO Men's Health Concerns Sourcebook, 3rd Edition, Urinary Tract and Kidney Diseases and Disorders Sourcebook, 2nd Edition

Prostate Cancer Sourcebook

Basic Consumer Health Information about Prostate Cancer, Including Information about the Associated Risk Factors, Detection, Diagnosis, and Treatment of Prostate Cancer

Along with Information on Non-Malignant Prostate Conditions, and Featuring a Section

Listing Support and Treatment Centers and a Glossary of Related Terms

Edited by Dawn D. Matthews. 340 pages. 2001. 978-0-7808-0324-4.

"Recommended reference source."
—*Booklist, Jan '02*

"A valuable resource for health care consumers seeking information on the subject. . . . All text is written in a clear, easy-to-understand language that avoids technical jargon. Any library that collects consumer health resources would strengthen their collection with the addition of the *Prostate Cancer Sourcebook.*"
—*American Reference Books Annual, 2002*

SEE ALSO *Cancer Sourcebook, 5th Edition, Men's Health Concerns Sourcebook, 3rd Edition*

Rehabilitation Sourcebook

Basic Consumer Health Information about Rehabilitation for People Recovering from Heart Surgery, Spinal Cord Injury, Stroke, Orthopedic Impairments, Amputation, Pulmonary Impairments, Traumatic Injury, and More, Including Physical Therapy, Occupational Therapy, Speech/Language Therapy, Massage Therapy, Dance Therapy, Art Therapy, and Recreational Therapy

Along with Information on Assistive and Adaptive Devices, a Glossary, and Resources for Additional Help and Information

Edited by Dawn D. Matthews. 519 pages. 2000. 978-0-7808-0236-0.

"This is an excellent resource for public library reference and health collections."
—*American Reference Books Annual, 2001*

"Recommended reference source."
—*Booklist, May '00*

Respiratory Disorders Sourcebook, 2nd Edition

Basic Consumer Health Information about Infectious, Inflammatory, and Chronic Conditions Affecting the Lungs and Respiratory System, Including Pneumonia, Bronchitis, Influenza, Tuberculosis, Sarcoidosis, Asthma, Cystic Fibrosis, Chronic Obstructive Pulmonary Disease, Lung Abscesses, Pulmonary Embolism, Occupational Lung Diseases, and Other Bacterial, Viral, and Fungal Infections

Along with Facts about the Structure and Function of the Lungs and Airways, Methods of Diagnosing Respiratory Disorders, and Treatment and Rehabilitation Options, a Glossary of Related Terms, and a Directory of Resources for Additional Help and Information

Edited by Sandra L. Judd. 638 pages. 2008. 978-0-7808-1007-5.

"A great addition for public and school libraries because it provides concise health information . . . readers can start with this reference source and get satisfactory answers before proceeding to other medical reference tools for more in depth information . . . A good guide for health education on lung disorders."
—*ARBAonline, Nov '08*

SEE ALSO *Lung Disorders Sourcebook*

Sexually Transmitted Diseases Sourcebook, 4th Edition

Basic Consumer Health Information about Chlamydial Infections, Gonorrhea, Hepatitis, Herpes, HIV/AIDS, Human Papillomavirus, Pubic Lice, Scabies, Syphilis, Trichomoniasis, Vaginal Infections, and Other Sexually Transmitted Diseases, Including Facts about Risk Factors, Symptoms, Diagnosis, Treatment, and the Prevention of Sexually Transmitted Infections

Along with Updates on Current Research Initiatives, a Glossary of Related Terms, and Resources for Additional Help and Information

Edited by Laura Larsen. 600 pages. 2009. 978-0-7808-1073-0.

SEE ALSO *AIDS Sourcebook, 4th Edition, Contagious Diseases Sourcebook, 2nd Edition, Men's Health Concerns Sourcebook, 3rd Edition, Women's Health Concerns Sourcebook, 3rd Edition*

Sleep Disorders Sourcebook, 2nd Edition

Basic Consumer Health Information about Sleep and Sleep Disorders, Including Insomnia, Sleep Apnea, Restless Legs Syndrome, Narcolepsy, Parasomnias, and Other Health Problems That Affect Sleep, Plus Facts about Diagnostic Procedures, Treatment Strategies,

Sleep Medications, and Tips for Improving Sleep Quality

Along with a Glossary of Related Terms and Resources for Additional Help and Information

Edited by Amy L. Sutton. 567 pages. 2005. 978-0-7808-0743-3.

"This book will be useful for just about everybody, especially the 40 million Americans with sleep disorders."
—American Reference Books Annual, 2006

"A welcome addition to public libraries and consumer health libraries."
—Medical Reference Services Quarterly, Summer '06

Smoking Concerns Sourcebook

Basic Consumer Health Information about Nicotine Addiction and Smoking Cessation, Featuring Facts about the Health Effects of Tobacco Use, Including Lung and Other Cancers, Heart Disease, Stroke, and Respiratory Disorders, Such as Emphysema and Chronic Bronchitis

Along with Information about Smoking Prevention Programs, Suggestions for Achieving and Maintaining a Smoke-Free Lifestyle, Statistics about Tobacco Use, Reports on Current Research Initiatives, a Glossary of Related Terms, and Directories of Resources for Additional Help and Information

Edited by Karen Bellenir. 595 pages. 2004. 978-0-7808-0323-7.

"Provides everything needed for the student or general reader seeking practical details on the effects of tobacco use."
—The Bookwatch, Mar '05

"Public libraries and consumer health care libraries will find this work useful."
—American Reference Books Annual, 2005

SEE ALSO Respiratory Disorders Sourcebook, 2nd Edition

Sports Injuries Sourcebook, 3rd Edition

Basic Consumer Health Information about Sprains and Strains, Fractures, Growth Plate Injuries, Overtraining Injuries, and Injuries to the Head, Face, Shoulders, Elbows, Hands, Spinal Column, Knees, Ankles, and Feet, and with Facts about Heat-Related Illness, Steroids and Sport Supplements, Protective Equipment, Diagnostic Procedures, Treatment Options, and Rehabilitation

Along with a Glossary of Related Terms and a Directory of Resources for Additional Help and Information

Edited by Sandra J. Judd. 623 pages. 2007. 978-0-7808-0949-9.

SEE ALSO Fitness and Exercise Sourcebook, 3rd Edition

Stress-Related Disorders Sourcebook, 2nd Edition

Basic Consumer Health Information about Stress and Stress-Related Disorders, Including Types of Stress, Sources of Acute and Chronic Stress, the Impact of Stress on the Body's Systems, and Mental and Emotional Health Problems Associated with Stress, Such as Depression, Anxiety Disorders, Substance Abuse, Posttraumatic Stress Disorder, and Suicide

Along with Advice about Getting Help for Stress-Related Disorders, Information about Stress Management Techniques, a Glossary of Stress-Related Terms, and a Directory of Resources for Additional Help and Information

Edited by Amy L. Sutton. 608 pages. 2007. 978-0-7808-0996-3.

"Accessible to the lay reader. Highly recommended for medical and psychiatric collections."
—Library Journal, Mar '08

"Well-written for a general readership, the 2nd Edition of Stress-Related Disorders Sourcebook is a useful addition to the health reference literature."
—American Reference Books Annual, 2008

SEE ALSO Mental Health Disorders Sourcebook, 4th Edition

Stroke Sourcebook, 2nd Edition

Basic Consumer Health Information about Stroke, Including Ischemic, Hemorrhagic, and Mini Strokes, as Well as Risk Factors, Prevention Guidelines, Diagnostic Tests, Medications and

Surgical Treatments, and Complications of Stroke

Along with Rehabilitation Techniques and Innovations, Tips on Staying Healthy and Maintaining Independence after Stroke, a Glossary of Related Terms, and a Directory of Resources for Stroke Survivors and Their Families

Edited by Amy L. Sutton. 626 pages. 2008. 978-0-7808-1035-8.

"An encyclopedic handbook on stroke that is written in a language the layperson can understand. . . . This is one of the most helpful, readable books on stroke. This volume is highly recommended and should be in every medical, hospital and public library; in addition, every family practitioner should have a copy in his or her office."
—ARBAonline Dec '08

SEE ALSO Hypertension Sourcebook

Surgery Sourcebook, 2nd Edition

Basic Consumer Health Information about Common Inpatient and Outpatient Surgeries, Including Critical Care and Trauma, Gastrointestinal, Gynecologic and Obstetric, Cardiac and Vascular, Neurologic, Ophthalmologic, Orthopedic, Reconstructive and Cosmetic, and Other Major and Minor Surgeries

Along with Information about Anesthesia and Pain Relief Options, Risks and Complications, Postoperative Recovery Concerns, and Innovative Surgical Techniques and Tools, a Glossary of Related Terms, and a Directory of Additional Resources

Edited by Amy L. Sutton. 645 pages. 2008. 978-0-7808-1004-4.

"Large public libraries and medical libraries would benefit from this material in their reference collections."
—ARBAonline Aug '08

SEE ALSO Cosmetic and Reconstructive Surgery Sourcebook, 2nd Edition

Thyroid Disorders Sourcebook

Basic Consumer Health Information about Disorders of the Thyroid and Parathyroid Glands, Including Hypothyroidism, Hyperthyroidism,

Graves Disease, Hashimoto Thyroiditis, Thyroid Cancer, and Parathyroid Disorders, Featuring Facts about Symptoms, Risk Factors, Tests, and Treatments

Along with Information about the Effects of Thyroid Imbalance on Other Body Systems, Environmental Factors That Affect the Thyroid Gland, a Glossary, and a Directory of Additional Resources

Edited by Joyce Brennfleck Shannon. 573 pages. 2005. 978-0-7808-0745-7.

"Recommended for consumer health collections."
—American Reference Books Annual, 2006

"Highly recommended pick for basic consumer health reference holdings at all levels."
—The Bookwatch, Aug '05

SEE ALSO Endocrine and Metabolic Disorders Sourcebook, 2nd Edition

Transplantation Sourcebook

Basic Consumer Health Information about Organ and Tissue Transplantation, Including Physical and Financial Preparations, Procedures and Issues Relating to Specific Solid Organ and Tissue Transplants, Rehabilitation, Pediatric Transplant Information, the Future of Transplantation, and Organ and Tissue Donation

Along with a Glossary and Listings of Additional Resources

Edited by Joyce Brennfleck Shannon. 610 pages. 2002. 978-0-7808-0322-0.

"Recommended for libraries with an interest in offering consumer health information."
—E-Streams, Jul '02

"This is a unique and valuable resource for patients facing transplantation and their families."
—Doody's Review Service, Jun '02

Traveler's Health Sourcebook

Basic Consumer Health Information for Travelers, Including Physical and Medical Preparations, Transportation Health and Safety, Essential Information about Food and Water, Sun Exposure, Insect and Snake Bites, Camping and Wilderness Medicine, and Travel with Physical or Medical Disabilities

Along with International Travel Tips, Vaccination Recommendations, Geographical Health Issues, Disease Risks, a Glossary, and a Listing of Additional Resources

Edited by Joyce Brennfleck Shannon. 619 pages. 2000. 978-0-7808-0384-8.

"Recommended reference source."
—Booklist, Feb '01

"This book is recommended for any public library, any travel collection, and especially any collection for the physically disabled."
—American Reference Books Annual, 2001

SEE ALSO Worldwide Health Sourcebook

Urinary Tract and Kidney Diseases and Disorders Sourcebook, 2nd Edition

Basic Consumer Health Information about the Urinary System, Including the Bladder, Urethra, Ureters, and Kidneys, with Facts about Urinary Tract Infections, Incontinence, Congenital Disorders, Kidney Stones, Cancers of the Urinary Tract and Kidneys, Kidney Failure, Dialysis, and Kidney Transplantation

Along with Statistical and Demographic Information, Reports on Current Research in Kidney and Urologic Health, a Summary of Commonly Used Diagnostic Tests, a Glossary of Related Terms, and a Directory of Resources for Additional Help and Information

Edited by Ivy L. Alexander. 621 pages. 2005. 978-0-7808-0750-1.

"A good choice for a consumer health information library or for a medical library needing information to refer to their patients."
—American Reference Books Annual, 2006

SEE ALSO Prostate and Urological Disorders Sourcebook

Vegetarian Sourcebook

Basic Consumer Health Information about Vegetarian Diets, Lifestyle, and Philosophy, Including Definitions of Vegetarianism and Veganism, Tips about Adopting Vegetarianism, Creating a Vegetarian Pantry, and Meeting Nutritional Needs of Vegetarians, with Facts Regarding Vegetarianism's Effect on Pregnant and Lactating Women, Children, Athletes, and Senior Citizens

Along with a Glossary of Commonly Used Vegetarian Terms and Resources for Additional Help and Information

Edited by Chad T. Kimball. 337 pages. 2002. 978-0-7808-0439-5.

"Organizes into one concise volume the answers to the most common questions concerning vegetarian diets and lifestyles. This title is recommended for public and secondary school libraries."
—E-Streams, Apr '03

"Invaluable reference for public and school library collections alike."
—Library Bookwatch, Apr '03

"The articles in this volume are easy to read and come from authoritative sources. The book does not necessarily support the vegetarian diet but instead provides the pros and cons of this important decision. . . . Recommended for public libraries and consumer health libraries."
—American Reference Books Annual, 2003

SEE ALSO Diet and Nutrition Sourcebook, 3rd Edition

Women's Health Concerns Sourcebook, 3rd Edition

Basic Consumer Health Information about Issues and Trends in Women's Health and Health Conditions of Special Concern to Women, Including Endometriosis, Uterine Fibroids, Menstrual Irregularities, Menopause, Sexual Dysfunction, Infertility, Cancer in Women, and Other Such Chronic Disorders as Lupus, Fibromyalgia, and Thyroid Disease

Along with Statistical Data, Tips for Maintaining Wellness, a Glossary, and a Directory of Resources for Further Help and Information

Edited by Sandra J. Judd. 600 pages. 2009. 978-0-7808-1036-5.

SEE ALSO Breast Cancer Sourcebook, 3rd Edition, Cancer Sourcebook for Women, 3rd Edition, Healthy Heart Sourcebook for Women, Osteoporosis Sourcebook

Workplace Health and Safety Sourcebook

Basic Consumer Health Information about Workplace Health and Safety, Including the Effect of Workplace Hazards on the Lungs,

Skin, Heart, Ears, Eyes, Brain, Reproductive Organs, Musculoskeletal System, and Other Organs and Body Parts

Along with Information about Occupational Cancer, Personal Protective Equipment, Toxic and Hazardous Chemicals, Child Labor, Stress, and Workplace Violence

Edited by Chad T. Kimball. 610 pages. 2000. 978-0-7808-0231-5.

"As a reference for the general public, this would be useful in any library."
—E-Streams, Jun '01

"Provides helpful information for primary care physicians and other caregivers interested in occupational medicine. . . . General readers; professionals."
—CHOICE, May '01

Worldwide Health Source-book

Basic Information about Global Health Issues, Including Malnutrition, Reproductive Health, Disease Dispersion and Prevention, Emerging Diseases, Risky Health Behaviors, and the Leading Causes of Death

Along with Global Health Concerns for Children, Women, and the Elderly, Mental Health Issues, Research and Technology Advancements, and Economic, Environmental, and Political Health Implications, a Glossary, and a Resource Listing for Additional Help and Information

Edited by Joyce Brennfleck Shannon. 597 pages. 2001. 978-0-7808-0330-5.

"Named an Outstanding Academic Title."
—CHOICE, Jan '02

"Yet another handy but also unique compilation in the extensive *Health Reference Series*, this is a useful work because many of the international publications reprinted or excerpted are not readily available. Highly recommended."
—CHOICE, Nov '01

SEE ALSO *Traveler's Health Sourcebook*

Teen Health Series

Complete Catalog

List price $69 per volume. School and library price $62 per volume.

Abuse and Violence Information for Teens

Health Tips about the Causes and Consequences of Abusive and Violent Behavior

Including Facts about the Types of Abuse and Violence, the Warning Signs of Abusive and Violent Behavior, Health Concerns of Victims, and Getting Help and Staying Safe

Edited by Sandra Augustyn Lawton. 411 pages. 2008. 978-0-7808-1008-2.

"A useful resource for schools and organizations providing services to teens and may also be a starting point in research projects."
—*Reference and Research Book News, Aug '08*

"Violence is a serious problem for teens. . . . This resource gives teens the information they need to face potential threats and get help—either for themselves or for their friends."
—*ARBAonline, Aug '08*

Accident and Safety Information for Teens

Health Tips about Medical Emergencies, Traumatic Injuries, and Disaster Preparedness

Including Facts about Motor Vehicle Accidents, Burns, Poisoning, Firearms, Natural Disasters, National Security Threats, and More

Edited by Karen Bellenir. 420 pages. 2008. 978-0-7808-1046-4.

SEE ALSO *Sports Injuries Information for Teens, 2nd Edition*

Alcohol Information for Teens, 2nd Edition

Health Tips about Alcohol and Alcoholism

Including Facts about Alcohol's Effects on the Body, Brain, and Behavior, the Consequences of Underage Drinking, Alcohol Abuse Prevention and Treatment, and Coping with Alcoholic Parents

Edited by Lisa Bakewell. 400 pages. 2009. 978-0-7808-1043-3.

SEE ALSO *Drug Information for Teens, 2nd Edition*

Allergy Information for Teens

Health Tips about Allergic Reactions Such as Anaphylaxis, Respiratory Problems, and Rashes

Including Facts about Identifying and Managing Allergies to Food, Pollen, Mold, Animals, Chemicals, Drugs, and Other Substances

Edited by Karen Bellenir. 410 pages. 2006. 978-0-7808-0799-0.

"This is a comprehensive, readable text on the subject of allergic diseases in teenagers. 5 Stars (out of 5)!"
—*Doody's Review Service, Jun '06*

"This authoritative and useful self-help title is a solid addition to YA collections, whether for personal interest or reports."
—*School Library Journal, Jul '06*

Asthma Information for Teens

Health Tips about Managing Asthma and Related Concerns

Including Facts about Asthma Causes, Triggers, Symptoms, Diagnosis, and Treatment

Edited by Karen Bellenir. 386 pages. 2005. 978-0-7808-0770-9.

"Highly recommended for medical libraries, public school libraries, and public libraries."
—*American Reference Books Annual, 2006*

"Although this volume is nearly 400 pages long, it is so clearly written and well organized that even hesitant readers will be able to find the facts they need, whether for reports or personal information. . . . A succinct but complete resource."
—*School Library Journal, Sep '05*

Body Information for Teens

Health Tips about Maintaining Well-Being for a Lifetime

Including Facts about the Development and Functioning of the Body's Systems, Organs, and Structures and the Health Impact of Lifestyle Choices

Edited by Sandra Augustyn Lawton. 458 pages. 2007. 978-0-7808-0443-2.

Cancer Information for Teens, 2nd Edition

Health Tips about Cancer Awareness, Symptoms, Prevention, Diagnosis, and Treatment

Including Facts about Common Cancers Affecting Teens, Causes, Detection, Coping Strategies, Clinical Trials, Nutrition and Exercise, Cancer in Friends or Family, and More

Edited by Karen Bellenir and Lisa Bakewell. 400 pages. 2009. 978-0-7808-1085-3.

Complementary and Alternative Medicine Information for Teens

Health Tips about Non-Traditional and Non-Western Medical Practices

Including Information about Acupuncture, Chiropractic Medicine, Dietary and Herbal Supplements, Hypnosis, Massage Therapy, Prayer and Spirituality, Reflexology, Yoga, and More

Edited by Sandra Augustyn Lawton. 407 pages. 2007. 978-0-7808-0966-6.

"This volume covers CAM specifically for teenagers but of general use also. It should be a welcome addition to both public and academic libraries."
—*American Reference Books Annual, 2008*

"This volume provides a solid foundation for further investigation of the subject, making it useful for both public and high school libraries."
—*VOYA: Voice of Youth Advocates, Jun '07*

Diabetes Information for Teens

Health Tips about Managing Diabetes and Preventing Related Complications

Including Information about Insulin, Glucose Control, Healthy Eating, Physical Activity, and Learning to Live with Diabetes

Edited by Sandra Augustyn Lawton. 410 pages. 2006. 978-0-7808-0811-9.

"A comprehensive instructional guide for teens. . . . some of the material may also be directed towards parents or teachers. 5 stars (out of 5)!"
—*Doody's Review Service, 2006*

"Students dealing with their own diabetes or that of a friend or family member or those writing reports on the topic will find this a valuable resource."
—*School Library Journal, Aug '06*

"This text is directed to the teen population and would be an excellent library resource for a health class or for the teacher as a reference for class preparation. It can, however, serve a much wider audience. The clinical educator on diabetes may find it valuable to educate the newly diagnosed client regardless of age. It also would be an excellent reference and education tool for a preventive medicine seminar on diabetes."
—*Physical Therapy, Mar '07*

Diet Information for Teens, 2nd Edition

Health Tips about Diet and Nutrition

Including Facts about Dietary Guidelines, Food Groups, Nutrients, Healthy Meals, Snacks, Weight Control, Medical Concerns Related to Diet, and More

Edited by Karen Bellenir. 432 pages. 2006. 978-0-7808-0820-1.

"A very quick and pleasant read in spite of the fact that it is very detailed in the information it gives. . . . A book for anyone concerned about diet and nutrition."
—*American Reference Books Annual, 2007*

SEE ALSO Eating Disorders Information for Teens, 2nd Edition

Drug Information for Teens, 2nd Edition

Health Tips about the Physical and Mental Effects of Substance Abuse

Including Information about Marijuana, Inhalants, Club Drugs, Stimulants, Hallucinogens,

Opiates, Prescription and Over-the-Counter Drugs, Herbal Products, Tobacco, Alcohol, and More
Edited by Sandra Augustyn Lawton. 468 pages. 2006. 978-0-7808-0862-1.

"As with earlier installments in Omnigraphics' **Teen Health Series, Drug Information for Teens** is designed specifically to meet the needs and interests of middle and high school students. . . . Strongly recommended for both academic and public libraries."
—*American Reference Books Annual, 2007*

"Solid thoughtful advice is given about how to handle peer pressure, drug-related health concerns, and treatment strategies."
—*School Library Journal, Dec '06*

SEE ALSO Alcohol Information for Teens, 2nd Edition, Tobacco Information for Teens

Eating Disorders Information for Teens, 2nd Edition
Health Tips about Anorexia, Bulimia, Binge Eating, And Other Eating Disorders
Including Information about Risk Factors, Diagnosis and Treatment, Prevention, Related Health Concerns, and Other Issues
Edited by Sandra Augustyn Lawton. 377 pages. 2009. 978-0-7808-1044-0.

SEE ALSO Diet Information for Teens, 2nd Edition

Fitness Information for Teens, 2nd Edition
Health Tips about Exercise, Physical Well-Being, and Health Maintenance
Including Facts about Conditioning, Stretching, Strength Training, Body Shape and Body Image, Sports Nutrition, and Specific Activities for Athletes and Non-Athletes
Edited by Lisa Bakewell. 432 pages. 2009. 978-0-7808-1045-7.

SEE ALSO Diet Information for Teens, 2nd Edition, Sports Injuries Information for Teens, 2nd Edition

Learning Disabilities Information for Teens
Health Tips about Academic Skills Disorders and Other Disabilities That Affect Learning
Including Information about Common Signs of Learning Disabilities, School Issues, Learning to Live with a Learning Disability, and Other Related Issues
Edited by Sandra Augustyn Lawton. 400 pages. 2006. 978-0-7808-0796-9.

"This book provides a wealth of information for any reader interested in the signs, causes, and consequences of learning disabilities, as well as related legal rights and educational interventions. . . . Public and academic libraries should want this title for both students and general readers."
—*American Reference Books Annual, 2006*

Mental Health Information for Teens, 2nd Edition
Health Tips about Mental Wellness and Mental Illness
Including Facts about Mental and Emotional Health, Depression and Other Mood Disorders, Anxiety Disorders, Conduct Disorder, Self-Injury, Psychosis, Schizophrenia, and More
Edited by Karen Bellenir. 424 pages. 2006. 978-0-7808-0863-8.

"This excellent overview of the psychological disorders that affect teens provides clear definitions and descriptions, and discusses resources, therapies, coping mechanisms, and medications."
—*School Library Journal Curriculum Connections, Fall '07*

"A well done reference for a specific, often under-represented group."
—*Doody's Review Service, 2006*

SEE ALSO Stress Information for Teens

Pregnancy Information for Teens
Health Tips about Teen Pregnancy and Teen Parenting
Including Facts about Prenatal Care, Pregnancy Complications, Labor and Delivery,

Postpartum Care, Pregnancy-Related Lifestyle Concerns, and More

Edited by Sandra Augustyn Lawton. 434 pages. 2007. 978-0-7808-0984-0.

SEE ALSO Sexual Health Information for Teens, 2nd Edition

Sexual Health Information for Teens, 2nd Edition

Health Tips about Sexual Development, Reproduction, Contraception, and Sexually Transmitted Infections

Including Facts about Puberty, Sexuality, Birth Control, Chlamydia, Gonorrhea, Herpes, Human Papillomavirus, Syphilis, and More

Edited by Sandra Augustyn Lawton. 430 pages. 2008. 978-0-7808-1010-5.

"This offering represents the most up-to-date information available on an array of topics including abstinence-only sexual education and pregnancy-prevention methods. . . . The range of coverage—from puberty and anatomy to sexually transmitted diseases—is thorough and extensive. Each chapter includes a bibliographic citation, and the three back sections containing additional resources, further reading, and the index are all first-rate. . . . This volume will be well used by students in need of the facts, whether for educational or personal reasons."

—School Library Journal, Nov '08

SEE ALSO Pregnancy Information for Teens

Skin Health Information for Teens, 2nd Edition

Health Tips about Dermatological Concerns and Skin Cancer Risks

Including Facts about Acne, Warts, Allergies, and Other Conditions and Lifestyle Choices, Such as Tanning, Tattooing, and Piercing, That Affect the Skin, Nails, Scalp, and Hair

Edited by Edited by Kim Wohlenhaus. 400 pages. 2009. 978-0-7808-1042-6.

Sleep Information for Teens

Health Tips about Adolescent Sleep Requirements, Sleep Disorders, and the Effects of Sleep Deprivation

Including Facts about Why People Need Sleep, Sleep Patterns, Circadian Rhythms, Dreaming, Insomnia, Sleep Apnea, Narcolepsy, and More

Edited by Karen Bellenir. 355 pages. 2008. 978-0-7808-1009-9.

SEE ALSO Body Information for Teens

Sports Injuries Information for Teens, 2nd Edition

Health Tips about Acute, Traumatic, and Chronic Injuries in Adolescent Athletes

Including Facts about Sprains, Fractures, and Overuse Injuries, Treatment, Rehabilitation, Sport-Specific Safety Guidelines, Fitness Suggestions, and More

Edited by Karen Bellenir. 429 pages. 2008. 978-0-7808-1011-2.

"An engaging selection of informative articles about the prevention and treatment of sports injuries. . . The value of this book is that the articles have been vetted and are often augmented with inserts of useful facts, definitions of technical terms, and quick tips. Sensitive topics like injuries to genitalia are discussed openly and responsibly. This revised edition contains updated articles and defines sport more broadly than the first edition."

—School Library Journal, Nov '08

"This work will be useful in the young adult collections of public libraries as well as high school libraries. . . . A useful resource for student research."

—ARBAonline, Aug '08

SEE ALSO Accident and Safety Information for Teens

Stress Information for Teens

Health Tips about the Mental and Physical Consequences of Stress

Including Information about the Different Kinds of Stress, Symptoms of Stress, Frequent Causes of Stress, Stress Management Techniques, and More

Edited by Sandra Augustyn Lawton. 392 pages. 2008. 978-0-7808-1012-9.

"Understanding what stress is, what causes it, how the body and the mind are impacted by it, and what teens can do are the general categories addressed here. . . . The chapters are brief but informative, and the list of community-help organizations is exhaustive. Report writers will find information quickly and easily, as will those who have personal concerns. The print is clear and the format is readable, making this an accessible resource for struggling readers and researchers."

—*School Library Journal, Dec '08*

"The articles selected will specifically appeal to young adults and are designed to answer their most common questions."

—*ARBAonline, Aug '08*

SEE ALSO *Mental Health Information for Teens, 2nd Edition*

Suicide Information for Teens

Health Tips about Suicide Causes and Prevention

Including Facts about Depression, Risk Factors, Getting Help, Survivor Support, and More

Edited by Joyce Brennfleck Shannon. 368 pages. 2005. 978-0-7808-0737-2.

"Highly Recommended for libraries serving teenagers as well as those who work with them."

—*E-Streams, Apr '06*

SEE ALSO *Mental Health Information for Teens, 2nd Edition*

Tobacco Information for Teens

Health Tips about the Hazards of Using Cigarettes, Smokeless Tobacco, and Other Nicotine Products

Including Facts about Nicotine Addiction, Immediate and Long-Term Health Effects of Tobacco Use, Related Cancers, Smoking Cessation, Tobacco Use Prevention, and Tobacco Use Statistics

Edited by Karen Bellenir. 440 pages. 2007. 978-0-7808-0976-5.

"A comprehensive resource. Each chapter is written to stand alone, so students can dip in and use the information in each section for reports or to answer personal questions without

having to read the entire book. . . . The book is packed full of statistics, with sources to help students look up more."

—*School Library Journal, Sep '07*

"Pulls together a wide variety of authoritative sources to provide a comprehensive overview of tobacco use for this age group. . . . This reasonably priced reference title should be considered a necessary purchase for all public libraries and school media centers, along with academic libraries supporting teacher education."

—*American Reference Books Annual, 2008*

SEE ALSO *Drug Information for Teens, 2nd Edition*

Health Reference Series